Neuropeptides and Psychiatric Disorders

PROGRESS IN PSYCHIATRY

Number 29

David Spiegel, M.D.
Series Editor

Neuropeptides and Psychiatric Disorders

Edited by
Charles B. Nemeroff, M.D., Ph.D.

American Psychiatric Press, Inc.

Washington, DC
London, England

Note: The authors have worked to ensure that all information in this book concerning drug dosages, schedules, and routes of administration is accurate as of the time of publication and consistent with standards set by the U.S. Food and Drug Administration and the general medical community. As medical research and practice advance, however, therapeutic standards may change. For this reason and because human and mechanical errors sometimes occur, we recommend that readers follow the advice of a physician who is directly involved in their care or the care of a member of their family.

Manufactured in the United States of America
First Printing 93 92 91 90 4 3 2 1

American Psychiatric Press, Inc.
1400 K Street, N.W., Washington, DC 20005

The paper used in this publication meets the minimum requirements of the American National Standard for Information Sciences—Permanence of Paper for Printed Library Materials, ANSI Z39.48–1984. ♾

Library of Congress Cataloging-in-Publication Data

Neuropeptides and psychiatric disorders / edited by Charles B. Nemeroff—1st ed.
p. cm. — (Progress in psychiatry : no. 29)
Includes bibliographical references.
ISBN 0-88048-185-4 (alk. paper)
1. Mental illness — Physiological aspects.
2. Neuropeptides — Pathophysiology. I. Nemeroff, Charles B. II. Series.
[DNLM: 1. Mental disorders — physiopathology.
2. Neuropeptides — physiology. WL 104 N494222]
RC455.4.B5N467 1990
616.89é07—dc20
DNLM/DLC
for Library of Congress 90-924
CIP

British Library Cataloguing in Publication Data

A CIP record is available from the British Library.

CONTENTS

Contributors

Garth Bissette, Ph.D.
Department of Psychiatry, Duke University Medical Center, Durham, North Carolina

Anders Bjartell, M.D.
Department of Psychiatry and Neurochemistry, University of Lund, Lund, Sweden

J. N. Crawley, Ph.D.
Clinical Neuroscience Branch, National Institute of Mental Health, Bethesda, Maryland

Candace L. Davis, B.S.
National Institute of Mental Health, Bethesda, Maryland

Kenneth L. Davis, M.D.
Department of Psychiatry, Mount Sinai Medical Center, New York, New York

Errol B. De Souza, Ph.D.
Laboratory of Neurobiology, Neuroscience Branch, Addiction Research Center, National Institute on Drug Abuse, Baltimore, Maryland

Carol A. Dudley, M.S.
Department of Physiology, The University of Texas Southwestern Medical Center, Dallas, Texas

Rolf Ekman, M.D., Ph.D.
Department of Psychiatry and Neurochemistry, University of Lund, Lund, Sweden

Dwight L. Evans, M.D.
Departments of Psychiatry and Medicine, University of North Carolina School of Medicine, Chapel Hill, North Carolina

Ede Frecska, M.D.
Department of Psychiatry, Mount Sinai Medical Center, New York, New York

Robert N. Golden, M.D.
Department of Psychiatry, University of North Carolina School of Medicine, Chapel Hill, North Carolina

John J. Haggerty, Jr., M.D.
Department of Psychiatry, University of North Carolina School of Medicine, Chapel Hill, North Carolina

Markus Heilig, M.D.
Department of Psychiatry and Neurochemistry, University of Lund, Lund, Sweden

Lakshmi S. Kamaraju, M.D.
Department of Psychiatry, Duke University Medical Center, Durham, North Carolina

S. Kuo, M.D.
Experimental Therapeutics Branch, National Institute of Neurological and Communicative Disorders and Stroke, Bethesda, Maryland

Beth Levant, Ph.D.
Department of Pharmacology, Duke University Medical Center, Durham, North Carolina

William M. McDonald, M.D.
Department of Psychiatry, Duke University Medical Center, Durham, North Carolina

Robert L. Moss, Ph.D.
Professor of Physiology and Neurology, Department of Physiology, The University of Texas Southwestern Medical Center, Dallas, Texas

Charles B. Nemeroff, M.D., Ph.D.
Departments of Psychiatry and Pharmacology, Duke University Medical Center, Durham, North Carolina

Cort A. Pedersen, M.D.
Department of Psychiatry, University of North Carolina School of Medicine, Chapel Hill, North Carolina

Diana O. Perkins, M.D.
Department of Psychiatry, University of North Carolina School of Medicine, Chapel Hill, North Carolina

Robert M. Post, M.D.
National Institute of Mental Health, Bethesda, Maryland

K. Ranga Rama Krishnan, M.D.
Department of Psychiatry, Duke University Medical Center, Durham, North Carolina

S. Craig Risch, M.D.
Department of Psychiatry, Emory University School of Medicine, Atlanta, Georgia

Peter N. Riskind, M.D., Ph.D.
Department of Neurology, Massachusetts General Hospital, Boston, Massachusetts

David R. Rubinow, M.D.
National Institute of Mental Health, Bethesda, Maryland

Jeffrey S. Simon, M.D.
Department of Psychiatry, University of Wisconsin, Mount Sinai Medical Center, Milwaukee, Wisconsin

Robert A. Stern, Ph.D.
Department of Psychiatry, University of North Carolina School of Medicine, Chapel Hill, North Carolina

C. A. Tamminga, M.D.
Experimental Therapeutics Branch, National Institute of Neurological and Communicative Disorders and Stroke, Bethesda, Maryland; Department of Psychiatry, MPRC, University of Maryland, Baltimore, Maryland

K. Tanimoto, M.D.
Experimental Therapeutics Branch, National Institute of Neurological and Communicative Disorders and Stroke, Bethesda, Maryland

Erik Widerlöv, M.D., Ph.D.
Department of Psychiatry and Neurochemistry, University of Lund, Lund, Sweeden

Andrew Winokur, M.D., Ph.D.
Departments of Psychiatry and Pharmacology, University of Pennsylvania, Philadelphia, Pennsylvania

Introduction to the Progress in Psychiatry Series

The Progress in Psychiatry Series is designed to capture in print the excitement that comes from assembling a diverse group of experts from various locations to examine in detail the newest information about a developing aspect of psychiatry. This series emerged as a collaboration between the American Psychiatric Association's (APA) Scientific Program Committee and the American Psychiatric Press, Inc. Great interest is generated by a number of the symposia presented each year at the APA Annual Meeting, and we realized that much of the information presented there, carefully assembled by people who are deeply immersed in a given area, would unfortunately not appear together in print. The symposia sessions at the Annual Meetings provide an unusual opportunity for experts who otherwise might not meet on the same platform to share their diverse viewpoints for a period of 3 hours. Some new themes are repeatedly reinforced and gain credence, while in other instances disagreements emerge, enabling the audience and now the reader to reach informed decisions about new directions in the field. The Progress in Psychiatry Series allows us to publish and capture some of the best of the symposia and thus provide an in-depth treatment of specific areas that might not otherwise be presented in broader review formats.

Psychiatry is by nature an interface discipline, combining the study of mind and brain, of individual and social environments, of the humane and the scientific. Therefore, progress in the field is rarely linear=mit often comes from unexpected sources. Further, new developments emerge from an array of viewpoints that do not necessarily provide immediate agreement but rather expert examination of the issues. We intend to present innovative ideas and data that will enable you, the reader, to participate in this process.

We believe the Progress in Psychiatry Series will provide you with an opportunity to review timely new information in specific fields of interest as they are developing. We hope you find that the excitement of the presentations is captured in the written word and that this book proves to be informative and enjoyable reading.

David Spiegel, M.D.
Series Editor
Progress in Psychiatry Series

Progress in Psychiatry Series Titles

The Borderline: Current Empirical Research (#1)
Edited by Thomas H. McGlashan, M.D.

Premenstrual Syndrome: Current Findings and Future Directions (#2)
Edited by Howard J. Osofsky, M.D., Ph.D., and Susan J. Blumenthal, M.D.

Treatment of Affective Disorders in the Elderly (#3)
Edited by Charles A. Shamoian, M.D.

Post-Traumatic Stress Disorder in Children (#4)
Edited by Spencer Eth, M.D., and Robert S. Pynoos, M.D., M.P.H.

The Psychiatric Implications of Menstruation (#5)
Edited by Judith H. Gold, M.D., F.R.C.P. (C)

Can Schizophrenia Be Localized in the Brain? (#6)
Edited by Nancy C. Andreasen, M.D., Ph.D.

Medical Mimics of Psychiatric Disorders (#7)
Edited by Irl Extein, M.D., and Mark S. Gold, M.D.

Biopsychosocial Aspects of Bereavement (#8)
Edited by Sidney Zisook, M.D.

Psychiatric Pharmacosciences of Children and Adolescents (#9)
Edited by Charles Popper, M.D.

Psychobiology of Bulimia (#10)
Edited by James I. Hudson, M.D., and Harrison G. Pope, Jr., M.D.

Cerebral Hemisphere Function in Depression (#11)
Edited by Marcel Kinsbourne, M.D.

Eating Behavior in Eating Disorders (#12)
Edited by B. Timothy Walsh, M.D.

Tardive Dyskinesia: Biological Mechanisms and Clinical Aspects (#13)
Edited by Marion E. Wolf, M.D., and Aron D. Mosnaim, Ph.D.

Current Approaches to the Prediction of Violence (#14)
Edited by David A. Brizer, M.D., and Martha L. Crowner, M.D.

Treatment of Tricyclic-Resistant Depression (#15)
Edited by Irl L. Extein, M.D.

Depressive Disorders and Immunity (#16)
Edited by Andrew H. Miller, M.D.

Depression and Families: Impact and Treatment (#17)
Edited by Gabor I. Keitner, M.D.

Depression in Schizophrenia (#18)
Edited by Lynn E. DeLisi, M.D.

Biological Assessment and Treatment of Posttraumatic Stress Disorder (#19)
Edited by Earl L. Giller, Jr., M.D., Ph.D.

Personality Disorders: New Perspectives on Diagnostic Validity (#20)
Edited by John M. Oldham, M.D.

Serotonin in Major Psychiatric Disorders (#21)
Edited by Emil F. Coccaro, M.D., and Dennis L. Murphy, M.D.

Amino Acids in Psychiatric Disease (#22)
Edited by Mary Ann Richardson, Ph.D.

Family Environment and Borderline Personality Disorder (#23)
Edited by Paul Skevington Links, M.D.

Biological Rhythms, Mood Disorders, Light Therapy, and the Pineal Gland (#24)
Edited by Mohammad Shafii, M.D., and Sharon Lee Shafii, R.N., B.S.N.

Treatment Strategies for Refractory Depression (#25)
Edited by Steven P. Roose, M.D., and Alexander H. Glassman, M.D.

Combined Pharmacotherapy and Psychotherapy for Depression (#26)
Edited by Donna Manning, M.D., and Allen J. Frances, M.D.

The Neuroleptic Nonresponsive Patient: Characterization and Treatment (#27)
Edited by Burt Angrist, M.D., and S. Charles Schulz, M.D.

Negative Schizophrenic Symptoms: Pathophysiology and Clinical Implications (#28)
Edited by John F. Greden, M.D., and Rajiv Tandon, M.D.

Neuropeptides and Psychiatric Disorders (#29)
Edited by Charles B. Nemeroff, M.D., Ph.D.

Chapter 1

The Neurobiology of Neuropeptides: An Introduction

Charles B. Nemeroff, M.D., Ph.D.

Chapter 1

The Neurobiology of Neuropeptides: An Introduction

This chapter provides the reader with a brief introduction to the neurobiology of neuropeptides, which will serve as a template for each of the chapters that follow.

More than 50 neuropeptides have thus far been isolated and sequenced (see Table 1-1). They range in size from small dipeptides (two amino acids joined by a single peptide bond) to large molecules, such as corticotropin-releasing factor (CRF), which is comprised of 41 amino acids. Several comprehensive reviews of the distribution and neurochemical, neurophysiological, neuropharmacological, and behavioral effects of the major neuropeptides have recently appeared. These data are briefly reviewed below, with special attention to the literature concerning the human central nervous system (CNS). In particular, the neurobiology of neuropeptides is compared with that of the previously described monoamine neurotransmitters. (See Figure 1-1 for a comparison of peptidergic neurons with monoaminergic neurons.)

With few exceptions, peptides have been discovered by a singular pattern. A crude brain extract is noted to possess some biological activity (e.g., hypotension). This activity is then found to be due to the presence of a peptide, and the peptide is eventually purified and sequenced. In 1931, substance P was discovered by von Euler and Gaddum (1931); however, 40 years elapsed prior to elucidation of its chemical identity as a undecapeptide. Some peptides, such as insulin, were discovered in pure form in the early 1950s; their presence in brain was not appreciated until approximately 20 years later. In the

The author's research is supported by grants MH-39415, MH-40159, and MH-40524 from the National Institute of Mental Health. The author is grateful to Shelia Walker for typing the manuscript.

1940s and 1950s, the vision of a select few investigators gave rise to the "new" multidisciplinary field of neuroendocrinology (McCann 1988).

In fact, for many years, the single greatest impetus for neuropeptide research was the realization that the endocrine axes are organized in

Table 1-1. Neuropeptides identified in mammalian brain

Adrenocorticotropin (ACTH)	Kytorphin
Alpha-endorphin	Leucine-enkephalin
Angiotensin	Luteinizing hormone (LH)
Atrial natriuretic hormone	α-Melanocyte-stimulating hormone (α-MSH)
Beta-endorphin	β-Melanocyte-stimulating hormone (β-MSH)
Bombesin	Melanocyte-stimulating hormone release–inhibiting factor (MIF-I)
Bradykinin	Methionine-enkephalin
Calcitonin	Motilin
Calcitonin-gene–related peptide	Neurokinin A
Carnosine	Neuromedin N
Cholecystokinin	Neuropeptide Y
Corticotropin-releasing factor (CRF)	Neurotensin
Delta-sleep–inducing peptide (DSIP)	Oxytocin
Dynorphin	Pancreatic polypeptide
Galanin	Peptide histidine isoleucine
Gamma-endorphin	Peptide YY
Gastric-inhibitory peptide (GIP)	Prolactin (PRL)
Gastrin	Relaxin
Gastrin-releasing peptide	Secretin
Glicentin	Somatostatin (SRIF, GHIH)
Glucagon	Substance P
Gonadotropin-releasing hormone (GnRH)	Thyroid-stimulating hormone (thyrotropin, TSH)
Growth hormone (GH)	Thyrotropin-releasing hormone (TRH)
Growth hormone–releasing factor (GHRF)	Vasoactive intestinal polypeptide (VIP)
Inhibin	Vasopressin
Insulin	Vasotocin
Kallikrein	

a hierarchical fashion, with the CNS at the nadir. The major physiological control of anterior pituitary hormone secretion is now known to be mediated by neuropeptides: the hypothalamic hypophysiotropic (release and release-inhibiting) factors. The elucidation of this hierarchical organization of neuroendocrine regulation had many contributors, but two groups must be mentioned here. Ernst and Berta Scharrer (Scharrer and Scharrer 1940), along with Bargmann (1975), demonstrated the presence of secretory

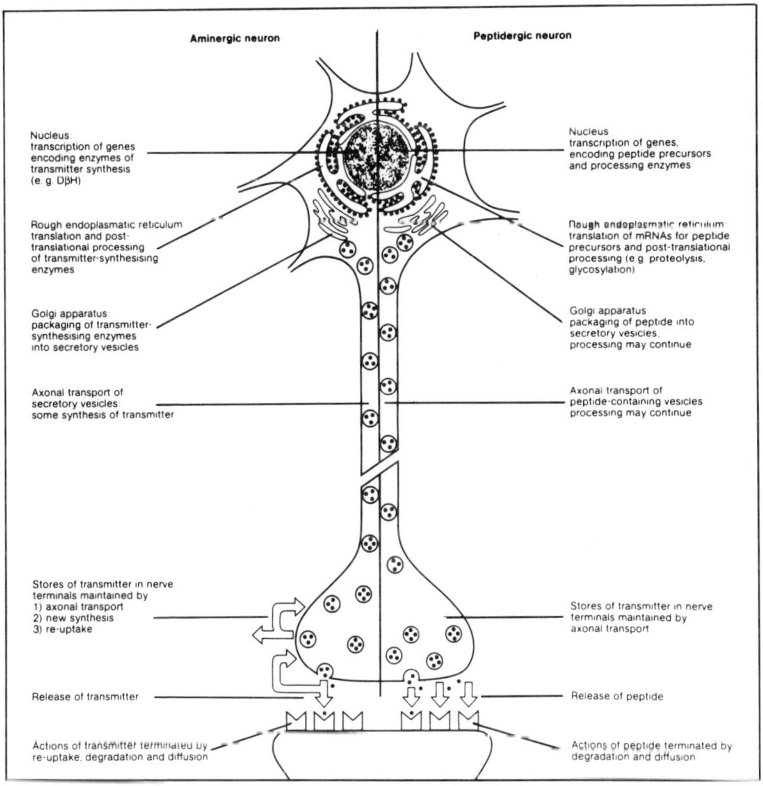

Figure 1-1. Schematic diagram illustrating the differences between peptidergic neurons and those containing classical neurotransmitters. Reprinted, with permission, from Harmar AJ, in *Transmitter Molecules in the Brain*. Edited by Fink G, McQueen J, Harmar AJ, et al. Berlin, Springer-Verlag, 1985, p. 20. Copyright 1985, Springer-Verlag.

granules within CNS neurons, giving rise to the entire concept of *neurosecretion.* Second, Harris (1955) formulated the *chemotransmitter-portal vessel hypothesis*, which proposed that neurohormones are released from nerve terminals in the median eminence of the hypothalamus and humorally transported from the primary capillary plexus to the adenohypophysis by the hypothalamo-hypophyseal venous portal system. We now know that once in the anterior pituitary, these releasing hormones bind to membrane receptors, which results in the release (or inhibition of release) of one or more pituitary trophic hormones. Millions of sheep (ovine) and pig (porcine) hypothalami were used to provide eventually a few precious milligrams of the first hypothalamic releasing factors to be discovered. These included the tripeptide *thyrotropin-releasing hormone* (TRH), the decapeptide *luteinizing hormone–releasing hormone* (LHRH), and the tetradecapeptide *somatostatin* (somatotropin-release–inhibiting factor [SRIF]).[1]

Not only have these findings resulted in diagnostic and treatment advances in endocrinology, but they have also had considerable impact in psychiatry (see below). It is now becoming more evident that particular psychiatric disorders are often associated with robust and reproducible neuroendocrine abnormalities. It is clear that neuropeptides are important chemical messengers in the CNS; they function as neurotransmitters or neuromodulators and, consequently, modulate behavior. Moreover, alterations of specific neuropeptide-containing neurons apparently occur in several neuropsychiatric diseases, including Alzheimer's disease, Parkinson's disease, mood disorders, schizophrenia, and Huntington's disease (Nemeroff and Bissette 1986).

Obviously, a comprehensive discussion of the evidence that supports a neurotransmitter role for each of the neuropeptides present in the mammalian CNS cannot be provided within the framework of this chapter. As with the monoamines, controversy still exists as to whether or not these chemical messengers fulfill *all* of the requisite neurotransmitter criteria. There is also evidence that neuropeptides can act as neuromodulators (substances that modulate the actions of classical neurotransmitters).

ANATOMIC LOCALIZATION OF NEUROPEPTIDES

Neuropeptides are heterogeneously distributed in the CNS, as ascertained from immunohistochemical and biochemical studies. The

[1]Interestingly, it has been reported that neuropeptides are present in unicellular organisms such as *E. coli*. Their structures have therefore been conserved through millions of years of evolution (Acher 1983).

pattern of distribution of each peptide is relatively unique. Thus in man and other mammals, neurotensin is found in high concentrations in the hypothalamus, amygdala, nucleus accumbens, and septum. In contrast, vasoactive intestinal polypeptide (VIP) and cholecystokinin are present in high concentrations in the cerebral cortex, as well as in the hippocampus. Other neuropeptides, such as LHRH or growth hormone–releasing factor (GHRF), have much more restricted patterns of distribution; they are found almost exclusively in the diencephalon.

Recent findings of Hökfelt and colleagues (1984), and of others (Nemeroff and Bissette 1986), have convincingly demonstrated colocalization of neuropeptides and monoamines. The colocalization of substance P and 5-hydroxytryptamine (5-HT) in descending spinal pathways has been perhaps the most closely scrutinized example of this phenomenon. Recently, compelling evidence for colocalization of cholecystokinin and dopamine has appeared. As noted above, the colocalization of dopamine and several neuropeptides in neurons of the tuberoinfundibular system of the hypothalamus, a circuit of certain significance in neuroendocrine regulation, is of particular importance.

SYNTHESIS

Again, it is of interest to compare the neurobiology of neuropeptides with that of the more well-studied monoamines (Figure 1-1). One major difference between these two classes of neurotransmitters is in their biosynthesis (see Eiden 1988 for review). Neuropeptides are synthesized in the perikaryon (typically as a large prohormone) via protein synthesis on polyribosomes by messenger RNA (mRNA) transcribed from DNA, and, after packaging, the neuropeptides are transported down the axon to the nerve terminal, where they are cleaved to yield the active form, which is subsequently released. The primary mRNA sequence contains the primary sequence of the prohormone interrupted by sequences known as introns. The mRNA is transported to the cytoplasm, where it binds to ribosomes, and translation ensues to yield the prohormone. In contrast, monoamines are synthesized primarily within the nerve terminal by a series of well-characterized enzymatic steps from an amino acid precursor (see above).

The mode of inactivation in each of these two classes of neuroregulators is also quite unique. Peptides are inactivated by enzymes (peptidases) that cleave peptide bonds; monoamines are removed from the synaptic cleft primarily by reuptake into the presynaptic terminal. The physiological consequences of monoamine release are brief, whereas the action of neuropeptides can be relatively long lived.

The prohormone molecules are considerably larger than the active peptides, and we know little about the process by which the active peptide is liberated from its large precursor. We do know that dibasic amino acid pairs are almost always present at the cleavage sites where neuropeptides are liberated from their prohormones. In addition, for at least some peptides, such as LHRH, the portion of the precursor that does not contain the active neuropeptide is not biologically inert—it contains a prolactin-inhibiting factor (Seeburg and Adelman 1984).

Posttranslation modifications of peptides, particularly large ones, have now been demonstrated, including glycosylation, amidation, phosphorylation, and acetylation (Eiden 1988).

Although we cannot yet reliably measure neuropeptide turnover, we can obtain estimates of neuropeptide biosynthesis. In situ hybridization using complementary DNA (cDNA) probes can be utilized to visualize mRNA in microscopic sections of the brain. This method has extraordinary anatomic resolution and can be quantified by computer-assisted methods. Biochemical methods to measure mRNA concentrations are also available.

RELEASE

Neuropeptide release occurs when neurons are depolarized. This process can be studied in the laboratory in brain slices or preparations of isolated nerve endings (synaptosomes). Release of neuropeptides can be induced by electrical stimulation or by the addition of depolarizing concentrations of potassium. As in the case of other neurotransmitters, neuropeptide release has been shown to be calcium-dependent (Smith et al. 1986). In certain brain regions, neuropeptide release is modified by monoamine neurotransmitters.

After being released from presynaptic nerve terminals, neuropeptides diffuse across the synapse and bind to high-affinity receptors located on the postsynaptic membrane. These receptors have been identified using iodinated or tritiated ligands coupled with autoradiography or "grind-and-bind" methods. Autoradiography is similar to in situ hybridization in providing exquisite anatomical resolution. In addition to postsynaptic receptors, there is also some evidence for the existence of presynaptic peptidergic receptors on nerve terminals, which may represent autoreceptors that modulate peptide release.

After neuropeptides bind to their receptors, they act via second-messenger systems to produce changes in the postsynaptic neurons.

The involvement of cyclic nucleotides such as cyclic AMP and cyclic GMP as second messengers in mediating the actions of certain neuropeptides such as SRIF and CRF, after they bind to their respective receptors, is well established (Northup 1989). More recently, another second-messenger system has been elucidated: phosphoinositide hydrolysis (Agranoff 1989). There is evidence that the action of certain peptides, such as TRH, is mediated by this pathway after the peptide binds to its postsynaptic receptor. It is also of interest to note the recent work on identification of third-messenger systems in signal transduction: these appear to be largely comprised of phosphorylation of specific membrane proteins mediated by protein kinases (Cain et al. 1988). Electrophysiological correlates of neuropeptide action at the receptors have also been described, especially for LHRH and CRF (Jan and Jan 1983).

The termination of peptide action by peptidases was briefly alluded to above. A number of peptidases have been described, including specific endopeptidases, a pyroglutamyl peptidase, carboxypeptidases, and others (Turner 1987). Certain of these peptidases are soluble, whereas others are membrane bound. We know virtually nothing about the regulation of the activity of these enzymes or in fact whether they are involved in physiologically regulating neuropeptide availability in the CNS.

One of the factors that has hindered neuropeptide research to a considerable extent is the lack of pharmacological agents that *specifically* alter the synaptic availability of neuropeptides. With the exception of naloxone and naltrexone, the opioid-receptor antagonists, there are few available neuropeptide-receptor antagonists. There are no drugs that specifically cause the degeneration or depletion of any one neuropeptide. Protein-synthesis inhibitors, such as cycloheximide, will inhibit the protein synthesis of all proteins, including neuropeptides, but they are relatively toxic agents and lack specificity. Lipophilic compounds that act as agonists at peptide receptors and that can readily enter the brain after peripheral administration are also lacking.

APPLICATIONS TO PSYCHIATRIC ILLNESS

In view of the large number of neuropeptides in the brain and their occurrence in brain regions thought to be involved in the pathogenesis of major psychiatric disorders, investigators have sought to determine whether alterations in neuropeptide systems are associated with schizophrenia, mood disorders, anxiety disorders, and neurodegenerative diseases. The major strategies employed to test these hypotheses are as follows. First, neuropeptides and neuropeptide receptors are measured in postmortem brain tissue from patients with one or another psychiatric disorder and from appropriate control subjects. In addition, cerebrospinal fluid (CSF) concentrations of neuropeptides have also been measured. A second strategy has been to administer neuropeptides or neuropeptide-receptor antagonists to patients and determine if any amelioration in symptoms occurs. A third approach has been the neuroendocrine "window" strategy, which, simply stated, is the attempt to elucidate endocrine alterations in psychiatric disease and determine their cause, (e.g., hypothalamic peptide or amine dysregulation). In the chapters that follow, each of these strategies is discussed in detail for each of the peptides described.

If one peruses the neuropeptide literature, the progress made in the last two decades must be considered impressive. Much of this can be attributed to technical advances in methodology—radioimmunoassay, high-pressure liquid chromatography, autoradiography, and in situ hybridization. Our clinical studies are also becoming better designed and more sophisticated. As advances in design of peptidomimetic compounds occur, the possibility for novel therapeutic agents increases substantially. As the reader will see in the chapters that follow, there is no longer any doubt that neuropeptide-containing neurons are altered in several neuropsychiatric disorders. The future for neuropeptides in psychiatry remains bright indeed.

REFERENCES

Acher R: Principles of evolution: the neural hierarchy model, in Brain Peptides. Edited by Krieger DT, Brownstein MJ, Martin JB. New York, John Wiley-Interscience, 1983, pp 136–163

Agranoff BW: Phosphoinositides, in Basic Neurochemistry, 4th Edition. Edited by Siegel G, Agranoff B, Albers RW, et al. New York, Raven, 1989, pp 333–347

Bargmann W: A marvelous region, in Pioneers in Neuroendocrinology, Vol 1. Edited by Meites J, Donovan BT, McCann SM. New York, Plenum, 1975, pp 37–43

Cain ST, Abramson M, Nemeroff CB: Neurotensin stimulates the phosphorylation of caudate nucleus synaptosomal proteins. Ann NY Acad Sci 537:488–490, 1988

Eiden LE: The cell biology of the peptidergic neuron: an overview, in Neuropeptides in Psychiatric and Neurological Disorders. Edited by Nemeroff CB. Baltimore, MD, Johns Hopkins University Press, 1988, pp 1–17

Harris GW: Neural Control of the Pituitary Gland. London, Arnold, 1955

Hökfelt T, Everitt BJ, Theodorsson-Norheim T, et al: Neurotensin and NPY-like immunoreactivities in central catecholamine neurons, in Catecholamines: Neuropharmacology and Central Nervous System: Theoretical Aspects. Edited by Usdin E, Carlsson A, Dahlstrom A, et al. New York, Alan R Liss, 1984, pp 231–237

Jan YN, Jan LY: Electrophysiological techniques, in Brain Peptides. Edited by Krieger DT, Brownstein MJ, Martin JB. New York, John Wiley-Interscience, 1983, pp 547–564

McCann SM: Saga of the discovery of hypothalamic releasing and inhibiting hormones, in Endocrinology: People and Ideas. Edited by McCann SM. Bethesda, MD, American Physiological Society, 1988, pp 41–62

Nemeroff CB, Bissette G: Neuropeptides in psychiatric disorders, in American Handbook of Psychiatry, Vol 8. Edited by Berger PA, Brodie HKH. New York, Basic Books, 1986, pp 64–110

Northup JK: Regulation of cyclic nucleotides in the nervous system, in Basic Neurochemistry, 4th Edition. Edited by Siegal G, Agranoff B, Albers RW, et al. New York, Raven, 1989, pp 349–363

Scharrer E, Scharrer B: Secretory cells within the hypothalamus. Res Publ Assoc Res Nerv Ment Dis 20:170–194, 1940

Seeburg PH, Adelman JP: Characterization of cDNA for precursor of human luteinizing hormone releasing hormone. Nature 311:666–668, 1984

Smith MA, Bissette G, Slotkin TA, et al: Release of corticotropin-releasing factor from rat brain regions in vitro. Endocrinology 118:1997–2001, 1986

Turner AJ (ed): Neuropeptides and Their Peptidases. Chichester, UK, Ellis Horwood, 1987

von Euler US, Gaddum JH: An unidentified depressor substance in certain tissue extracts. J Physiol (Lond) 72:74–81, 1931

Watson SJ, Khachaturian H, Lewis ME, et al: Chemical neuroanatomy as a basis for biological psychiatry, in American Handbook of Psychiatry, Vol 8. Edited by Berger PA, Brodie HKH. New York, Basic Books, 1986, pp 3–33

Chapter 2

The Relevance of Thyrotropin-Releasing Hormone to Psychiatric Disorders

Andrew Winokur, M.D., Ph.D.

Chapter 2

The Relevance of Thyrotropin-Releasing Hormone to Psychiatric Disorders

This chapter serves as an overview of the relevance of thyrotropin-releasing hormone (TRH) to psychiatric disorders. The major areas to be considered include preclinical studies examining behavioral effects of TRH and clinical studies on TRH in depression and schizophrenia. Before discussing these topics, however, it seems appropriate to provide a brief overview regarding some basic aspects of TRH in the central nervous system (CNS).

TRH was the first of the hypothalamic releasing hormones to be isolated and characterized. Its structure, which was first reported in 1969, was identified as a tripeptide, pyroglutamylhistidylprolinamide (Bowers et al. 1970; Burgus et al. 1970). TRH was soon synthesized in biologically active form, and it rapidly became widely available both for research studies and for use clinically as a neuroendocrine provocative agent of value in the assessment of thyroid axis dysfunction. In 1972, a sensitive and specific radioimmunoassay procedure for TRH was developed (Bassiri and Utiger 1972). This assay allowed several investigators to examine the regional distribution of TRH throughout the CNS. In 1974, reports from three different laboratories established that TRH was widely distributed throughout the CNS and not, as might previously have been imagined, exclusively localized in the hypothalamus (Jackson and Reichlin 1974; Oliver et al. 1974; Winokur and Utiger 1974). Immediately following this discovery, many investigations focused on the hypothesis that TRH may function as a neurotransmitter or neuromodulator in the CNS.

Supported by a National Institute of Mental Health Research Scientist Award (MH-00044).

Subsequent studies have established, for example, that TRH is highly concentrated in the nerve terminal region and apparently stored in synaptic vesicles (Winokur et al. 1977), that enzymes are available in the brain that can inactivate the tripeptide (Griffiths et al. 1983), and that receptors for TRH are widely and selectively localized throughout the CNS (Manaker et al. 1986). Moreover, studies employing neurophysiological techniques have provided evidence that TRH is capable of directly altering neuronal activity (Renaud and Martin 1975) and that interactive effects between TRH and several other neurochemical systems (e.g., norepinephrine, acetylcholine, glutamate) can be demonstrated (Renaud et al. 1979; Winokur and Beckman 1978; Yarbrough 1976). Thus, a considerable amount of research supports the involvement of TRH in a wide range of CNS functions.

BEHAVIORAL EFFECTS OF TRH

Examination of behavioral effects produced by TRH evolved from a series of studies on hormones of the thyroid axis in depression carried out in the 1960s at the University of North Carolina by Prange, Lipton, and coworkers (Prange 1974). In particular, they reported interactive effects between thyroid hormones and tricyclic antidepressant compounds in animals (Breese et al. 1974b), subsequently demonstrating that small doses of a thyroid hormone preparation could potentiate the effects of tricyclic antidepressants (TCAs) in depressed subjects (Wilson et al. 1974). With the availability of TRH for experimentation in the early 1970s, it was of interest to determine whether this CNS component of the thyroid axis could produce effects of relevance to the antidepressant compounds.

In collaboration with N. P. Plotnikoff of Abbott Laboratories, the North Carolina investigators administered TRH (10 mg intraperitoneally) to mice in the dopa potentiation test, an animal model used to screen for putative antidepressant effects (Plotnikoff et al. 1972). In this model, mice are pretreated with a priming dose of a monoamine oxidase inhibitor (MAOI) and a threshold dose of L-dopa. Administration of a clinically effective antidepressant compound such as the TCA imipramine results in a marked increase in spontaneous motor activity in animals pretreated in this manner. When a novel compound is demonstrated to enhance motor activity in the dopa potentiation test, it is considered to be a candidate for having antidepressant efficacy. In the study by Plotnikoff et al. (1972), TRH was reported to produce significant enhancement of motor activity in appropriately pretreated mice. The effects produced by TRH administration were similar to those observed in imipramine-treated mice. Moreover, the effects produced by TRH were still seen in mice that had previously been hypophysectomized. Thus, this study produced two striking findings. First, the efficacy of TRH in the dopa potentiation test suggested that this tripeptide might have efficacy as an antidepressant compound. Second, the observation that TRH exerted comparable effects in hypophysectomized mice indicated that these effects were not accounted for by mobilization of the pituitary-thyroid axis (i.e., the classic hypophysiotropic effects of TRH), but rather reflected direct CNS actions of the tripeptide. (As a follow-up to this study, two investigators [Kastin et al. 1972; Prange et al. 1972] examined the effects of TRH administration in depressed patients. The findings obtained from these clinical trials will be described later in this chapter.)

As noted above, the report of Plotnikoff et al. (1972) provided strong evidence that TRH was capable of exerting direct effects on the CNS. With the subsequent reports that this hypothalamic releasing hormone was actually distributed widely throughout the CNS (Jackson and Reichlin 1974; Oliver et al. 1974; Winokur and Utiger 1974), considerable interest was directed to the hypothesis that TRH functioned as a neurotransmitter or neuromodulator in the CNS. While neuropeptides are now commonly recognized to subserve varied, diverse roles both in the CNS and in the periphery, such insights were quite novel in the early 1970s. Spurred on by these early reports, many investigators undertook studies to elucidate the CNS effects of TRH, and, indeed, administration of TRH was soon linked to a variety of physiological and behavioral effects (Griffiths 1985; Yarbrough 1979). Physiological effects associated with TRH administration included (among many others) alterations in cardiovascular function, respiratory rate, body temperature, gastric secretion, colonic motility, and electroencephalographic activity. A variety of behavioral effects were also demonstrated following TRH administration. A complete compilation of these effects is not possible in this chapter, but a few specific examples will be discussed.

One of the most widely studied behavioral effects of TRH involves its ability to reverse the sedative and hypothermic effects of a number of CNS-depressant compounds. Initially reported with respect to the sedating effects of ethanol and pentobarbital (Breese et al. 1974a; Prange et al. 1974), TRH has subsequently been shown to exert analeptic properties in animals treated with barbiturate compounds, opiates, minor tranquilizers (i.e., benzodiazepines), and major tranquilizers (i.e., phenothiazines) (Kalivas and Horita 1979). Kalivas and Horita (1979) attempted to identify the anatomic substrates of the analeptic properties of TRH by examining its efficacy following microinjection into discrete brain regions of pretreated rats. A pronounced pattern of regional anatomic sensitivity was identified, with areas of highest responsitivity to TRH administration being localized in the ventromedial septum. These findings prompted the investigators to speculate that TRH produced its analeptic properties by modulating septohippocampal neurons, with actions presumed to involve alteration of cholinergic neurons (Kalivas et al. 1981).

Stanton and coworkers (1980) extended this line of investigation by examining the effects of TRH in an animal in a "natural" state of CNS depression—the hibernating ground squirrel (*Citellus lateralis*). Microinjection of TRH bilaterally into the dorsal hippocampus resulted in full physiological and behavioral arousal from hibernation. Strikingly, TRH was active in doses as low as 100 picograms (0.32 pM). The regional specificity of the effects produced by TRH was evidenced by the finding that microinjection of higher doses (up to 1,000 ng) into other regions, including the cerebral cortex, brain stem, and hypothalamus, did not produce alterations in the state of hibernation. Moreover, chemical specificity for the effects of TRH was indicated by the finding that administration of TRH-OH, the biologically inactive free acid metabolite of TRH, into the dorsal hippocampus in doses up to 1,000 ng was ineffective in altering the state of hibernation.

Stanton and coworkers (1981) then examined the effects of TRH microinjection into the dorsal hippocampus of ground squirrels studied while euthermic but in a state of slow-wave sleep. In this case, TRH produced effects that were similar in direction, although smaller in magnitude, to those seen in hibernating animals. Thus, there was a modest increase in brain temperature and metabolic rate following administration of TRH during slow-wave sleep. In this study, electromyographic activity and electroencephalographic activity were also recorded throughout the period of observation. Administration of TRH during slow-wave sleep produced an increase in electromyographic activity and an activation of electroencephalographic activity.

In the next series of studies, TRH was microinjected into the dorsal hippocampus of ground squirrels studied while euthermic and awake (Stanton et al. 1981). Interestingly, in this case, TRH produced effects that were *opposite* in direction to those observed in both the hibernating and the euthermic sleeping ground squirrels. Thus, microinjection of TRH to active ground squirrels produced a decrease in brain temperature, metabolic rate, and electromyographic activity and a slowing of electroencephalographic activity, with the appearance of sleep spindles being evident in some cases. Moreover, more potent effects following TRH administration were observed in behaviorally active ground squirrels than in quiescent animals. Based upon the findings obtained in this line of studies with the ground squirrel, Stanton et al. (1981) speculated that TRH might play a role in the regulation of CNS activity states. Thus, TRH might serve to protect a homeostatically regulated set point for CNS activity, which would consequently counteract swings in either direction (depression or excitation).

If TRH does play a role in the regulation of CNS activity states, it might also be anticipated that profound changes in CNS activity would produce significant alterations in some TRH neuronal systems. To examine this hypothesis, Stanton and coworkers (1982) examined endogenous concentrations of TRH in various brain regions of ground squirrels during different seasons or in the winter season while the squirrels were hibernating or awake. A significant reduction in the concentration of TRH was observed in the hypothalamus and preoptic-septal area of hibernating ground squirrels as compared with euthermic ground squirrels studied during the same season (i.e., winter). Examination of TRH concentrations in the pineal gland during different phases of hibernation revealed a striking fourfold increase from early to late in the hibernation bout. This finding raises the possibility that TRH plays a role as an endogenous agent of arousal from the state of hibernation, consistent with its demonstrated potency in producing arousal from hibernation following microinjection into the hippocampus.

Another opportunity to investigate the relationship between TRH and CNS activity states was provided by studies with the African lungfish (*Protopterus annectans*). During the dry season, the lungfish enters a state of torpor referred to as "estivation" (a form of "summer hibernation"). The state of estivation can be induced in the laboratory, allowing examination of the effect of this profound state of CNS depression on TRH levels in various brain regions. Kreider et al. (1987a) observed a significant decrease in TRH concentrations in the diencephalon (the region containing the hypothalamus) of estivating lungfish. Lungfish that were maintained in a state of starvation for a comparable period of time did not demonstrate any alterations in TRH concentrations, supporting the interpretation that the changes observed in the estivating animals were due to alterations in CNS activity state and not due to the effects of starvation per se.

The studies described to this point involved assessment of the relationship between TRH and states of CNS depression. It is also of interest to consider the converse situation: TRH and heightened CNS activity. Kubek and Sattin (1984) examined the effects of electroconvulsive shock (ECS), administered in a manner to simulate electroconvulsive therapy (ECT) for psychiatric patients, on regional brain TRH levels. A single ECS treatment did not alter TRH levels in any brain region examined. However, administration of ECS on an alternate-day schedule for 5 days produced pronounced increases in TRH concentration in various limbic regions, including the amygdala and hippocampus. The administration of a subconvulsant electrical current did not alter TRH levels, indicating that the induction of a seizure was essential to produce effects on TRH. The responsiveness of TRH in limbic regions to repeated ECS administration raises the possibility that TRH is involved in mediating the antidepressant effects of ECT.

Other forms of seizure induction in addition to ECS have been demonstrated to produce effects on TRH. For example, Kreider et al. (1987b) utilized kainic acid administration to induce limbic seizures in rats. They observed pronounced increases in TRH concentration in limbic brain areas, including the hippocampus, the amygdala, and regions of cortex. Up to 27-fold increases in TRH concentration were observed following administration of kainic acid. The effectiveness of seizure-induction agents to increase TRH levels in discrete brain regions raises the possibility that TRH is involved in the pathophysiological mechanisms of seizure disorders. Interestingly, administration of TRH in animal models of seizure disorder (Sato et al. 1984) and to patients with the disorder of infantile spasm (Matsumoto et al. 1987) has been reported to reduce the intensity and duration of seizures. Thus, an area for further investigation involves assessment of the efficacy of TRH or TRH analogues in the treatment of seizure disorders.

To summarize, studies utilizing a variety of animal models have produced evidence that TRH is capable of exerting a wide range of physiological and behavioral effects. Potential clinical implications of these studies include the possible utility of TRH in treating sedative-hypnotic overdosage, depression, and epilepsy. Moreover, the data reviewed above suggest that TRH may play a role in the regulation of CNS activity. Thus, further studies on the basic mechanisms of regulation of TRH may lead to new insights about its clinical utility.

TRH IN PSYCHIATRIC DISORDERS

TRH and Depression

As described above, the study by Plotnikoff et al. (1972) generated interest in the potential antidepressant properties of TRH. In 1972, two reports described results of TRH administration in depressed patients (Kastin et al. 1972; Prange et al. 1972). In these studies, administration of TRH (500 μg by bolus intravenous infusion) produced a significant reduction in ratings of depression compared with saline infusion. Antidepressant effects were observed within a few hours of TRH administration, a finding that was particularly striking in light of the widely recognized observation that the standard antidepressant agents typically require a period of several weeks to be effective. Consistent with the short half-life of TRH, the antidepressant effects observed following administration of the tripeptide were generally transient in nature. Itil et al. (1975) reported that TRH was effective in ameliorating motivational deficits observed in depressed patients. In the same study, electroencephalographic activity was monitored following administration of TRH. Interestingly, TRH produced an activation of electroencephalographic patterns similar to the effects produced by psychostimulants such as dextroamphetamine, MAOIs, and protriptyline.

The antidepressant effects reported for TRH in the early 1970s attracted a great deal of interest and attention. A number of studies were subsequently carried out to evaluate the efficacy of TRH in the treatment of depression. In the majority of these studies, TRH was *not* demonstrated to be an effective treatment for depression. Thus, at the present time, TRH does not appear to have a relevant role in the treatment of depression. Nevertheless, the reported rapid mood-elevating effects of this tripeptide remain an issue of potential conceptual interest. Moreover, it remains to be established whether a long-acting, centrally potent analogue of TRH may be of value in the treatment of depression.

Two studies have examined TRH levels in CSF obtained from depressed patients (Bánki et al. 1988; Kirkegaard et al. 1979). When compared with neurological patients, the depressed groups in both studies demonstrated significantly higher concentrations of TRH. In their study, Bánki et al. (1988) included 16 control subjects (12 patients diagnosed as having only peripheral neurological disease and four patients having a DSM-III diagnosis of somatization disorder) and 17 patients with major depression (the majority of whom met DSM-III diagnostic criteria for major depression with melancholia or with psychotic features). None of the depressed patients or control subjects had been treated with psychotropic medications for at least 2 weeks prior to start of the study. The mean CSF TRH concentration for the combined control group was 4.4 ± 1.8 pg/ml, while the concentration in the depressed group was 12.8 ± 5.7 pg/ml, almost a threefold elevation. The findings from the studies of Kirkegaard et al. (1979) and of Bánki et al. (1988) raise the possibility that elevated TRH levels represent a biological marker of depression. Moreover, as these authors point out, the finding of elevated CSF TRH levels may reflect hypersecretion of TRH in the CNS of depressed patients.

In studies involving depressed patients, TRH has also proven to be of interest with regard to its traditional role as a neuroendocrine provocative agent. From the initial studies involving TRH administration in depressed patients (Kastin et al. 1972; Prange et al. 1972), it has consistently been reported that a subset of depressed patients demonstrate a diminished or "blunted" thyroid-stimulating hormone (TSH) response to TRH administration (Loosen 1985; Loosen and Prange 1982). This finding has repeatedly been observed in approximately 25% of depressed patients examined. To date, the mechanism underlying the blunted TSH response has not been clarified. More recently, a second TSH response abnormality has been observed in depressed patients. Gold et al. (1981) reported that 8% to 10% of depressed patients demonstrate an exaggerated TSH response to TRH, a finding that they suggested was indicative of the presence of clinical or "subclinical" hypothyroidism. They presented preliminary, uncontrolled data indicating that patients with an exaggerated TSH response to TRH often benefited from short periods of thyroid hormone replacement therapy. Further controlled studies are needed to evaluate the efficacy of thyroid hormone treatment—either alone or in combination with TCAs—in depressed patients with an exaggerated TSH response to TRH.

The finding of a blunted TSH response to TRH in depression has prompted a number of suggestions regarding the clinical utility of this biological marker. Some interest has been directed to the possibility that the TRH stimulation test is of diagnostic value with regard to depression. However, this application has not proven to be of value because the TRH stimulation test lacks both sensitivity and specificity for depression (Loosen 1985). Indeed, a number of other psychiatric diagnoses, including schizophrenia, borderline personality disorder, anorexia nervosa, bulimia, panic disorder, obsessive-compulsive disorder, and alcoholism, have been reported to be associated with a higher than expected incidence of blunted TSH responses (Garbutt et al. 1983; Kiriike et al. 1987; Larsen et al. 1985; Levy et al. 1988; Loosen 1985; Sauer et al. 1984; Wolkin et al. 1984).

Although the TRH stimulation test has not proven to be of diagnostic validity with respect to depression, two other proposals have been advanced for its utility. First, Langer et al. (1986) have presented evidence to suggest that a change in the TSH response from blunted to normal predicts a positive response to antidepressant therapy. Additionally, Kirkegaard (1981) has emphasized the prognostic value of the TSH response in predicting long-term clinical outcome (remission or relapse) following completion of antidepressant drug therapy or ECT. While the results presented in these studies are of considerable potential interest, contradictory findings have been obtained in other investigations. Thus, further studies are needed to clarify the potential clinical utility of the TRH stimulation test in the treatment of depression.

TRH and Schizophrenia

While the majority of studies on TRH in psychiatric disorders have focused on affective disorders, some interest has been directed to schizophrenia as well. Several studies have examined the therapeutic benefits of TRH or TRH analogues in patients with schizophrenia (Brambilla et al. 1986; Inanaga et al. 1978; Mizuki et al. 1985; Wilson et al. 1973). Interestingly, the majority of studies to date have reported beneficial effects associated with TRH administration in schizophrenic patients. It should be emphasized that these studies have largely been carried out as open clinical trials, and, thus, further studies employing more rigorously controlled research designs are needed to assess the therapeutic potential for TRH in schizophrenia. In contrast to the rational conceptual linkage between basic and clinical studies of TRH in depression, no strong conceptual framework currently exists to underpin the empirical clinical findings derived from studies of TRH administration in schizophrenic patients.

Another approach to exploring the relevance of TRH to schizophrenia has involved examination of TRH and TRH receptors in postmortem brain specimens from patients with schizophrenia. Nemeroff et al. (1983) examined the concentration of TRH in various regions of schizophrenic brain tissue. No differences in TRH concentration were observed between schizophrenic and control specimens in any of the subcortical regions examined, including the amygdala, nucleus accumbens, caudate nucleus, and hypothalamus. However, significant reductions in TRH concentration were observed in cerebral cortical regions of schizophrenic brain, including Brodmann's areas 12 and 32. A recent preliminary investigation carried out in our own laboratory (unpublished data) employed the technique of quantitative autoradiography to examine the distribution of TRH receptors in various regions of schizophrenic brain. Significantly elevated concentrations of TRH receptors were observed in the hippocampus of schizophrenic brains, particularly in the molecular layer of the dentate gyrus, whereas significant decreases in TRH receptors were observed in several discrete nuclei of the amygdala. Of course, postmortem studies of schizophrenic brain tissue are potentially complicated by the confounding effects of neuroleptic medications. In the present preliminary study, however, two of the patients in the schizophrenia group had never received neuroleptic drug treatment. Moreover, in this study, postmortem brain specimen from neuroleptic-treated patients with Huntington's disease did not show increases in TRH concentrations in the hippocampus, as was observed in the schizophrenic brain specimen. Although preliminary in nature, these findings provide further support for the possible relevance of TRH to schizophrenia. The specific mechanisms underlying the increase in the number of TRH receptors in the hippocampus of schizophrenic brains remain to be established. An increase in postsynaptic receptors (i.e., "up-regulation") frequently occurs as a consequence of diminished availability of the presynaptic neurotransmitter agent. Thus, one might speculate that schizophrenia is associated with diminished TRH activity in certain neuronal systems of relevance to hippocampal function. Whether such hypothesized deficits would involve TRH pathways intrinsic to the hippocampus or projection pathways from extrinsic sites (as would pertain, for example, in the case of the septo-hippocampal pathway) remains to be established. Of course, other explanations for the elevated TRH receptor concentrations in the hippocampus must also be explored.

As noted above, studies on TRH in schizophrenia have been much more limited than have studies of affective disorders. Clearly, a more compelling rationale currently motivates studies of TRH in depression than in schizophrenia. Nevertheless, some interesting findings have emerged in the studies focusing on schizophrenia—in particular, observations of positive therapeutic effects associated with TRH administration to schizophrenic patients, and the finding of significantly elevated concentrations of TRH receptors in the hippocampus and decreases in these concentrations in nuclei of the amygdala of schizophrenic brains. Thus, this area has considerable promise for further exploration.

SUMMARY

Interest in the role of TRH in the CNS has expanded markedly over the past 20 years from the initial focus on its function as a hypothalamic hypophysiotropic agent. The study of Plotnikoff et al. (1972) provided compelling early evidence that administration of TRH could produce behavioral effects, that these effects are mediated through direct CNS mechanisms, and that the effects produced by TRH may be relevant to human psychiatric disorders. Further preclinical studies have strengthened and extended understanding of the physiological and behavioral effects exerted by TRH. Clinically directed studies of TRH in depression and schizophrenia have yielded both promising and disappointing results. To date, findings emerging from these studies have not clarified a specific role for TRH in the treatment of any psychiatric disorder. It should be emphasized, however, that a more definitive assessment of this issue may await the availability of TRH analogues that are safe, long acting, and centrally potent. On another level, data emerging from both preclinical and clinical studies may provide conceptual bases for implicating TRH as a component in the pathophysiological mechanisms of depression and/or schizophrenia.

REFERENCES

Bánki CM, Bissette G, Arato M, et al: Elevation of immunoreactive CSF TRH in depressed patients. Am J Psychiatry 145:1526–1531, 1988

Bassiri RM, Utiger RD: The preparation and specificity of antibody to thyrotropin releasing hormone. Endocrinology 90:722–727, 1972

Bowers CY, Schally AV, Schalch DS, et al: Activity and specificity of synthetic thyrotropin-releasing hormone in man. Biochem Biophys Res Commun 39:352–355, 1970

Brambilla F, Aguglia E, Massironi R, et al: Neuropeptide therapies in chronic schizophrenia: TRH and vasopressin administration. Neuropsychobiology 15:114–121, 1986

Breese GR, Cott JM, Cooper BR, et al: Antagonism of ethanol narcosis by thyrotropin-releasing hormone. Life Sci 14:1053–1063, 1974a

Breese GR, Prange AJ Jr, Lipton MA: Pharmacological interactions of thyroid-imipramine interactions in animals, in The Thyroid Axis, Drugs, and Behavior. Edited by Prange AJ Jr. New York, Raven, 1974b, pp 29–48

Burgus R, Dunn TE, Desideris D, et al: Characterization of ovine hypothalamic hypophysiotropic TSH-releasing factor. Nature 226:321–325, 1970

Garbutt JC, Loosen PT, Tipermas A, et al: The TRH test in patients with borderline personality disorder. Psychiatry Res 9:107–113, 1983

Gold MS, Pottash ALC, Mueller EA, et al: Grades of thyroid failure in 100 depressed and anergic patients. Am J Psychiatry 138:253–255, 1981

Griffiths EC: Thyrotrophin releasing hormone: endocrine and central effects. Psychoneuroendocrinology 10:225–235, 1985

Griffiths EC, McDermott JR, Visser TJ: Mechanisms of TRH inactivation: physiological significance of TRH degrading enzymes, in Thyrotropin-Releasing Hormone. Edited by Griffiths EC, Bennett GW. New York, Raven, 1983, pp 85–94

Inanaga K, Nakano T, Nagata T, et al: Behavioral effects of protirelin in schizophrenia. Arch Gen Psychiatry 35:1011–1014, 1978

Itil TM, Patterson CD, Polvan N, et al: Clinical and CNS effects of oral and intravenous thyrotropin-releasing hormone. Psychopharmacol Bull 1:29–37, 1975

Jackson IMD, Reichlin S: Thyrotropin releasing hormone (TRH): distribution in hypothalamic and extrahypothalamic brain tissues of mammalian and submammalian chordates. Endocrinology 95:854–862, 1974

Kalivas PW, Horita A: Thyrotropin-releasing hormone: central site of action in antagonism of pentobarbital narcosis. Nature 278:461–463, 1979

Kalivas PW, Simasko SM, Horita A: Effect of septohippocampal lesions on thyrotropin-releasing hormone antagonism of pentobarbital narcosis. Brain Res 222:253–265, 1981

Kastin AJ Jr, Schalch DS, Ehrensing RH, et al: Improvement in mental depression with decreased thyrotropin response after administration of thyrotropin-releasing hormone. Lancet 2:740–742, 1972

Kiriike N, Nishiwaki S, Izumiya Y, et al: Thyrotropin, prolactin, and growth hormone responses to the thyrotropin-releasing hormone in anorexia nervosa and bulimia. Biol Psychiatry 22:167–176, 1987

Kirkegaard C: The thyrotropin response to thyrotropin-releasing hormone in endogenous depression. Psychoneuroendocrinology 6:189–212, 1981

Kirkegaard C, Faber J, Hummer L, et al: Increased levels of TRH in cerebrospinal fluid from patients with endogenous depression. Psychoneuroendocrinology 4:227–235, 1979

Kreider MS, Winokur A, Pack AI, et al: Changes in the concentration of TRH in lungfish brain during estivation. Federation Proceedings 46:839, 1987a

Kreider MS, Wolfinger BL, Winokur A: Effect of systemic kainic acid on regional TRH concentrations in rat central nervous system. Neuroscience Abstracts 13:1656, 1987b

Kubek MJ, Sattin A: Effect of electroconvulsive shock on the content of thyrotropin-releasing hormone in rat brain. Life Sci 34:1149–1152, 1984

Langer G, Koinig G, Hatzinger R, et al: Response of thyrotropin to thyrotropin-releasing hormone as predictor of treatment outcome. Arch Gen Psychiatry 43:861–868, 1986

Larsen JK, Bjorum N, Kirkegaard C, et al: Dexamethasone suppression test,

TRH test and Newcastle II depression rating in the diagnosis of depressive disorders. Acta Psychiatr Scand 71:499–505, 1985

Levy AB, Dixon KN, Malarkey WB: Pituitary response to TRH in bulimia. Biol Psychiatry 23:476–484, 1988

Loosen PT: The TRH-induced TSH response in psychiatric patients: a possible neuroendocrine marker. Psychoneuroendocrinology 10:237–260, 1985

Loosen PT, Prange AJ Jr: Serum thyrotropin response to thyrotropin-releasing hormone in psychiatric patients: a review. Am J Psychiatry 239:405–416, 1982

Manaker S, Rainbow TC, Winokur A: Thyrotropin releasing hormone (TRH) receptors: localization in rat and human central nervous system, in Quantitative Receptor Autoradiography. Edited by Boast C, Snowhill EW, Altar CA. New York, Alan R Liss, 1986, pp 105–135

Matsumoto A, Kumagai T, Takeuchi T, et al: Clinical effects of thyrotropin-releasing hormone for severe epilepsy in children: a comparative study with ACTH therapy. Epilepsia 28:49–55, 1987

Mizuki Y, Nishikori S, Kajimura N, et al: A treatment trial with an analog of thyrotropin-releasing hormone (DN-1417) in schizophrenia. Biol Psychiatry 20:1030–1035, 1985

Nemeroff CB, Youngblood WW, Manberg PJ, et al: Regional brain concentrations of neuropeptides in Huntington's chorea and schizophrenia. Science 221:972–975, 1983

Oliver C, Eskay RL, Ben-Jonathan N, et al: Distribution and concentration of TRH in the rat brain. Endocrinology 96:540–546, 1974

Plotnikoff NP, Prange AJ Jr, Breese GR, et al: Thyrotropin releasing hormone: enhancement of DOPA activity by a hypothalamic hormone. Science 178:417–418, 1972

Prange AJ Jr: The Thyroid Axis, Drugs, and Behavior. New York, Raven, 1974

Prange AJ Jr, Wilson IC, Lara PP, et al: Effects of thyrotropin-releasing hormone in depression. Lancet 1:999–1002, 1972

Prange AJ Jr, Breese GR, Cott JM, et al: Thyrotropin-releasing hormone: antagonism of pentobarbital in rodents. Life Sci 14:447–455, 1974

Renaud LP, Martin JB: Thyrotropin-releasing hormone: depressant action on central neuronal activity. Brain Res 86:150–154, 1975

Renaud LP, Blume HW, Pittman QJ, et al: Thyrotropin-releasing hormone selectively depresses glutamate excitation of cerebral cortical neurons. Science 205:1275–1277, 1979

Sato M, Morimoto K, Wada JA: Antiepileptic effects of thyrotropin-releasing hormone and its new derivative, DN-1417, examined in feline amygdaloid kindling preparation. Epilepsia 25:537–544, 1984

Sauer H, Köhler KG, Sass H, et al: The dexamethasone suppression test and thyroid stimulating hormone response to TRH in RDC schizoaffective patients. Eur Arch Psychiatry Neurol Sci 234:264–267, 1984

Stanton TL, Winokur A, Beckman AL: Reversal of natural CNS depression by TRH action in the hippocampus. Brain Res 137:470–475, 1980

Stanton TL, Winokur A, Beckman AL: TRH effects in the CNS: dependence on arousal state. Science 214:678–681, 1981

Stanton TL, Winokur A, Beckman AL: Seasonal variation in TRH content of different brain regions and the pineal in the mammalian hibernator, *Citellus lateralis.* Regul Pept 3:135–144, 1982

Wilson IC, Lara PP, Prange AJ Jr: Thyrotropin-releasing hormone in schizophrenia. Lancet 2:43–44, 1973

Wilson IC, Prange AJ Jr, Lara PP: L-Triiodothyronine alone and with imipramine in the treatment of depressed women, in The Thyroid Axis, Drugs, and Behavior. Edited by Prange AJ Jr. New York, Raven, 1974, pp 49–62

Winokur A, Beckman AL: Effects of thyrotropin-releasing hormone, norepinephrine and acetylcholine on the activity of neurons in the hypothalamus, septum and cerebral cortex of the rat. Brain Res 150:205–209, 1978

Winokur A, Utiger RD: Thyrotropin-releasing hormone regional distribution in rat brain. Science 185:265–267, 1974

Winokur A, Davies R, Utiger RD: Subcellular distribution of thyrotropin-releasing hormone (TRH) in rat brain and hypothalamus. Brain Res 120:423–434, 1977

Wolkin A, Peselow ED, Smith M, et al: TRH test abnormalities in psychiatric disorders. J Affective Disord 6:273–281, 1984

Yarbrough GG: TRH potentiates excitatory actions of acetylcholine on cerebral cortical neurons. Nature 263:523–524, 1976

Yarbrough GG: On the neuropharmacology of thyrotropin releasing hormone (TRH). Prog Neurobiol 12:291–312, 1979

Chapter 3

Somatostatin

David R. Rubinow, M.D.
Robert M. Post, M.D.
Candace L. Davis, B.S.

Chapter 3

Somatostatin

Early efforts to identify the hypothalamic stimulating factor for growth hormone release from the pituitary inadvertently resulted in the discovery of a hypothalamic inhibitor of growth hormone release (Krulich et al. 1968). Despite much initial skepticism regarding its existence, this inhibiting factor, somatostatin (growth hormone release–inhibiting factor, somatotropin release–inhibiting factor [SRIF]), was subsequently isolated and structurally characterized in 1973 (Brazeau et al. 1973). As has been the case for most of the brain neuropeptides identified over the past two decades, the known neuroregulatory effects of the tetradecapeptide somatostatin have expanded the role of this peptide far beyond its originally discovered role. In this chapter we will review the evidence that alterations in brain or CSF somatostatin might reflect or contribute to the pathophysiology of several neuropsychiatric disorders, particularly Alzheimer's disease and depression. In addition, we will summarize the observations that support a role for somatostatin as a modulator of central nervous system (CNS) activity.

DISEASE-RELATED ALTERATIONS IN SOMATOSTATIN

The first report of disease-related alterations in cerebrospinal fluid (CSF) somatostatin concentration was that of Patel et al. (1977), who observed increased levels of CSF somatostatin in inflammatory or destructive neurological disorders (spinal cord disease, nerve root compression, cerebral tumor, meningitis, metabolic encephalopathy) when compared with those of neurological control subjects. These findings were subsequently confirmed by Beal et al. (1985). However, decreased levels of CSF somatostatin also have been noted in several neuropsychiatric disorders, including Parkinson's disease (Dupont et al. 1982), multiple sclerosis (during relapse) (Beal et al. 1985; Sorensen et al. 1980), and senile dementia (Oram et al. 1981) and Alzheimer's disease (Cramer et al. 1985; Gomez et al. 1986; Serby et al. 1984; Wood et al. 1982). Both decreased and normal CSF somatostatin levels have been reported in patients with Huntington's disease (Beal et al. 1986; Cramer et al. 1981) and multi-infarct dementia (Beal et al. 1986; Cramer et al. 1985). The results of human postmortem studies parallel those of CSF, with decreased somatostatin concentrations observed in the cortex and hippocampus in Parkinson's disease (Epelbaum et al. 1983) and in a variety of cortical and subcortical sites in Alzheimer's disease (Arai et al. 1984; Candy et al. 1985; Davies and Terry 1981; Nemeroff et al. 1983a; Rossor et al. 1980). In contrast, increased levels of somatostatin have been observed in several brain regions in Huntington's disease (Aronin et al. 1983).

The decreased levels of CSF and brain somatostatin in Alzheimer's disease constitute, along with evidence of degeneration of cholinergic neurons, the most commonly observed biochemical lesion in this disorder. The clinical relevance of altered somatostatin function in Alzheimer's disease is also suggested by 1) reports of correlations between the degree of cognitive impairment and reduction of somatostatin levels in brain (Francis et al. 1987) or CSF (Soininen et al. 1984); 2) reports of the colocalization of somatostatin neurons with neurofibrillary tangles and plaques (Morrison et al. 1985; Roberts et al. 1985); and 3) the demonstration that the brain areas showing the greatest reduction in somatostatin are those that are most markedly hypometabolic as determined by positron-emission tomography (PET) (Tamminga et al. 1985). While the decreased brain and CSF somatostatin in Alzheimer's disease is believed to be a product of neuronal degeneration, Karlsson et al. (1985) and Widerlöv et al. (in press) have described a relative increase in CSF somatostatin concentration in association with reversal of dementia symptoms in Alzheimer's patients exposed to intensive environmental stimulation. Therapeutic trials that have attempted to manipulate central somatostatin levels have been performed by administering a somatostatin analogue to patients with Alzheimer's disease (Cutler et al. 1985) or a somatostatin-depleting agent (cysteamine) to patients with Huntington's disease (Shults et al. 1986). No significant change in disease symptoms was noted with either trial, although the effects of these treatments on central somatostatin function in these studies can only be inferred.

Among the psychiatric disorders studied, evidence is clearest for an alteration in central somatostatin function and/or concentration in affective illness. Gerner and Yamada (1982) and Rubinow et al. (1983) reported significant decreases in CSF somatostatin levels in depressed patients compared with normal control subjects. Subsequent studies have confirmed these initial findings. Ågren and

Lundqvist (1984) described significantly lower somatostatin levels in a group of depressed patients studied during these patients' worst week of depression compared with depressed patients studied more than 2 months following their most depressed week. Black et al. (1986) reported lower levels of somatostatin in the ventricular CSF of depressed patients studied prior to cingulotomy compared with ventricular CSF values in hydrocephalic patients and lumbar CSF values in healthy control subjects. Sunderland et al. (1987) described decreased CSF somatostatin in elderly depressed patients compared with age-matched control subjects, with the values in the depressed group not significantly different from those obtained in a group of patients with Alzheimer's disease. Finally, significantly lower CSF somatostatin values in depressed patients compared with control subjects have been observed in studies by Bissette et al. (1986), Davis et al. (1988), and Rubinow (1986), in an extension of his earlier findings. In the latter study, 49 medication-free depressed patients had significantly decreased CSF somatostatin levels compared with 47 nondepressed volunteers and 23 patients with affective illness in the improved or euthymic state. Thus, it appears that the decreases in CSF somatostatin levels are state-related and normalize with recovery from depression.

In contrast to the consistency of findings in studies of depressed patients, alterations of CSF somatostatin in other psychiatric disorders have not been reliably observed. Whereas Bissette et al. (1986) found lower CSF somatostatin levels in 11 schizophrenic patients compared with control subjects, Doran et al. (1986) reported normal somatostatin levels in 44 schizophrenic patients. In mania, both increased (Gerner and Yamada 1982) and normal (Rubinow et al. 1983) CSF somatostatin values have been described. Decreased somatostatin values were observed in anorexic patients by Gerner and Yamada (1982) but not by Kaye et al. (1988). In the latter study, a small but significant increase in CSF somatostatin occurred in patients with bulimia during abstinence from binge eating compared with the same patients when actively binge eating. Finally, Vecsei and Widerlöv (1988) found normal CSF somatostatin levels in patients with panic disorder and observed no effect of menstrual cycle phase on somatostatin levels in patients with premenstrual syndrome. Several postmortem studies of brain somatostatin concentrations in patients with psychiatric illness have been performed, although no consistent findings have been demonstrated to date. Thus, in schizophrenic patients, reductions in somatostatin concentration in the frontal cortex (Nemeroff et al. 1983b) and in the hippocampus in a subgroup of patients (Ferrier et al. 1983) have been described. In addition, preliminary observations (D. R. Rubinow, manuscript in preparation) suggest no difference in somatostatin concentration in the frontal cortex, caudate, or amygdala in schizophrenic and affectively ill suicide victims compared with accident victim control subjects.

The potential importance of disease-related alterations in somatostatin is best revealed by the substantial evidence suggesting that somatostatin may have a role as a modulator of CNS activity. First, somatostatin neurons are distributed in a widespread and selective fashion throughout the brain, appearing in the median eminence (the source of anterior pituitary regulation), the posterior pituitary (Patel et al. 1979; Van Leeuwen et al. 1979), the limbic system, the cortex, the hippocampus, and the hypothalamus and hypothalamic projections to the brain stem and spinal cord (Krisch 1981). The greatest amount of somatostatin appears in the cortex, while somatostatin is most *concentrated* in the hypothalamus. Several distinct somatostatin pathways have been identified, with the periventricular nucleus the primary source of somatostatin input to the median eminence (Reichlin 1983). Second, somatostatin receptors are selectively distributed throughout the brain (Leroux and Pelletier 1984; Leroux et al. 1985; Srikant and Patel 1985; Tran et al. 1984). Several forms of the somatostatin-14 receptor identified in human brain display different localization and affinity characteristics (Reubi et al. 1987; Tran et al. 1985), although Epelbaum has suggested that other factors (e.g., manganese) mediate differences in affinity of a single somatostatin receptor (Beaudet et al. 1988). Finally, as is the case with most neuropeptides, what is referred to as somatostatin is actually a family of peptides, with somatostatin-14 a C-terminal cleavage product of a larger prohormone. Several N-terminal extensions of this tetradecapeptide, such as somatostatin-28, prosomatostatin (92 amino acids), and pre-prosomatostatin (116 amino acids), have been identified (Benoit et al. 1982, 1984; Goodman et al. 1983), as has the convertase responsible for the proteolytic cleavage of somatostatin-28 to somatostatin-14 (Glushankof et al. 1984). The N-terminal extension precursors of somatostatin-14 (which are recognized by antibodies directed toward the midregion or C-terminal of somatostatin-14) appear in the CSF (Reichlin 1982) and possess biological activities and potencies as well as patterns of distribution in the CNS that differ from those of somatostatin-14 (Meyers et al. 1980; Morrison et al. 1982, 1983; Srikant and Patel 1985). Although distinct roles for the somatostatin-related peptides in neuropsychiatric disorders cannot currently be assigned, Gomez et al. (1986) have reported that the decreased somatostatin concentration in the CSF of patients with Alzheimer's disease consists of a decrease in somatostatin-14 and an increase in the concentration of the 15-kd precursor, thus suggesting a posttranslational dysfunction as the source for decreased somatostatin concentration observed. Further study of the somatostatin-related peptide profiles in neuropsychiatric disorders is clearly indicated.

SOMATOSTATIN AS A MODULATOR OF CENTRAL NERVOUS SYSTEM ACTIVITY

In addition to its widespread CNS localization, several other described properties of somatostatin suggest its ability to act as a neurotransmitter or neuromodulator. First, both inhibitory and excitatory neuronal effects have been observed following somatostatin application, with a dose-related, biphasic effect on neuronal action-potential generation (Delfs and Dichter 1983; Dodd and Kelly 1978; Olpe et al. 1980). Second, as reviewed elsewhere (Reichlin 1983), somatostatin displays mutual regulatory interactions with many classical neurotransmitters and neuropeptides. While the effects of somatostatin on neurotransmitter turnover and release are neurotransmitter- and site-specific, somatostatin has a strikingly uniform inhibitory effect on the secretion of a variety of hormones, such that McCann (1982) suggested that somatostatin should be called "panhibin."

Several mechanisms have been proposed by which somatostatin may interfere with stimulated hormonal secretion, including inhibition of adenylate cyclase through G-protein activation (Reisine 1984), reduction of cytosolic free calcium, interference with calcium mobilization (Schlegel et al. 1984), enhancement of the permeability of cells to potassium (Pace and Tarvin 1981), and inhibition of protein phosphorylation (Dokas et al. 1983). While somatostatin totally inhibits growth hormone stimulated by growth hormone–releasing factor (GHRF), it decreases GHRF-stimulated cyclic adenosine monophosphate (cAMP) by only 50% (Sheppard et al. 1985), thus suggesting that the inhibitory effects of somatostatin on hormonal secretion cannot be explained solely in terms of inhibition of adenylate cyclase. In contrast, somatostatin totally inhibits GHRF-stimulated calcium efflux (Logan and Judd 1986) and blocks the stimulating effects on growth hormone release of the calcium ionophore A23187 (Kraicer and Spence 1981).

Finally, the effect of somatostatin on CNS activity is further demonstrated by the alterations in behavior or vegetative function observed following intracerebroventricular or intracerebral administration. Several of the behaviors affected by somatostatin are disturbed in depression. For example, depression is characterized by decreased total and slow-wave sleep and shortened REM latency (Gillin et al. 1983), increased or decreased appetite and/or locomotor activity, decreased pain sensitivity (Davis et al. 1982), and impaired cognition (Weingartner and Silberman 1983). Decreased total, slow-wave, and REM sleep have been observed following central somatostatin administration (Havlicek et al. 1976; Rezek et al. 1976); more recently, however, Danguir (1986) described a significant increase in REM sleep in rats following intracerebroventricular somatostatin infusion, as well as suppression of REM sleep following intracerebroventricular administration of cysteamine, a somatostatin depletor. Central somatostatin administration has also been associated with dose-related, biphasic alterations in locomotor activity (stimulation with low doses and inhibition with high doses) (Rezek et al. 1977) and with eating disturbances (increased or dose-related, biphasic food consumption) (Aponte et al. 1984; Lotter and Woods 1977; Rezek et al. 1976). Intrathecal administration of somatostatin produces a non-naloxone–reversible analgesia in both animals and man (Havlicek et al. 1977; Meynadier et al. 1985). Finally, Vecsei et al. (1984) and Walsh et al. (1985) have demonstrated that somatostatin may enhance learning and reverse learning deficits, whereas somatostatin depletion (with cysteamine) diminishes performance.

A variety of indirect evidence reviewed elsewhere (Reichlin 1983) suggests that CSF somatostatin in large part reflects brain secretion, although the significance of the depression state–related decreases in CSF somatostatin is currently uncertain. While the elevated levels of CSF somatostatin observed in inflammatory or destructive neurological disorders were presumably the result of "leakage" from damaged or anoxic neurons, the decreased levels observed in other neuropsychiatric disorders seem more suggestive of functional neuronal alterations. Given the existence of several neuropsychiatric disorders that are characterized by decreased CSF somatostatin, it is unlikely that somatostatin dysregulation plays a central etiologic role in depression, although it may reflect or contribute to syndromal or symptomatic aspects of this and other neuropsychiatric disorders. Thus, decreases in levels of CSF somatostatin may occur secondary to a primary central neuroregulator disturbance or appear as a result of depression-related shifts in circadian rhythms (Wehr 1984). We observed no significant circadian rhythm effect on CSF somatostatin levels in depressed patients or in volunteers who underwent both morning and evening lumbar punctures. However, in contrast to A.M. differences, highly similar evening somatostatin values were noted in both patients and healthy volunteer groups (Rubinow 1986). Thus, detection of decreased CSF somatostatin levels in depressed patients relative to control volunteers appears to be dependent on the time of day at which the samples are obtained, and therefore these differences may represent disturbed circadian rather than total somatostatin secretion. Of interest in this regard is the recent report by Sorensen et al. (1987) of the loss of diurnal variation of CSF somatostatin in patients with multiple sclerosis (MS) during relapse compared with MS patients in the stable phase or control subjects.

Finally, it is possible that decreased CSF somatostatin, in the disorders characterized by this abnormality, reflects a common central neuroregulatory disturbance or mediates common manifestations of these disorders (e.g., cognitive impairment or cortisol hypersecretion). As described above, central somatostatin administration appears to facilitate learning and memory (delay extinction of a learned avoidance response and reverse electric shock–induced learning impairment), and depletion of somatostatin results in impaired performance in the same learning paradigms (Vecsei et al. 1983, 1984; Walsh et al. 1985). Consistent with these findings is the observation that some degree of cognitive impairment is a common manifestation of neuropsychiatric disorders associated with decreased CSF somatostatin (i.e., Alzheimer's disease, depression, MS, Parkinson's disease, Cushing's disease). Further, correlations have been reported between the extent of the decrease in CSF (or brain) somatostatin and the degree of cognitive impairment in patients with Alzheimer's disease (Cramer et al. 1985; Francis et al. 1987; Soininen et al. 1984, 1988; Sunderland et al. 1987), Parkinson's disease (Epelbaum et al. 1983), and alcoholic dementia (Martin et al., in press).

SOMATOSTATIN IN DEPRESSION

The possibility that alterations in somatostatin function may mediate some of the physiologic disturbances described in depression also has been explored. Observations of the ability of somatostatin to inhibit stimulated adrenocorticotropin (ACTH) secretion (Heisler et al. 1982; Petraglia et al. 1986) and stress-induced corticotropin-releasing factor (CRF) secretion (Brown et al. 1984) allowed for the possibility that decreased CSF somatostatin might contribute to disinhibition of hypothalamo-pituitary-adrenal (HPA) axis activity, the most commonly reported biological abnormality in depression (Carroll et al. 1976). Consistent with this possibility was the observation by Doran et al. (1986) that depressed and schizophrenic patients who escaped from dexamethasone suppression displayed significantly lower levels of CSF somatostatin. While this relationship was not observed by Ågren and Lundqvist (1984) or Bissette et al. (1986), a remarkably similar negative correlation between CSF somatostatin and response to dexamethasone was reported by Serby et al. (1986) in patients with Alzheimer's disease and by Kaye et al. (1988) in underweight anorexic individuals. Recent evidence suggests that hypercortisolemia may produce, rather than reflect, the decreased somatostatin levels observed. Wolkowitz et al. (1987), for example, observed that 5 days of prednisone administration (80 mg per day) significantly reduced CSF somatostatin levels in healthy volunteers. Kling et al. (in press) reported decreased CSF somatostatin in patients with ACTH-dependent Cushing's syndrome. In cell culture studies, Cote et al. (1986) demonstrated dramatic reductions in somatostatin messenger RNA (mRNA) and somatostatin secretion following application of dexamethasone. Should it be demonstrated that decreased CSF somatostatin in depression reflects, rather than causes, HPA axis disinhibition, a variety of evidence suggests that the relationship between somatostatin and the HPA axis may nonetheless be physiologically meaningful and may provide a useful means for exploring those disorders characterized by dysregulation of this axis. In addition to that already cited, this evidence includes reports of CRF-stimulated somatostatin secretion (Aguilla and McCann 1985; Katakami et al. 1985; Rivier and Vale 1985) as well as observations of a significant positive correlation between CSF somatostatin and CRF in several patient populations, including acute and abstinent bulimic patients (Kaye et al. 1988), euthymic bipolar patients (Berrettini et al. 1983), Cushing's disease patients (Kling et al., in press), and healthy volunteers (Berrettini et al., unpublished observations; Kaye et al. 1988).

Although the precise role of somatostatin in depression and other neuropsychiatric disorders is unknown, the relevance of alterations in somatostatin secretion to CNS activity and seizure development is increasingly apparent. Evidence of a close relationship includes the following:

1. Long-term increases in somatostatin in brain regions (amygdala and sensorimotor, piriform, and entorrhinal cortices) following kindling (Kato et al. 1983).
2. Kindling-related down-regulation of somatostatin receptors in the hippocampus (Higuchi et al. 1984).
3. Periventricular somatostatin release following electrical stimulation of several limbic sites (Kato et al. 1986).
4. Precipitation of seizures following intracerebroventricular or intracerebral injection of somatostatin (Havlicek and Friesen 1979; Ioffe et al. 1977).

5. Inhibition of kindled seizures following administration of cysteamine or somatostatin antiserum (Higuchi et al. 1983).
6. Selective increases in somatostatin and pre-prosomatostatin mRNA (but not glutamic acid decarboxylase [GAD] or GAD mRNA) in the striatum and neocortex in stage-5 kindled rats (Shinoda et al., in press).
7. Increases in somatostatin-14 in focal (epileptic) compared with nonfocal (nonepileptic) regions of the temporal cortex in 33 of 35 patients with intractable seizures (Nadi et al., in press).
8. Increases of somatostatin in stage-3 kindled rats, with the elevation seen in the stage-5 kindled rats 1 hour after the seizure and persisting up to 2 weeks following the last seizure (Nadi 1988).

Pitkanen et al. (1987), however, observed no acute change in CSF somatostatin levels in humans following a generalized seizure. Further, Cottrell and Robertson (1987) have suggested that cysteamine produces long-term inhibition of kindled seizures by inducing myoclonic seizures and not as a result of somatostatin depleting effects.

Nonetheless, additional evidence for a potential role for somatostatin in seizure disorders can be found in reports on the effects of several anticonvulsants on somatostatin. We described significant decreases in CSF somatostatin in patients with affective illness during treatment with the anticonvulsant carbamazepine compared with baseline values obtained under medication-free conditions (Rubinow et al. 1985). Depression ratings were comparable during the paired lumbar punctures, so changes in CSF somatostatin were not attributable to changes in mood state. Significant carbamazepine-induced decreases in CSF somatostatin were also reported by Steardo et al. (1986) in patients with temporal lobe epilepsy. Carbamazepine has been found to blunt kindled elevations in brain somatostatin in rats (Higuchi et al. 1986), although Weiss et al. (1987) reported an absence of effect on basal somatostatin in several brain regions. Finally, Stryker et al. (1986) reported that benzodiazepine-induced stimulation of the $GABA_B$ receptor inhibits somatostatin secretion in vitro, which is manifested in vivo by increased growth hormone secretion.

CONCLUSIONS

At present, somatostatin is the peptide with the best delineated involvement in neuropsychiatric illnesses, including Alzheimer's disease, depression, MS (in relapse), Parkinson's disease, and Cushing's disease. Whereas decreases in brain and CSF somatostatin concentrations in Alzheimer's disease appear to reflect an irreversible, degenerative neurological process, the somatostatin dysregulation seen in depression, like that in MS, is transient and reversible and appears to represent a consequence of functional alterations in somatostatin secretion and/or metabolism. Studies of somatostatin mRNA should help differentiate these possibilities.

Future attempts to chromatographically characterize CSF and brain somatostatin may identify specific somatostatin-related peptide fragments that are selectively dysregulated in different neuropsychiatric disorders. Further, passive immunization studies, and investigations employing somatostatin antagonists and agonists that gain access to the brain, will permit precise determination of the role of somatostatin in CNS activity. Through these and other means of altering the activity of somatostatin and somatostatin-related peptides, it is hoped that a clearer understanding will emerge of the significance of somatostatin decreases in depression and in other neuropsychiatric disorders.

REFERENCES

Ågren H, Lundqvist G: Low levels of somatostatin in human CSF mark depressive episodes. Psychoneuroendocrinology 9:233–248, 1984

Aguilla MC, McCann SM: The influence of hCRF, CRF, TRH and LHRH on the SRIF release from median eminence fragments. Brain Res 348:180–182, 1985

Aponte G, Leung P, Gross D, et al: Effects of somatostatin on food intake in rats. Life Sci 35:741–746, 1984

Arai H, Moroji T, Kosaka K: Somatostatin and vasoactive intestinal polypeptide in postmortem brains from patients with Alzheimer-type dementia. Neurosci Lett 53:73–78, 1984

Aronin N, Cooper PE, Lorenz LJ, et al: Somatostatin is increased in the basal ganglia in Huntington's disease. Ann Neurol 13:519–526, 1983

Beal MF, Mazurek MF, Black PM, et al: Human cerebrospinal fluid somatostatin in neurologic disease. J Neurol Sci 71:91–104, 1985

Beal MF, Growdon JH, Mazurek MF, et al: CSF somatostatin-like immunoreactivity in dementia. Neurology 36:294–297, 1986

Beaudet A, Moyse E, Tannenbaum G, et al: Association of SRIF binding sites with GRF containing neurons in rat arcuate nucleus. Society for Neuroscience Abstracts 14 (abstr no 426.12):1059, 1988

Benoit R, Ling N, Alford B, et al: Seven peptides derived from prosomatostatin in rat brain. Biochem Biophys Res Commun 107:944–950, 1982

Benoit R, Bohlen P, Esch F, et al: Neuropeptides derived from prosomatostatin that do not contain the somatostatin-14 sequence. Brain Res 311:23–29, 1984

Berrettini WB, Nurnberger J, Nadi NS, et al: CSF studies in euthymic bipolar patients, in Scientific Program for the 38th Annual Convention of the Society for Biological Psychiatry, Abstr no 49. New York, Society for Biological Psychiatry, May 1983

Bissette G, Widerlöv E, Walléus H, et al: Alterations in cerebrospinal fluid concentrations of somatostatin-like immunoreactivity in neuropsychiatric disorders. Arch Gen Psychiatry 43:1148–1151, 1986

Black PM, Ballantine HT Jr, Carr DB, et al: Beta-endorphin and somatostatin concentrations in the ventricular cerebrospinal fluid of patients with affective disorder. Biol Psychiatry 21:1077–1081, 1986

Brazeau P, Vale W, Burgus R, et al: Hypothalamic polypeptide that inhibits the secretion of immunoreactive pituitary growth hormone. Science 197:77–79, 1973

Brown MR, Rivier C, Vale W: Central nervous system regulation of adrenocorticotropin secretion: role of somatostatin. Endocrinology 114:1546–1549, 1984

Candy JM, Gascoigne AD, Biggins JA, et al: Somatostatin immunoreactivity in cortical and some subcortical regions in Alzheimer's disease. J Neurol Sci 71:315–323, 1985

Carroll BJ, Curtis GC, Davis BM, et al: Urinary free cortisol excretion in depression. J Psychol Med 6:43–50, 1976

Cote GJ, Palmer WN, Leonhart K, et al: The regulation of somatostatin production in human medullary thyroid carcinoma cells by dexamethasone. J Biol Chem 261:12930–12935, 1986

Cottrell GA, Robertson HA: Prevention of cysteamine-induced myoclonus blocks the long-term inhibition of kindled seizures. Brain Res 412:161–164, 1987

Cramer H, Kohler J, Oepen G, et al: Huntington's chorea: measurements of somatostatin, substance P and cyclic nucleotides in the cerebrospinal fluid. J Neurol 225:183–187, 1981

Cramer H, Schaudt D, Rissler K, et al: Somatostatin-like immunoreactivity and substance-P–like immunoreactivity in the CSF of patients with senile dementia of Alzheimer type, multi-infarct syndrome and communicating hydrocephalus. J Neurol 232:346–351, 1985

Cutler NR, Haxby JV, Narang PR, et al: Evaluation of an analogue of somatostatin (L363,586) in Alzheimer's disease. N Engl J Med 312:725, 1985

Danguir J: Intracerebroventricular infusion of somatostatin selectively increases paradoxical sleep in rats. Brain Res 367:26–30, 1986

Davies P, Terry RD: Cortical somatostatin-like immunoreactivity in cases of Alzheimer's disease and senile dementia of the Alzheimer type. Neurobiology 2:9–14, 1981

Davis GC, Buchsbaum MS, Naber D, et al: Altered pain perception and CSF endorphins in psychiatric illness. Ann NY Acad Sci 398:366–373, 1982

Davis KL, Davidson M, Yang RT, et al: CSF somatostatin in Alzheimer's disease, depressed patients, and controls. Biol Psychiatry 24:710–712, 1988

Delfs JR, Dichter MA: Effects of somatostatin on mammalian cortical neurons in culture: physiological actions and unusual dose response characteristics. J Neurosci 3:1176–1188, 1983

Dodd J, Kelly JS: Is somatostatin an excitatory transmitter in the hippocampus? Nature 273:674–675, 1978

Dokas LA, Kliss M, Liauw A, et al: Evidence that (D-Trp^{8}) somatostatin inhibits synaptic plasma membrane protein phosphorylation by interaction with a specific membrane binding site. Society for Neuroscience Abstracts 9 (abstr no 171.4):589, 1983

Doran A, Rubinow DR, Roy A, et al: CSF somatostatin and abnormal response to dexamethasone administration in schizophrenic and depressed patients. Arch Gen Psychiatry 43:365–369, 1986

Dupont E, Christensen SE, Hansen AP, et al: Low cerebrospinal fluid somatostatin in Parkinson's disease: an irreversible abnormality. Neurology 32:312–314, 1982

Epelbaum J, Ruberg M, Moyse E, et al: Somatostatin and dementia in Parkinson's disease. Brain Res 278:376–379, 1983

Ferrier IN, Cross AJ, Johnson JA, et al: Neuropeptides in Alzheimer type dementia. J Neurol Sci 62:159–170, 1983

Francis PT, Bowen DM, Lowe SL, et al: Somatostatin content and release measured in cerebral biopsies from demented patients. J Neurol Sci 78:1–16, 1987

Gerner RH, Yamada T: Altered neuropeptide concentrations in cerebrospinal fluid of psychiatric patients. Brain Res 238:298–302, 1982

Gillin JC, Sitaram N, Wehr T, et al: Sleep and affective illness, in Neurobiology of Mood Disorders. Edited by Post RM, Ballenger JC. Baltimore, MD, Williams & Wilkins, 1983, pp 157–189

Glushankof P, Morel A, Gomez S, et al: Enzymes processing somatostatin precursors: an Arg-Lys esteropeptidase from the rat brain cortex converting somatostatin-28 into somatostatin-14. Proc Natl Acad Sci USA 81:6662–6666, 1984

Gomez S, Puymirat J, Valade P, et al: Patients with Alzheimer's disease show an increased content of 15 Kdalton somatostatin precursor and a lowered level of tetradecapeptide in their cerebrospinal fluid. Life Sci 39:623–627, 1986

Goodman RH, Aron DC, Roosa BA: Rat pre-prosomatostatin structure and processing by microsomal membranes. J Biol Chem 258:5570–5573, 1983

Havlicek V, Friesen HG: Comparison of behavioral effects of SRIF and β-endorphin in animals, in Central Nervous System Effects of Hypothalamic Hormones and Other Peptides. Edited by Collu R, Barbeau A, Rochefort JG, et al. New York, Raven, 1979, pp 381–402

Havlicek V, Rezek M, Friesen H: Somatostatin and thyrotropin releasing hormone: central effect on sleep and motor system. Pharmacol Biochem Behav 4:455–459, 1976

Havlicek V, Rezek M, Leybin L, et al: Analgesic effect of cerebral ventricular administration of somatostatin (SRIF). Federation Proceedings 36:363, 1977

Heisler S, Reisine T, Hook V, et al: Somatostatin inhibits multireceptor stimulation of cyclic AMP formation and corticotrophin secretion in mouse pituitary tumor cells. Proc Natl Acad Sci USA 79:6502–6507, 1982

Higuchi T, Sikand GS, Kato N, et al: Profound suppression of kindled seizures by cysteamine: possible role of somatostatin to kindled seizures. Brain Res 288:359–362, 1983

Higuchi T, Kokubu T, Sikand GS, et al: A study of somatostatin receptors in amygdaloid-kindled rat brain. J Neurochem 43:1271–1276, 1984

Higuchi T, Kato N, Noguchi T, et al: Kindling and somatostatin, in Kindling, Vol 3. Edited by Wada JA. New York, Raven, 1986, pp 349–360

Ioffe S, Havlicek V, Friesen HG, et al: Effect of iontophoretically applied somatostatin (SRF) on cortical neurons in awake unanesthetized animals. Federation Proceedings 36:364, 1977

Karlsson I, Widerlöv E, Melin EV, et al: Changes of CSF neuropeptides after environmental stimulation in dementia. Nordic Psychiatric Journal 39 (suppl 11):75–81, 1985

Katakami H, Arimura A, Frohman LA: Involvement of hypothalamic somatostatin in the suppression of growth hormone secretion by central corticotropin-releasing factor in conscious male rats. Neuroendocrinology 41:390–393, 1985

Kato N, Higuchi T, Friesen HG, et al: Changes in immunoreactive somatostatin and β-endorphin content in rat brain after amygdaloid kindling. Life Sci 32:2415–2422, 1983

Kato M, Kakegawa T, Suzuki M: Electrical stimulation of several limbic areas suppressed the growth hormone (GH) release induced by human pancreatic GH-releasing factor in pentobarbital-anesthetized rats. Endocrinology 118:955–960, 1986

Kaye W, Rubinow DR, Gwirtsman H, et al: CSF somatostatin in anorexia nervosa and bulimia: relationship to the hypothalamic-pituitary-adrenal cortical axis. Psychoneuroendocrinology, 13:265–272, 1988

Kling MA, Doran AR, Rubinow DR, et al: The cerebrospinal fluid neurohormonal milieu in Cushing's disease, major depression, and normal volunteers: pathophysiologic and diagnostic relevance. N Engl J Med (in press)

Kraicer J, Spence JW: Release of growth hormone from purified somatotrophs: use of high K^+ and the ionophore A23187 to elucidate interrelations among Ca^{++}, adenosine 3′,5′-monophosphate and somatostatin. Endocrinology 108:651–657, 1981

Krisch B: Somatostatin-immunoreactive fiber projections into the brainstem and the spinal cord of the rat. Cell Tissue Res 217:531–532, 1981

Krulich L, Dhariwal APS, McCann SM: Stimulatory and inhibitory effects of purified hypothalamic extracts on growth hormone release from rat pituitary in vitro. Endocrinology 83:783–790, 1968

Leroux P, Pelletier G: Radioautographic localization of somatostatin-28 binding sites in the rat brain. Peptides 5:503–506, 1984

Leroux P, Quirion R, Pelletier G: Localization and characterization of brain somatostatin receptors as studied with somatostatin-14 and somatostatin-28 receptor radioautography. Brain Res 347:74–84, 1985

Logan IW, Judd ALM: Trophic effects of somatostatin on calcium flux: dynamic analysis and correlation with pituitary hormone release. Endocrinology 119:1703–1707, 1986

Lotter EC, Woods SC: Somatostatin decreases food intake. Diabetes 26 (suppl 1):358, 1977

Martin PR, Adinoff B, Eckardt MJ, et al: Effective pharmacotherapy of alcoholic amnestic disorder with fluvoxamine: preliminary findings. Arch Gen Psychiatry (in press)

McCann SM: Physiology and pharmacology of LHRH and somatostatin. Annu Rev Pharmacol Toxicol 22:491–515, 1982

Meyers CA, Murphy WA, Redding TW, et al: Synthesis and biological actions of prosomatostatin. Proc Natl Acad Sci USA 77:6171–6174, 1980

Meynadier J, Chrubasik J, Dubar M, et al: Intrathecal somatostatin in terminally ill patients: a report of two cases. Pain 23:9–12, 1985

Morrison JH, Benoit R, Magistretti PJ, et al: Immunohistochemical distribution of pro-somatostatin–related peptides in hippocampus. Neurosci Lett 34:137–142, 1982

Morrison JH, Benoit R, Magistretti PJ, et al: Immunohistochemical distribution of pro-somatostatin–related peptides in cerebral cortex. Brain Res 262:344–351, 1983

Morrison JH, Rogers J, Scherr S, et al: Somatostatin immunoreactivity in neuritic plaques of Alzheimer's patients. Nature 314:90–92, 1985

Nadi NS: The time course of chemical changes in the kindled rat brain, in 18th Annual Society for Neuroscience Meeting, Abstr no 411.4. Toronto, Society for Neuroscience, November 1988

Nadi NS, Port RJ, Wyler AR: Somatostatin levels in the spiking and nonspiking epileptic human. J Neurochem (in press)

Nemeroff CB, Bissette G, Busby WH, et al: Regional brain concentrations of neurotensin, thyrotropin releasing hormone and somatostatin in Alzheimer's disease. Society for Neuroscience Abstracts 9:1052, 1983a

Nemeroff CB, Youngblood WW, Manberg PJ, et al: Regional brain concentrations of neuropeptides in Huntington's chorea and schizophrenia. Science 221:972–975, 1983b

Olpe HR, Balcar VJ, Bittiger H, et al: Central actions of somatostatin. Eur J Pharmacol 63:127–133, 1980

Oram JJ, Edwardson J, Millard PH: Investigation of cerebrospinal fluid neuropeptides in idiopathic senile dementia. Gerontology 27:216–223, 1981

Pace CS, Tarvin JT: Somatostatin: mechanism of action in pancreatic islet B-cells. Diabetes 30:836–842, 1981

Patel YC, Rao K, Reichlin S: Somatostatin in human cerebrospinal fluid. N Engl J Med 296:529–533, 1977

Patel YC, Hoyte K, Martin JB: Effect of anterior hypothalamic lesions on neurohypophysial and peripheral tissue concentration of somatostatin in the rat brain. Endocrinology 105:712–715, 1979

Petraglia F, Facchinetti F, D'Ambrogio G, et al: Somatostatin and oxytocin infusion inhibits the rise of plasma β-endorphin, β-lipotrophin and cortisol induced by insulin hypoglycemia. Clin Endocrinol 24:609–616, 1986

Pitkanen A, Jolkkonen J, Riekkinen P: β-Endorphin, somatostatin, and prolactin levels in cerebrospinal fluid of epileptic patients after generalized convulsion. J Neurol Neurosurg Psychiatry 50:1294–1297, 1987

Reichlin S: Somatostatin in the nervous system, in Molecular Genetic Neuroscience. Edited by Schmitt FO, Bird SJ, Bloom FE. New York, Raven, 1982, pp 359–372

Reichlin S: Somatostatin, in Brain Peptides. Edited by Krieger DT, Brownstein MJ, Martin JB. New York, Wiley, 1983, pp 711–752

Reisine T: Somatostatin inhibition of cyclic AMP accumulation and adrenocorticotropin release: mechanisms of action and mode of self-regulation. Clin Neuropharmacol 7 (suppl 1):56–57, 1984

Reubi JC, Probsta A, Cortes R, et al: Distinct topographical localisation of two somatostatin receptor subpopulations in the human cortex. Brain Res 406:391–396, 1987

Rezek M, Havlicek V, Hughes KR, et al: Cortical administration of somatostatin (SRIF): effect on sleep and motor behavior. Pharmacol Biochem Behav 5:73–77, 1976

Rezek M, Havlicek V, Hughes KR, et al: Behavioural and motor excitation and inhibition induced by the administration of small and large doses of somatostatin into the amygdala. Neuropharmacology 16:157–162, 1977

Rivier C, Vale W: Involvement of corticotropin-releasing factor and somatostatin in stress-induced inhibition of growth hormone secretin in the rat. Endocrinology 117:2478–2482, 1985

Roberts GW, Crow TJ, Polak JM: Localization of neuronal tangles in somatostatin neurones in Alzheimer's disease. Nature 314:92–94, 1985

Rossor MN, Emson PC, Mountjoy CQ, et al: Reduced amounts of immunoreactive somatostatin in the temporal cortex in senile dementia of Alzheimer type. Neurosci Lett 20:373–377, 1980

Rubinow DR: Cerebrospinal fluid somatostatin and psychiatric illness. Biol Psychiatry 21:341–365, 1986

Rubinow DR, Gold PW, Post RM, et al: CSF somatostatin in affective illness. Arch Gen Psychiatry 40:409–412, 1983

Rubinow DR, Post RM, Gold PW, et al: Effect of carbamazepine on cerebrospinal fluid somatostatin. Psychopharmacology (Berlin) 85:210–213, 1985

Schlegel W, Wuarin F, Wollheim CB, et al: Somatostatin lowers the cytosolic free CA_2^{++} concentration in clonal rat pituitary cells (Gh3 cells). Cell Calcium 5:223–236, 1984

Serby M, Richardson SB, Twente S, et al: CSF somatostatin in Alzheimer's disease. Neurobiol Aging 5:187–189, 1984

Serby M, Richardson SB, Rypma B, et al: Somatostatin regulation of the CRF-ACTH-cortisol axis. Biol Psychiatry 21:971–974, 1986

Sheppard S, Moor B, Kraicer J: Release of growth hormone (GH) from purified somatotrophs: interaction of GH-releasing factor and somatostatin and role of adenosine 3′,5′-monophosphate. Endocrinology 117:2364–2374, 1985

Shinoda H, Schwartz JP, Nadi NS: Amygdaloid kindling of rats increases preprosomatostatin mRNA and somatostatin without affecting glutamic acid decarboxylase (GAD) nRMA or GAD. Mol Brain Res (in press)

Shults C, Steardo L, Barone P, et al: Huntington's disease: effect of cysteamine, a somatostatin-depleting agent. Neurology 36:1099–1102, 1986

Soininen HS, Jolkkonen JT, Reinikainen KJ, et al: Reduced cholinesterase activity and somatostatin-like immunoreactivity in the cerebrospinal fluid of patients with dementia of the Alzheimer type. J Neurol Sci 63:167–172, 1984

Soininen H, Riekkinen PJ, Partanen J, et al: Cerebrospinal fluid somatostatin correlates with spectral EEG variables and with parietotemporal cognitive dysfunction in Alzheimer patients. Neurosci Lett 85:131–136, 1988

Sorensen KV, Christensen SE, Dupont E, et al: Low somatostatin content in cerebrospinal fluid in multiple sclerosis. Acta Neurol Scand 61:186–191, 1980

Sorensen KV, Alslev T, Christensen SE, et al: CSF somatostatin in multiple sclerosis: reversible loss of diurnal oscillation in relapses. Neurology 37:1050–1053, 1987

Srikant CB, Patel YC: Somatostatin receptors. Adv Exp Med Biol 188:291–301, 1985

Steardo L, Barone P, Hunnicutt E: Carbamazepine lowering effect on CSF somatostatin-like immunoreactivity in temporal lobe epileptics. Acta Neurol Scand 74:140–144, 1986

Stryker T, Conlin T, Reichlin S: Influence of a benzodiazepine, midazolam, and gamma-aminobutyric acid (GABA) on basal somatostatin secretion from cerebral and diencephalic neurons in dispersed cell culture. Brain Res 362:339–343, 1986

Sunderland T, Rubinow DR, Tariot PN, et al: CSF somatostatin in dementia, elderly depression and age-matched controls. Am J Psychiatry 144:1313–1316, 1987

Tamminga CA, Foster NL, Chase TN: Reduced brain somatostatin levels in Alzheimer's disease. N Engl J Med 13:1294–1295, 1985

Tran VT, Uhl GR, Petty DC, et al: Autoradiographic localization of somatostatin receptors in rat brain. Eur J Pharmacol 101:307–309, 1984

Tran VT, Beal MF, Martin JB: Two types of somatostatin receptors differentiated by cyclic somatostatin analogs. Science 288:492–495, 1985

Van Leeuwen FW, Deraay C, Swaab DR, et al: The localization of oxytocin, vasopressin, somatostatin and luteinizing hormone releasing hormone in the rat neurohypophysis. Cell Tissue Res 202:189–201, 1979

Vecsei L, Widerlöv E: Brain and CSF somatostatin concentrations in patients with psychiatric or neurological illness: an overview. Acta Psychiatr Scand 78:657, 1988

Vecsei L, Bollok I, Teledgy G: Intracerebroventricular somatostatin attenuates electroconvulsive shock-induced amnesia in rats. Peptides 4:293–295, 1983

Vecsei L, Kiraly C, Bollok I, et al: Comparative studies with somatostatin and cysteamine in different behavior tests on rats. Pharmacol Biochem Behav 21:833–837, 1984

Walsh TJ, Emerich DF, Winokur A, et al: Intrahippocampal injection of cysteamine depletes somatostatin and produces cognitive impairments in the rat. Society for Neuroscience Abstracts 11:621, 1985

Wehr TA: Biological rhythms and manic-depressive illness, in Neurobiology of Mood Disorders. Edited by Post RM, Ballenger JC. Baltimore, MD, Williams & Wilkins, 1984, pp 190–206

Weingartner H, Silberman EK: Cognitive changes in depression, in Neurobiology of Mood Disorders. Edited by Post RM, Ballenger JC. Baltimore, MD, Williams & Wilkins, 1983, pp 121–135

Weiss SRB, Nguyen T, Rubinow DR: Lack of effect of chronic carbamazepine on brain somatostatin in the rat. J Neural Transm 68:325–333, 1987

Widerlöv E, Brane GAM, Ekman R, et al: Elevated CSF somatostatin concentrations in demented patients parallel improved psychomotoric functions induced by integrity-promoting care. Acta Psychiatr Scand (in press)

Wolkowitz OM, Rubinow DR, Breier A, et al: Prednisone decreases CSF somatostatin in healthy humans: implications for neuropsychiatric illness. Life Sci 41:1929–1933, 1987

Wood PL, Etienne P, Lal S, et al: Reduced lumbar CSF somatostatin in Alzheimer's disease. Life Sci 31:2073–2079, 1982

Chapter 4

Gonadotropin-Releasing Hormone and Human Sexual Behavior

Robert L. Moss, Ph.D.
Carol A. Dudley, M.S.
Peter N. Riskind, M.D., Ph.D.

Chapter 4

Gonadotropin-Releasing Hormone and Human Sexual Behavior

More than a quarter of a century has passed since the concept that the secretion of the gonadotropins luteinizing hormone (LH) and follicle-stimulating hormone (FSH) from the anterior pituitary gland is governed by regulating factors localized within and released by the hypothalamus was first recognized (McCann 1962). Subsequently, a number of low–molecular-weight hypothalamic substances (peptides) have been structurally identified and synthesized. These include thyrotropin-releasing hormone (TRH), growth hormone–inhibiting factor (GHIF, also called somatostatin), growth hormone–releasing factor (GHRF, also called GHRH), and corticotropin-releasing factor (CRF, also called CRH). Some of these peptides promote the secretion (releasing hormones) and others inhibit the secretion (inhibiting hormones) of anterior pituitary hormones (for current review see Krieger et al. 1983; Martin et al. 1977; Riskind and Martin 1989). Among the most studied of these hypothalamic regulating peptides is gonadotropin-releasing hormone (GnRH, also called luteinizing hormone–releasing hormone [LHRH]). GnRH is a decapeptide (pyro-Glu^{1}-His^{2}-Trp^{3}-Ser^{4}-Tyr^{5}-Gly^{6}-Leu^{7}-Arg^{8}-Pro^{9}-Gly^{10}-NH_2) and a key integrator between the sensory, cortical, and circadian signals that input to the hypothalamus and the coordination of hypothalamic output controlling the secretion of LH and FSH from the anterior pituitary gland. This peptide is synthesized in hypothalamic neurons, then released in

The authors are indebted to Dr. Eileen Hollingsworth for aiding in the literature review and to Lisa L. Todd for typing and reviewing the chapter. The research presented in this chapter from the authors' laboratory is supported by National Institutes of Health Grants HD-09988 and MH-41784.

a pulsatile pattern into the hypothalamo-hypophyseal portal circulation. This pattern provokes the secretion of the gonadotropins from the anterior pituitary gland (Hazum and Conn 1988; Lincoln 1989). The gonadotropins, in turn, control the function of the gonads: LH stimulates ovulation and corpus luteum formation in females and androgen secretion in males, while FSH stimulates growth and maturation of ovarian follicles in females and spermatogenesis in males.

Paralleling the structural identification and synthesis of the hypothalamic releasing and inhibiting hormones was the demonstration that many of these peptide hormones also possessed the capability of initiating and/or modifying a variety of extrapituitary behaviors, including mating, feeding (i.e., eating and drinking), mood, drive, learning, and memory (for review see Krieger et al. 1983; Moss et al. 1989; Riskind and Martin 1989; Zadina and Kastin 1986). The decapeptide GnRH has been clearly established as the physiological regulator of LH and FSH secretion from specific trophic cells of the anterior pituitary gland and has also been implicated in the initiation and modulation of reproductive-sexual behavior in a variety of species ranging from reptiles to man (for current reviews see Moss and Dudley 1988, 1989; Moss et al. 1989). Thus, in addition to its *classical endocrine action* at the level of the anterior pituitary gland, GnRH has also been demonstrated to have an *extrapituitary behavioral action.* GnRH has been shown to act on multiple extrapituitary central nervous system (CNS) sites to regulate various aspects of sexual reproductive behavior.

The purpose of this chapter is to provide an overview of the literature concerning the potential role of GnRH as a physiological neuromodulator (enhancer) of human sexual behavior. Special attention is focused on the direct effects of GnRH on the enhancement of human sexual behavior. In addition, some discussion is included on the reproductive behavioral signs that have been associated with disorders in the GnRH–hypothalamic-endocrine system (e.g., hyperprolactinemia, hypothalamic amenorrhea, anorexia nervosa, and hypogonadism). A summary of the aforementioned data provides evidence to support the notion that GnRH is involved in the process of human sexual behavior, although the precise nature of this involvement remains ill defined.

BACKGROUND

The animal studies crucial to the concept that hypothalamic GnRH possesses extraendocrine (extrapituitary) CNS action were first reported by two independent laboratories (Moss and McCann 1973,

1975; Pfaff 1973). Collectively these studies demonstrated that GnRH, when administered subcutaneously in small nanogram quantities, potentiates sexual behavior (as measured by lordosis behavior) in ovariectomized, estrogen-primed rats in the absence of the adrenal and pituitary glands. The rationale for these studies was based on 1) a clear temporal relationship between the gonadotropin surge, ovarian cyclicity, and rhythms of sexual receptivity in the female rat (Kuehn and Beach 1963), and 2) the CNS localization of GnRH to neurons in specific areas that participate in the regulation of both gonadotropin secretion and sexual receptivity in the female rat (for review see Johnson and Everitt 1980; Moss and Dudley 1984, 1988; Moss et al. 1979).

Subsequently, infusion of the decapeptide into CNS sites implicated in the control of mating behavior was observed to facilitate the receptive component (lordosis) of mating behavior in the female rat (Dorsa and Smith 1980; Foreman and Moss 1977; Modianos and Pfaff 1976; Moss et al. 1975a, 1975b; Myers and Baum 1980; Riskind and Moss 1979; Rodriguez-Sierra and Komisaruk 1977; Tennent et al. 1982). However, neither the proceptive component (hopping, darting, and ear-wiggling) nor the motivational component (ability to seek out or solicit the sexually active male) of reproductive behavior was affected by GnRH treatment (Dudley and Moss 1985). Thus, the GnRH-induced behavioral effect appears to be limited to facilitating only the reflexive posturing component of mating behavior and not behavioral patterns of higher complexity. In contrast, the administration of progesterone in combination with estrogen to ovariectomized female rats initiates the complete reproductive behavioral repertoire, that is, proceptive, receptive, and motivational components of behavior (Dudley and Moss 1985; Fadem et al. 1979; Tennent et al. 1982). In agreement with the observed behavioral differences among the hormones, the CNS sites of action of these hormones have been reported to be different (Tennent et al. 1982).

Although GnRH does not appear to recruit all aspects of the female mating behavior pattern, the GnRH-induced response appears to be specific in that the other hypothalamic-hypophysiotropic hormones do not facilitate lordosis behavior. The physiological importance of GnRH in the induction of sexual receptivity in the female rat has been demonstrated in studies in which infusion of an anti-GnRH antibody resulted in disruption of lordosis (Kozlowski and Hostetter 1978; Sakuma and Pfaff 1980). As seen in Figure 4-1, administration of a potent, long-acting LHRH antagonist analog reduced lordosis behavior in estrogen-, progesterone-, or estrogen-GnRH–treated female rats (Dudley et al. 1982). The antagonist analog probably diminishes lordosis behavior by binding to GnRH receptors, recently localized in the CNS (Badr and Pelletier 1987), thereby reducing the number of GnRH-responsive receptor sites.

The nature of GnRH action upon hormonally mediated male sexual behavior in the rat was first reported in sexually experienced male rats that were castrated and treated daily with testosterone propionate in doses (10 μg) too low to initiate consistent copulatory behavior (Moss et al. 1975b). Following 3 weeks of testosterone therapy, the castrated male rats were injected with either saline or 500 ng of GnRH.

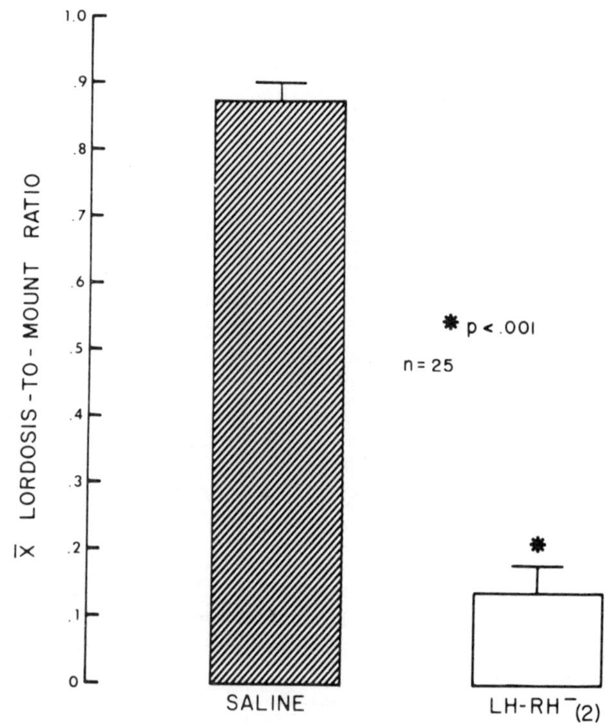

Figure 4-1. The effect of Ac-dehydro-Pro^1-pC1,D-Phe^2,D-Trp^{3,6} (LH-RH$^-_{(2)}$)$^{LH\text{-}RH}$ antagonist analogue on lordosis behavior following infusion of 50 ng into the third ventricle of ovariectomized, estrogen- and progesterone-primed female rats. Reprinted, with permission, from Dudley et al. 1982. Copyright 1982, Pergamon Press.

Injection of a single dose of GnRH was found to decrease significantly the time to achieve the first intromission and ejaculation, whereas a single injection of saline had no effect (see details in Figure 4-2). Similar data have been observed in the intact male rat treated with GnRH—that is, a decrease in the time to achieve the first intromission and ejaculation. It should be noted that the castrated male rat requires some testosterone for the GnRH to be effective under the conditions tested. This is similar to the ovariectomized female rat, which requires some estrogen for the GnRH to potentiate lordosis behavior.

Animal behavioral studies investigating the effects of GnRH have been conducted in a variety of species. Sexual behavior has been reported to be facilitated by GnRH in the male and female mouse (Gray and Luttge 1978; Luttge and Sheets 1977) and the male and

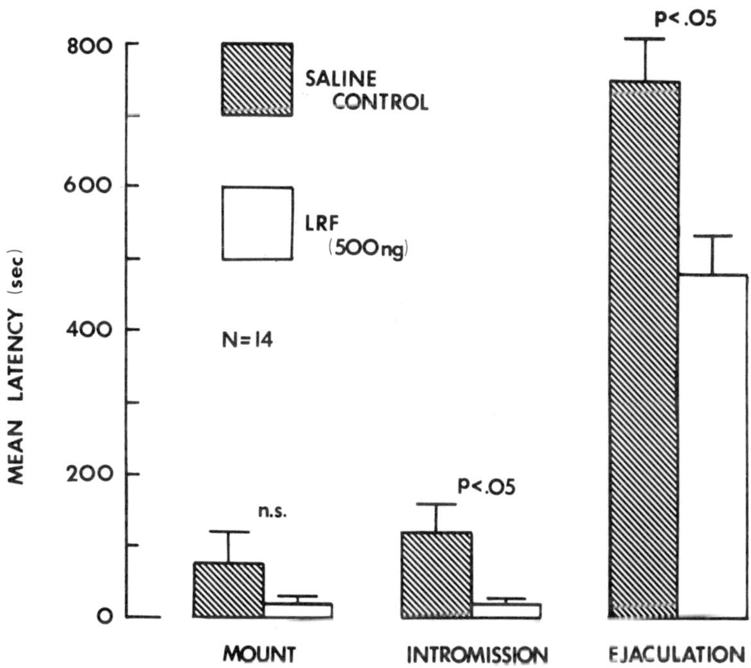

Figure 4-2. Paired comparison of mean latency to first mount, first intromission, and first ejaculation under saline and LH-RH treatments. Reprinted, with permission, from Moss et al. 1975b. Copyright 1975, Elsevier Science Publishers.

female dove (Cheng 1977; McDonald 1979). Reproductive behavior is also potentiated by GnRH in the lizard (Alderette et al. 1980; Crews 1979) and the frog (Kelley 1982). Increases in friendliness and sociability have been reported following GnRH administration in the chimpanzee (C. H. Doering, personal communication, 1978).

Thus, the overall picture that emerges from the animal literature is that GnRH is capable of facilitating specific aspects of sexual behavior in a variety of species. The enhancing effect of GnRH is dependent on the presence of gonadal steroids, but the behavioral effect is exerted in the CNS. Based on experiments in female rats, GnRH-facilitated sexual behavior appears to be a receptor-mediated event.

CHANGES IN HUMAN SEXUAL BEHAVIOR PATTERNS ASSOCIATED WITH DYSFUNCTIONS IN THE GnRH–HYPOTHALAMO-PITUITARY AXIS

Similarities in the pituitary effects of GnRH on subhuman and human species and the emergence of the concept that GnRH serves as an extrapituitary modulator of sexual behavior in a variety of subhuman species have led to speculation that GnRH may regulate human sexual behavior. The tendency to extrapolate to humans from the aforementioned animal data is strong; however, several important species differences are present (Bancroft 1978). Mating behavior patterns and sexual arousal in the female rat are dependent on the secretion of the ovarian steroids. The onset, maintenance, and intensity of sexual behavior in the female rat are time-locked to the secretion of estrogen and progesterone. The intact animal is sexually receptive for approximately 8 hours only during the proestrous phase of the estrous cycle (Beach 1976; Feder 1978, 1981; Johnson and Everitt 1980). Removal of the ovaries results in a total lack of sexual receptivity. On the other hand, sexual behavior in the human female can occur at any stage of the menstrual cycle. In humans, initiation of sexual encounters is more dependent on an interaction with one's partner, the environmental surroundings, and mental state; hormones appear to have an important, but not critical, role (Adler 1981; Goy and Resko 1972; Johnson and Everitt 1980; Johnson and Phoenix 1978; Matteo and Rissman 1984; Udry and Morris 1968). In male rats and in men, castration may eventually be followed by a reduction in sexual activity, but the time course ranges from weeks (in rat) to years (in men), and often the reduction in man does not proceed to a total loss of sexual behavior. Interestingly, testosterone therapy to "castrates" (rat and man) has been shown to effectively reverse the changes following castration, restoring sexual behavior to previous levels (for review see Johnson and Everitt 1980).

Support for the hypothesis that GnRH is involved in human sexual behavior can be found throughout the clinical literature, particularly in studies in which the relationship between copulatory behavior, sexual arousal, and endocrine gonadotropin secretion and function has been studied. A number of studies have reported a consistent relationship between peaks of sexual arousal and/or coitus and the midcycle (between the follicular and luteal) phase of the menstrual cycle (Adams et al. 1978; Gold and Adams 1981; Matteo and Rissman 1984; Sanders and Bancroft 1982). The mid–follicular-luteal phase of the menstrual cycle is a time when the plasma levels of the gonadotropins (LH and FSH) are rising and the estrogen levels are declining. Because the secretion of LH and FSH is regulated by GnRH release from hypothalamic-limbic system nerve cells, one can assume that CNS GnRH levels are high or progressively increasing at this time. Although a correlative relationship may exist between hormonal fluctuations and sexual arousal in the human female, it is generally accepted that ovariectomy in women does not normally result in changes in libido (i.e., the desire for sexual activity). Estrogen-replacement therapy may be necessary to ensure vaginal lubrication and to prevent atrophic changes in the reproductive tract. Hypogonadism in females usually results in amenorrhea, a disorder that is characterized by sexual dysfunction (a decrease in sexual behavior) and other affective behavioral abnormalities (Martin et al. 1977, 1987; Segal 1985). Adult female hypogonadal mice, in which the hypogonadism was secondary to a genetic deficiency in hypothalamic GnRH, have been shown to be infertile (Gibson et al. 1984a, 1984b, 1987). Gibson et al. further demonstrated that *mating*, pregnancy, and delivery of healthy litters occurred after the transplantation of normal fetal preoptic area tissue, a major site of GnRH-containing cell bodies, into the third ventricle. Thus, introduction of GnRH into the brain reversed mating deficiencies in hypogonadal female mice.

Additional observations supporting a possible role of GnRH in human sexual behavior have been derived in patients with hypothalamic or "central" disorders of sexual function and gonadotropin secretion. Patients with chronic elevations of plasma prolactin levels (hyperprolactinemia) typically have marked impairment of gonadotropin and gonadal hormone (testosterone or estrogen) secretion, as well as severe reductions in libido and sexual potency. These effects of excessive prolactin are believed to result, at least in part, from an inhibition of hypothalamic GnRH release. Interestingly, libido can be dramatically restored by medical or surgical normalization of prolactin levels (Schwartz et al. 1982). In contrast, testosterone treatment is generally ineffective in overcoming the impotence caused by hyperprolactinemia. These observations suggest that the CNS effects of prolactin, including the inhibition of GnRH release, may underlie the loss of libido seen in both men and women with hyperprolactinemia. A recent study by Fabbri et al. (1988) supports the notion that GnRH release may be important in some cases of psychogenic impotence. Men with psychogenic impotence were found to have subtle reduction of bioactive LH levels in plasma, which is consistent with a possible reduction of pulsatile GnRH secretion. Similarly, women with anorexia nervosa experience chronic reductions of gonadotropin secretion, loss of libido, and amenorrhea, presumably on the basis of a hypothalamic, or "central," abnormality (for a complete review see Bancroft 1978; Segal 1985). Although not conclusive, these observations suggest that there may be a role for GnRH in human sexual behavior.

It is of interest to note that in the animal models of hyperprolactinemia, a direct relationship has been observed between the high levels of prolactin, low LH and FSH levels (assumed low GnRH levels), and decreased sexual activity in both the male (Kalra and Clark 1986) and female (Moss et al. 1985) rat. Furthermore, plasma testosterone and testicular weight *are not* affected but the adrenal weights are slightly increased in the hyperprolactinemic rat with a marked reduction of copulatory behavior (Bartke 1978; Kupperman 1982; MacLeod 1976; MacLeod and Fontham 1970). Collectively, evidence from a variety of animal experiments has been thought to indicate a direct neurohumoral effect of LHRH on the CNS regulation of sexual behavior in the nonhuman species. These findings have provided a stimulus for the clinical investigations into the role of the releasing hormones on human sexual behavior.

DIRECT EFFECTS OF GnRH ON HUMAN SEXUAL BEHAVIORAL PATTERNS

Various efforts have been made over the years to correlate human sexual dysfunction with the gonadotropin–hypothalamo-pituitary axis. The early experiments in man were based on the fact that gonadal function was demonstrated to be regulated, via feedback mechanisms, by the pituitary hormones LH and FSH. The aforementioned endocrine finding, along with the already well-established interrelationship between gonadal function and sexual behavior, led many investigators to consider whether sexual dysfunction could be reflected in part by circulating levels of the gonadotropins LH and FSH. However, the majority of these studies have obtained findings that are suggestive at best. To date, the results of studies correlating plasma levels of LH and FSH and sexual dysfunction are inconclusive (Benkert and Holsboer 1976; Benkert et al. 1985; Davies et al. 1976, 1977; Delitala et al. 1977; Legros et al. 1973, 1978, 1980; Pirke et al. 1979).

Early studies were also conducted to determine whether sexual behavior in human patients could be influenced by the hypothalamic-hypophysiotropic releasing hormones (e.g., TRH and GnRH). TRH and GnRH are found in areas of the CNS that have been shown to regulate and/or modify reproductive behavior. Thus, localization studies supported the notion that these releasing hormones could be involved in the extrapituitary regulation of behavior. Experiments designed to compare the action of TRH, GnRH, and placebo in depressive patients using a double-blind, cross-over technique demonstrated that neither of the two hypothalamic releasing hormones appeared to be behaviorally active (i.e., to modify existing nonsexual behaviors) in depressed patients (Benkert and Holsboer 1985; Benkert et al. 1974, 1975). However, in subsequent studies, whereas TRH was found to be inactive in sexually impotent male patients, GnRH was demonstrated to facilitate libido in these same patients (Benkert 1975).

The universality of the GnRH-induced behavioral response in the nonhuman species (from lizard to monkey) and the endocrine-pituitary actions of GnRH in pituitary secretion of LH and FSH, coupled with the possible relationship between human sexual behavior deficits and gonadotropin dysfunction, provided good justification to proceed with further investigation into the behavioral effects of GnRH on human sexual behavior. A number of clinical experiments were designed specifically to evaluate the therapeutic effects of GnRH on human sexual behavior in men who were classified as being 1) normal and healthy, 2) sexually impotent, or 3) hypogonadal with hypothalamic or pituitary dysfunction.

GnRH and Sexual Activities in Healthy Men

The administration of GnRH to healthy males was reported to decrease self-reported fatigue and drowsiness relative to a placebo control (McAdoo et al. 1978). The effect was first observed 6 hours post GnRH injection. These psychological effects are interesting but extremely difficult to interpret. Other psychological effects were observed between viewing a sexually explicit film and correlating the observed increases in plasma LH and FSH levels with sexual arousal (LaFerla et al. 1978). The most complete study on the effects of GnRH on human sexual behavior in physiologically normal individuals was conducted by Evans and Distiller (1979). They observed increases in penile tumescence in response to a free-fantasy period in healthy male volunteers treated with GnRH (see Figure 4-3). In fact, intramuscular injections of 500 μg of GnRH initiated a shorter onset latency for tumescence to occur than did a comparable placebo treatment (control injection). These findings are somewhat consistent with the findings observed in the male rat in that the administration of GnRH decreased the time to first intromission and to ejaculation (Moss et al. 1975b). Evans and Distiller (1979) also measured heart rate and collected blood samples for radioimmunoassay of plasma LH,

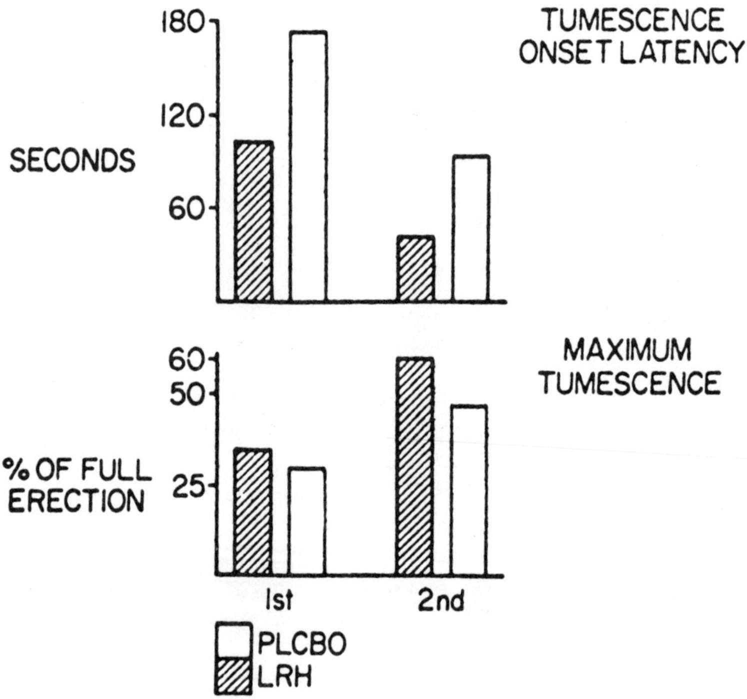

Figure 4-3. Mean penile tumescence levels obtained during free-fantasy period. Reprinted, with permission, from Evans and Distiller 1979. Copyright 1979, Plenum Publishing Corporation.

FSH, and testosterone levels. No significant correlation between plasma hormone levels and measurements of penile tumescence was observed. (It should be noted at this point that the subjects utilized in the aforementioned study were healthy volunteers.) Therefore, the GnRH-induced effect is an enhancement or a potentiation of a system that is normally functional, and its occurrence or appearance is independent of any sexual dysfunction.

GnRH and Sexual Activities in Male Patients With Psychogenic Impotence

Several laboratories have explored the action of GnRH in male patients presenting with secondary impotence, that is, a decrease in libido (drive and/or arousal) and/or a decrease in sexual behavior as a function of psychogenic origin with no known clinical pathology. One such clinical study investigated the effect of GnRH or placebo control on 10 male patients presenting secondary impotence in a double-blind, cross-over design (Davies et al. 1976). The administration of GnRH was found to enhance the subjective measures of general sexual interest but did not influence the quality of erection. In another clinical study, GnRH was found to induce a better therapeutic effect than was observed with placebo; however, the effect was not apparent until 4 to 6 weeks after cessation of the GnRH medication (Benkert et al. 1975). This experiment, performed on male patients presenting with secondary sexual impotence with no known clinical pathology, was a double-blind study designed to compare the effects of GnRH (administered via nasal spray) and placebo on human sexual behavior.

In our own studies (Moss et al. 1979) we investigated the therapeutic effect of the subcutaneous administration of GnRH (500 μg per day by injection) to eight male psychogenically impotent (secondary) patients with no known pathology and who displayed various levels of pretest masturbatory activity. The data are summarized in Figure 4-4. All patients selected for these studies were referred to our research group by a local urologist. The male subjects ranged in age between 25 and 45 years of age and were living with their spouse (female partner) throughout both studies (I and II). In addition to interviewing the male subject, the female partner was also interviewed separately as well as together with her spouse. Both partners were required to independently fill out daily questionnaires.

In Study I, the patients were tested for a total of 20 days in a double-blind, cross-over study such that the individual collecting the questionnaires and administering the agent had no prior knowledge of the questionnaire content or the specific agent that was being

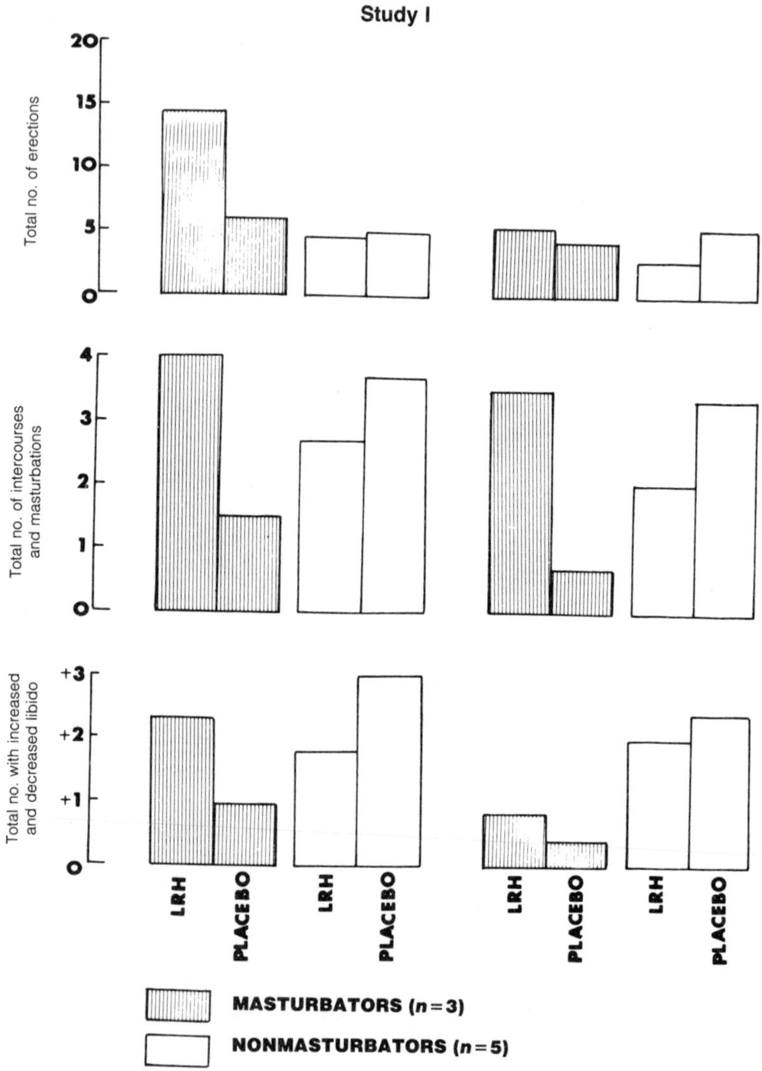

Figure 4-4. GnRH (LH-RH) and placebo tests in eight patients suffering from secondary sexual impotency. Study I consisted of a double-blind, crossover study with 10 days of LH-RH and placebo. Study II consisted of 1 week of placebo, 2 weeks of LH-RH, and 1 week of no treatment. Reprinted, with permission, from Moss et al. 1979. Copyright 1979, Raven Press.

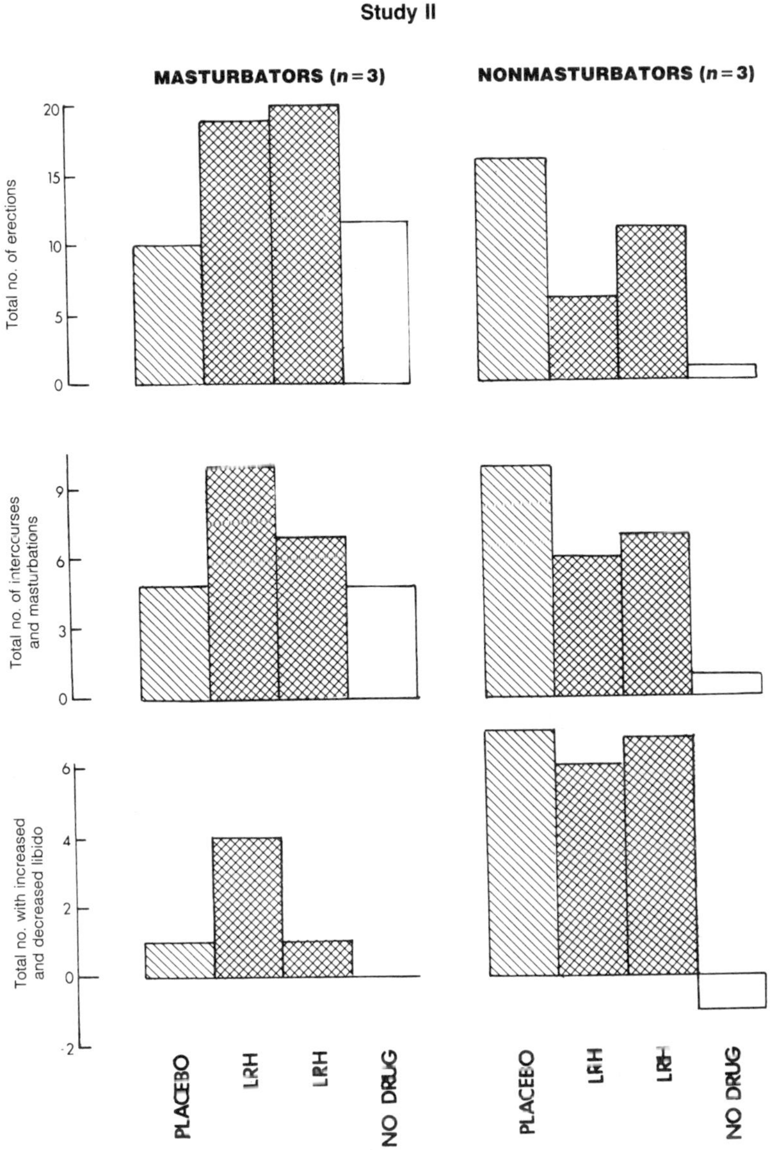
Study II
MASTURBATORS (n=3)
NONMASTURBATORS (n=3)
Total no. of erections
20
15
10
5
0
Total no. of intercourses and masturbations
9
6
3
0
Total no. with increased and decreased libido
6
4
2
0
-2
PLACEBO
LRH
LRH
NO DRUG
PLACEBO
LRH
LRH
NO DRUG

injected. The agents were coded by the Ayerst Laboratories (New York, NY), and the patients received 10 days of either GnRH or placebo followed by 10 days of the other agent. The experimenters broke the code and evaluated the questionnaires at the end of Study I and subsequently divided the data based on whether the patients had prior masturbatory activity. In Study II, the same subjects and their spouses as in Study I were tested under a different design. Study II was designed so that each subject received 1 week of placebo administration, followed by 2 weeks of GnRH administration and, finally, 1 week of no treatment. Again, as in Study I, both the subject and his spouse filled out independent daily questionnaires. The drug code was broken at the end of the study, and subsequent analysis of the data and questionnaires was performed.

Interestingly, GnRH administration in both Study I and Study II was found to improve the overall arousal level in the male subjects with some prior masturbatory activity under all conditions tested (see Figure 4-4). The subjects ($n = 3$) who showed a GnRH-induced effect also reported numerous anecdotes about the sexual side effects (erections feeling stronger and/or firm tumescence) that occurred during the period of GnRH administration. It should be noted that the spouse's report, in most cases, showed a positive correlation with the verbal and written reports by the husband. Even subjects (nonmasturbators) who did not display GnRH-induced potentiation of sexual desire or activities reported a feeling of euphoria on more than one occasion under the period of GnRH administration.

Not all clinical trials studying the effects of GnRH on male sexual behavior yield positive results. In a study by Ehrensing and coworkers (1981), prolonged treatment with GnRH at high dosages produced a small trend toward improvement. The authors suggested that because there was a slight GnRH-induced action on the improvement of libido, clinical trials with GnRH analogues should be explored.

GnRH and Sexual Activities in Male Patients With Other Endocrine Disorders

The administration of GnRH was found to increase sexual potency in hypogonadal males with hypothalamic or pituitary dysfunction (Mortimer et al. 1974). Schwarzstein and coworkers (1975) also described an increase of libido in four GnRH-treated oligospermic men; however, interest in sexual activity might be a natural consequence of treatment for infertility. Van Loon and Brown (1975) reported a case of a 49-year-old man with hypogonadotropic hypogonadism who was not impotent but who nevertheless showed an increased incidence of erections following daily administration of GnRH. Interestingly, although there were no significant effects on self-reported quality of erection, subjective measures of general sexual interest were marginally increased by GnRH.

CONCLUDING REMARKS AND FUTURE DIRECTIONS

It is clear in certain animal models, and perhaps even in man, that neuroendocrine function (hormone secretion), as well as specific behavioral patterns, is regulated or at least modulated by the activity of neuropeptides. This dual endocrine-behavioral action of the neuropeptides is even more striking when considering the CNS origin of these peptides and the fact that the limbic system and hypothalamo-pituitary axis appear to be critical to both the endocrine and behavioral events. Intriguing is the prominent relationship that exists between the hypothalamus, limbic system structures, endocrine function, and behavior. However, the neurobiological mechanism(s) underlying specific behavioral disorders and profiles of anterior pituitary hormone secretion, as well as the clinical significance of these hormonal changes during sexual dysfunction, is not clear. In fact, the majority of peptides employed in psychiatric research have previously been shown to have more promise as diagnostic tools than as therapeutic agents (Brambilla et al. 1979, 1985; Cohen and Cohen 1981; Prange and Loosen 1984).

In this chapter the emphasis has been placed on GnRH-induced changes in sexual activity in man. As noted throughout the chapter there are excellent and comprehensive reviews available that cover the role of hormones in sexual behavior from the basic science as well as the clinical perspective. (See, for example, the comprehensive reviews by Bancroft [1978], Martin et al. [1977, 1987], and Segal [1985].)

Like so many areas involving human behavior, the execution of effective sexual behavioral patterns is a complex event that involves the interplay between hormones, neurotransmitters, and nerve cells, as well as unknown, or at best ill-defined, psychological factors. Interpretation of the aforementioned clinical trials with GnRH is difficult because of lack of ability to control all of the variables involved. Certainly, there is a common thread that is apparent in all the reported human studies, namely, that while GnRH may not induce changes in penile erection, it does have an effect on libido. The strength of this effect depends on the clinical status of the subject. It appears that the action of GnRH is most prominent in healthy volunteers and in subjects that have "some on-going" level of sexual behavior still present. Thus, the GnRH positive data suggest that long-term administration of GnRH potentiates (either directly or indirectly via an unknown mechanism) sexual behavior providing that some sexual behavioral patterns are still present or elicitable in the individuals being studied. This factor could possibly account for the discrepancies in the reported clinical trials with GnRH. (Some studies report a GnRH-potentiation, whereas others report little, if any, effect.) Subjects with some sexual behavioral patterns still present may respond to the exogenous administration of GnRH differently than do subjects with no capability to initiate normal sexual behavioral patterns.

REFERENCES

Adams DB, Gold AR, Burt AD: Rise in female-initiated sexual activity by ovulation and its suppression by oral contraceptives. N Engl J Med 229:1145–1150, 1978

Adler NT: Neuroendocrinology of Reproduction: Physiology and Behavior. New York, Plenum, 1981

Alderette MR, Tokarz RR, Crews D: Luteinizing hormone–releasing hormone induction of female sexual receptivity in the lizard, *Anolis carolinensis.* Neuroendocrinology 30:200–205, 1980

Badr M, Pelletier G: Characterization and autoradiographic localization of LHRH receptors in the rat brain. Synapse 1:567–571, 1987

Bancroft J: The relationship between hormones and sexual behaviour in humans, in Biological Determinants of Sexual Behavior. Edited by Hutchison JB. New York, John Wiley, 1978, pp 493–519

Barkte A: Hyperprolactinemia and impotence. Andrology 1:2, 1978

Beach FA: Sexual attractivity, proceptivity, and receptivity in female mammals. Horm Behav 7:105–138, 1976

Benkert O: Clinical studies of the effects of neurohormones on sexual behavior, in Sexual Behavior: Pharmacology and Biochemistry. Edited by Sandler M, Gessa GL. New York, Raven, 1975, pp 297–305

Benkert O, Holsboer F: Sexual dysfunction in male patients: biological indices and classification, in Psychopharmacology of Sexual Disorders. Edited by Segal M. London, John Libbey, 1985, pp 133–144

Benkert O, Gordon A, Martschke D: The comparison of thyrotropin releasing hormone, luteinizing hormone–releasing hormone and placebo in depressive patients using a double-blind cross-over technique. Psychopharmacology (Berlin) 40:191–198, 1974

Benkert O, Jordon R, Dahlen HG, et al: Sexual impotence: a double blind study of LHRH nasal spray versus placebo. Neuropsychobiology 1: 203–210, 1975

Benkert O, Horn K, Pickardt CR, et al: Sexual impotence: studies of the hypothalamic-pituitary-thyroid axis and the effect of oral thyrotropin-releasing factor. Arch Sex Behav 5:275–281, 1976

Brambilla F, Smeraldi E, Sacchetti E, et al: Abnormal anterior pituitary responsiveness to hypothalamic hormones in depression, in Neuroendocrine Correlates in Neurology and Psychiatry. Edited by Muller EE, Agnoli A. Amsterdam, Elsevier North-Holland, 1979, pp 239–253

Brambilla F, Pugnetti L, Scarone S, et al: Abnormal anterior pituitary responsiveness to hypothalamic hormones in depression: neurophysiological correlates and psychopharmacological effects, in Chronic Treatments in Neuropsychiatry. Edited by Kemali D, Racagni G. New York, Raven, 1985, pp 69–80

Cheng M: Role of gonadotrophin releasing hormones in the reproductive behavior of female ring doves (*Streptopelia risoria*). J Endocrinol 74:37–45, 1977

Cohen RM, Cohen MR: Peptide challenges in affective illness. J Clin Psychopharmacol 1:214–222, 1981

Crews D: Endocrine control of reptilian reproductive behavior, in Endocrine Control of Sexual Behavior. Edited by Beyer C. New York, Raven, 1979, pp 167–222

Davies TF, Mountjoy CQ, Gomez-Pam A, et al: A double blind crossover trial of gonadotropin releasing hormone (LHRH) in sexually impotent men. Clin Endocrinol 5:601–607, 1976

Davies TF, Gomez-Pam A, Watson MJ, et al: Reduced gonadotropin response to releasing hormone after chronic administration to impotent men. Clin Endocrinol 6:213–218, 1977

DeGroot LJ: Endocrinology, Vol 1–3, 2nd Edition. Philadelphia, PA, WB Saunders, 1989

Delitala G, Masala A, Alagna S, et al: Luteinizing hormone, follicle stimulating hormone and testosterone in normal and impotent men following LHRH and HCG stimulation. Clin Endocrinol 6:11–15, 1977

Dorsa DM, Smith ER: Facilitation of mounting behavior in male rats by intracranial injection of luteinizing hormone releasing hormone. Regul Pept 1:147–155, 1980

Dudley CA, Moss RL: LHRH and mating behavior: sexual receptivity versus sexual preference. Pharmacol Biochem Behav 22:967–972, 1985

Dudley CA, Vale W, Rivier J, et al: The effect of LHRH antagonist analogs and an antibody to LHRH on mating behavior in female rats. Peptides 2:393–396, 1982

Ehrensing RH, Kastin AJ, Schally AV: Behavioral and hormonal effects of prolonged high doses of LHRH in male impotency. Peptides 2:115–121, 1981

Evans IM, Distiller LA: Effects of luteinizing hormone–releasing hormone on sexual arousal in normal men. Arch Sex Behav 8:385–395, 1979

Fabbri A, Jannini EA, Ulisse S, et al: Low serum bioactive luteinizing hormone in nonorganic male impotence: possible relationship with altered gonadotropin-releasing hormone pulsatility. J Clin Endocrinol Metab 67:867–875, 1988

Fadem BH, Barfield RJ, Whalen RE: Dose-response and time-response relationships between progesterone and the display of patterns of receptive and proceptive behavior in the female rat. Horm Behav 13:40–48, 1979

Feder HH: Specificity of steroid hormone activation of sexual behavior in rodents, in Biological Determinants of Sexual Behavior. Edited by Hutchinson JB. New York, John Wiley, 1978, pp 395–424

Feder HH: Estrous cyclicity in mammals, in Neuroendocrinology of Reproduction. Edited by Adler NT. New York, Plenum, 1981, pp 279–329

Foreman MM, Moss RL: Effects of subcutaneous injection and intrahypothalamic infusion of releasing hormones upon lordotic response to repetitive coital stimulation. Horm Behav 8:219–234, 1977

Gibson MJ, Charlton HM, Perlow MJ, et al: Preoptic area brain grafts in hypogonadal (hpg) female mice abolish effects of congenital hypothalamic gonadotropin-releasing hormone (GNRH) deficiency. Endocrinology 114:1938–1940, 1984a

Gibson MJ, Krieger DT, Charlton HM, et al: Mating and pregnancy can occur in genetically hypogonadal mice with preoptic area brain grafts. Science 225:949–951, 1984b

Gibson MJ, Moscovitz HC, Kokoris GJ, et al: Female sexual behavior in hypogonadal mice with GnRH-containing brain grafts. Horm Behav 21:211–222, 1987

Gold AR, Adams DB: Motivational factors affecting fluctuations of female sexual activity at menstruation. Psychiatric Women Quarterly 5 (suppl): 670–680, 1981

Goy RW, Resko JA: Gonadal hormones and behavior of normal and pseudohermaphroditic nonhuman female primates, in Recent Progress in Hormone Research. Edited by Astwood EB. New York, Academic, 1972, pp 707–733

Gray HE, Luttge WG: Apparent involvement of protein synthesis and LHRH in the inhibition by dihydrotestosterone of estrogen-induced sexual receptivity in the ovariectomized mouse. Physiol Behav 21:973–977, 1978

Hazum E, Conn PM: Molecular mechanism of gonadotropin releasing hormone (GnRH) action, I: the GnRH receptor. Endoc Rev 9:379–385, 1988

Johnson DF, Phoenix CH: Sexual behavior and hormone levels during the menstrual cycle of rhesus monkeys. Horm Behav 11:160–174, 1978

Johnson MH, Everitt BJ: Essential Reproduction. Oxford, UK, Blackwell Scientific Publications, 1980

Kalra PS, Clark JT: Dopamine, hyperprolactinemia, and sexual behavior, in Andrology: Male Fertility and Sterility. Edited by Paulson JD. New York, Academic, 1986, pp 125–147

Kelley DB: Female sex behaviors in the South African clawed frog, *Xenopus loenis*: gonadotropin-releasing, gonadotropic and steroid hormones. Horm Behav 16:158–174, 1982

Kozlowski GP, Hostetter G: Cellular and subcellular localization and behavioral effects of gonadotropin-releasing hormone (Gn-RH) in the rat, in Brain-Endocrine Interaction, III: Neural Hormones and Reproduction. Edited by Scott DE, Kozlowski GP, Weindl A. Basel, S Karger, 1978, pp 138–153

Krieger DT, Brownstein MJ, Martin JB: Brain Peptides. New York, John Wiley, 1983

Kuehn RE, Beach FA: Quantitative measurement of sexual receptivity in female rats. Behavior 21:282–299, 1963

Kupperman HS: The role of prolactin in impotence. Medical Aspects of Human Sexuality 16:9, 1982

LaFerla JJ, Anderson DL, Schalch DS: Psychoendocrine response to sexual arousal in human males. Psychosom Med 40:166–172, 1978

Legros JJ, Franchimont P, Palem-Vliers M, et al: FSH-LH and testosterone blood level in patients with psychogenic impotence. Endocrinol Exp (Bratisl) 7:59, 1973

Legros JJ, Mormont C, Servais J: A psychoendocrine study of erectile "psychogenic impotence": a comparison between normal patients and patients with abnormal glucose tolerance tests, in Clinical Psychoneuroendocrinology in Reproduction. Edited by Carenza L, Pancheri P, Zichella L. New York, Academic, 1978, pp 301–319

Legros JJ, Chiodera P, Mormont C, et al: Hormones and sexual impotence, in Hormones and the Brain. Edited by DeWied D, VanKeep PA. Baltimore, MD, University Park Press, 1980, pp 205–217

Lincoln DW: Luteinizing hormone–releasing hormone, in Endocrinology, Vol 1, 2nd Edition. Edited by DeGroot LJ. Philadelphia, PA, WB Saunders, 1989, pp 142–151

Luttge WG, Sheets CS: Further studies on the restoration of estrogen-induced sexual receptivity in ovariectomized mice treated with dihydrotestosterone: effects of progesterone, dihydroprogesterone and LHRH. Pharmacol Biochem Behav 7:563–566, 1977

MacLeod RM: Regulation of prolactin secretion, in Frontiers in Neuroendocrinology, Vol 4. Edited by Martini JC, Ganong WF. New York, Raven, 1976, pp 169–194

MacLeod RM, Fontham FM: Influence of ionic environment on the *in vitro* synthesis and release of pituitary hormones. Endocrinology 86:863–869, 1970

Martin JB, Reichlin S, Brown GM: Clinical Neuroendocrinology. Philadelphia, PA, FA Davis, 1977

Martin JB, Reichlin S, Brown GM: Clinical Neuroendocrinology, 2nd Edition. Philadelphia, PA, FA Davis, 1987

Matteo S, Rissman EF: Increased sexual activity during the midcycle portion of the human menstrual cycle. Horm Behav 18:249–255, 1984

McAdoo BC, Doering CH, Kraemer HC, et al: A study of the effects of gonadotropin-releasing hormone therapy in hypogonadal males with hypothalamic or pituitary dysfunction. Br Med J 4:617–621, 1978

McCann SM: A hypothalamic luteinizing-hormone–releasing factor. Am J Physiol 202:395–400, 1962

McDonald PA: Luteinizing hormone-releasing factor (LRF) and reproductive behavior in male doves exposed to long and short photoperiods. Neuroendocrinology 28:151–154, 1979

Modianos D, Pfaff D: Steroid and peptide hormones and the neural mechanisms for reproductive behavior. Excerpta Medica International Congress on Steroids 402:67–71, 1976

Mortimer CH, McNeilly AS, Fisher RA, et al: Gonadotropin-releasing hormone therapy in hypogonadal males with hypothalamic or pituitary dysfunction. Br Med J 4:617–621, 1974

Moss RL, Dudley CA: The challenge of studying the behavioral effects of neuropeptides, in Handbook of Psychopharmacology, Vol 18. Edited by Iversen LL, Iversen SD, Snyder SH. New York, Plenum, 1984, pp 397–454

Moss RL, Dudley CA: Luteinizing hormone–releasing hormone (LHRH): peptidergic signals in the neural integration of female reproductive behavior, in Neural Control of Reproductive Function. Edited by Lakoski JM, Perez-Polo RJ, Rassin DK. New York, John Wiley, 1988, pp 485–499

Moss RL, Dudley CA: Neuropeptides and the social aspects of female reproductive behavior, in Advances in Environmental and Comparative Physiology: Molecular and Cellular Basis of Social Behavior in Vertebrates. Edited by Balthazart J. Heidelberg, Springer-Verlag, 1989, pp 209–237

Moss RL, McCann SM: Induction of mating behavior in rats by luteinizing hormone releasing hormone. Science 181:177–179, 1973

Moss RL, McCann SM: Action of luteinizing hormone releasing factor (LRF) in the initiation of lordosis behavior in the estrone-primed ovariectomized female rat. Neuroendocrinology 17:309–318, 1975

Moss RL, Kelly MJ, Foreman MM, et al: Luteinizing hormone–releasing hormone (LRH) regulation of neural events controlling mating behavior. Physiologist 18:326, 1975a

Moss RL, McCann SM, Dudley CA: Releasing hormones and sexual behavior, in Progress in Brain Research, Vol 42: Hormones, Homeostasis, and the Brain. Edited by Gispen WH, Martini L. Amsterdam, Elsevier, 1975b, pp 37–46

Moss RL, Riskind P, Dudley CA: Effects of LHRH in sexual activity in animal and man, in Central Nervous System Effects of Hypothalamic Hormones and Other Peptides. Edited by Collu R, Barbeau A, Ducharme JR. New York, Raven, 1979, pp 345–366

Moss RL, Chan A, Dudley CA: Hyperprolactinemia: its electrophysiologic and pharmacologic effect on neurons of the ventromedial nucleus of the hypothalamus. Brain Res 346:301–309, 1985

Moss RL, Dudley CA, Gosnell BA: Behavior and the hypothalamus, in Endocrinology, Vol 1, 2nd Edition. Edited by DeGroot LJ. Philadelphia, PA, WB Saunders, 1989, pp 254–263

Myers BM, Baum MJ: Facilitation of copulatory performance in male rats by naloxone: effects of hypophysectomy, 17α-estradiol, and luteinizing hormone releasing hormone. Pharmacol Biochem Behav 12:365–370, 1980

Pfaff DW: Luteinizing hormone releasing factor (LRF) potentiates lordosis behavior in hypophysectomized, ovariectomized female rats. Science 182:1148–1149, 1973

Pirke KM, Kockutt G, Aldenhoff J, et al: Pituitary gonadal system function in patients with erectile impotence and premature ejaculation. Arch Sex Behav 8:41–48, 1979

Prange AJ, Loosen PT: Peptides in depression, in Frontiers in Biochemical and Pharmacological Research in Depression. Edited by Usdin E, et al. New York, Raven, 1984, pp 127–145

Riskind PN, Martin JB: Functional anatomy of the hypothalamic-anterior pituitary complex, in Endocrinology, Vol 1, 2nd Edition. Edited by DeGroot LJ. Philadelphia, PA, WB Saunders, 1989, pp 97–107

Riskind P, Moss RL: Midbrain central gray:LHRH infusion enhances lordotic behavior in estrogen-primed ovariectomized rats. Brain Res Bull 4:203–205, 1979

Rodriguez-Sierra JF, Komisaruk BR: Effects of prostaglandin E2 and indomethacin on sexual behavior in the female rat. Horm Behav 9:281–289, 1977

Sakuma Y, Pfaff DW: LH-RH in the mesencephalic central gray can potentiate lordosis reflex of female rats. Nature 283:566–567, 1980

Sanders D, Bancroft J: Hormones and the sexuality of women: the menstrual cycle. Clin Endocrinol Metab 11:639–659, 1982

Schwartz MF, Bauman JE, Masters WH: Hyperprolactinemia and sexual disorders in men. Biol Psychiatry 17:861–876, 1982

Schwarzstein L, Aparicio NJ, Turner D, et al: Use of synthetic luteinizing hormone–releasing hormone in treatment of oligospermic men: a preliminary report. Fertil Steril 26:331–340, 1975

Segal M: Psychopharmacology of Sexual Disorders. London, John Libbey, 1985

Tennent BJ, Smith ER, Dorsa DM: Comparison of some CNS effects of luteinizing hormone–releasing hormone and progesterone. Horm Behav 16:76–86, 1982

Udry JR, Morris NM: Distribution of coitus in the menstrual cycle. Nature 220:593–596, 1968

Van Loon GR, Brown CM: Secondary drug failure occurring during chronic treatment with LHRH: appearance of an antibody. J Clin Endocrinol Metab 41:640–643, 1975

Zadina JE, Kastin AJ: Multi-independent actions of peptides in the brain: LHRH, MIF-1 and CRF. American Zoologist 26:951–964, 1986

Chapter 5

Corticotropin-Releasing Factor

Charles B. Nemeroff, M.D., Ph.D.

Chapter 5

Corticotropin-Releasing Factor

In the past 15 years the chemical structures of the hypothalamic-hypophysiotropic hormones that regulate the secretion of the adenohypophysiotropic hormones have been elucidated. These include thyrotropin-releasing hormone (TRH), gonadotropin-releasing hormone (GnRH or LHRH), growth hormone-release-inhibiting factor (somatostatin, SRIF), growth hormone–releasing factor (GHRF), and corticotropin-releasing factor (CRF). The latter was first detected in 1955 by Saffran and Schally in hypothalamic extracts. More than 25 years elapsed before Vale and his colleagues (1981) determined the amino acid sequence of ovine CRF (Figure 5-1). This delay was largely due to the fact that 1) the amino acid sequence of CRF is considerably larger than that of most other hypothalamic hormones (e.g., TRH is a tripeptide); 2) the biological potency of CRF is markedly reduced by deletion of even a small portion of the sequence; and 3) numerous endogenous substances (e.g., vasopressin, oxytocin, epinephrine) also possess CRF-like activity and therefore obscured the identity of the endogenous CRF. Human and rat CRF differ from ovine CRF only in 7 of the 41 amino acids, and the substitutions are homologous. Several lines of experimental evidence have conclusively demonstrated that CRF is the major physiological mediator of adrenocorticotropin (ACTH) and other pro-opiomelanocortin–related peptides from the anterior pituitary (Rivier et al. 1982).

However, the emphasis of this chapter is not on the neuroendocrine role of CRF but on its putative role in the pathogenesis of psychiatric disorders. The impetus for evaluating the involvement of CRF in neuropsychiatric disorders was provided by a number of studies that resulted in data concordant with the hypothesis that CRF is a neurotransmitter in the mammalian central nervous system (CNS). Once the structure of CRF was elucidated, antisera were raised in rabbits against the peptide, and these antisera were then used for

The author's research is supported by National Institutes of Health Grant MH-42088.

immunohistochemical and radioimmunoassay studies. Such studies clearly demonstrated a heterogeneous distribution of CRF in the CNS of mammals, including man (Sawchenko and Swanson 1985). Consistent with CRF's role as a hypothalamic releasing factor regulating pituitary-adrenal activity, CRF neurons have been localized in the parvocellular region of the paraventricular nucleus (PVN) of the hypothalamus, whose main projection is to the median eminence, the site of the primary plexus of the hypothalamo-hypophyseal portal system.

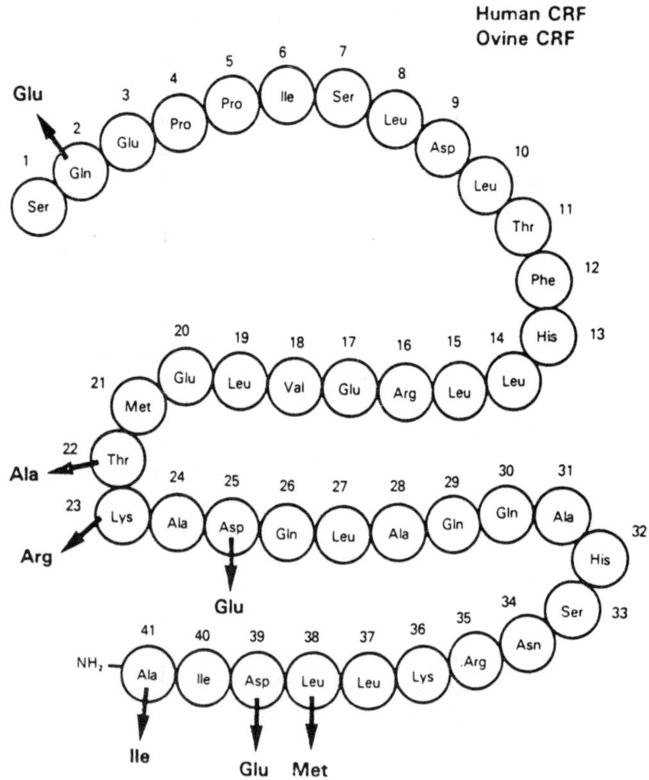

Figure 5-1. Comparison of the structures of ovine CRF (oCRF) and human CRF (hCRF). The basic structure is that of oCRF. The arrows indicate the locations and specific amino acid substitutions that distinguish hCRF from oCRF. Reprinted from Gold and Chrousos 1985, with permission of Pergamon Press. Copyright 1985, Pergamon Press.

Immunohistochemical and radioimmunoassay studies have shown that CRF-like immunoreactivity is also found in a number of extrahypothalamic areas. The extrahypothalamic distribution of CRF is compatible with an involvement in stress responses and emotionality because it is found in such forebrain limbic areas as the central and medial nuclei of the amygdala, the bed nucleus of the stria terminalis, the substantia innominata, septum, preoptic area, and lateral hypothalamus, and in brain-stem nuclei involved in stress responses and regulation of the autonomic nervous system, such as the locus coeruleus, the parabrachial nucleus, and the dorsal vagal complex. In addition, the distribution of high-affinity CRF receptors in the mammalian CNS, as demonstrated by both autoradiographic and radioligand-binding techniques, is also heterogeneous (De Souza et al. 1984). Exposure of brain slices to depolarizing concentrations of potassium results in CRF release; this release is calcium-dependent (Smith et al. 1986). Moreover, the use of modern molecular biological techniques has permitted elucidation of the prohormone for CRF and the sequence of the gene that encodes the prohormone (Furutani et al. 1983). In situ hybridization methods have been utilized to visualize CRF messenger RNA (mRNA) in CNS perikarya such as the PVN of the hypothalamus (Young et al. 1986). Taken together these findings reveal the presence of the cellular machinery for synthesis, release, and action (via receptors) of CRF. Furthermore, once CRF binds to its receptors, it acts, at least partly, by activation of adenylate cyclase, although evidence for an action on phosphoinositide hydrolysis has also been obtained (Bilezikjian and Vale 1983; Kilts et al. 1987). Finally, direct injection of CRF into the lateral cerebral ventricles produces a number of striking behavioral effects, including decreased food consumption (Levine et al. 1983), altered locomotor activity (Britton et al. 1986), diminished sexual behavior (Sirinathsinghji et al. 1983), sleep disruption (Ehlers et al. 1983), and anxiety (Butler et al. 1990), as well as neurochemical changes such as increased catecholamine utilization (Dunn and Berridge 1987). Many of these effects are similar to the signs and symptoms observed in patients with major depression (Table 5-1).

AFFECTIVE DISORDERS

Because CRF is the major cephalic representative of the hypothalamo-pituitary-adrenal (HPA) axis and because it is well established that drug-free patients who fulfill criteria for major depression are, as a group, hypercortisolemic when compared to control subjects (Evans and Nemeroff 1987), it was plausible to investigate whether CRF hypersecretion is, in part, responsible for this hyperactivity of the HPA

Table 5-1. Similarities between signs and symptoms of major depression (DSM-III-R criteria) and the behavioral effects of centrally administered CRF in laboratory animals

DSM-III-R Major Depression	Effects of CRF
At least five of the following are present for at least 2 weeks:	
1. Depressed mood (irritable mood in children and adolescents) most of the day, nearly every day, as indicated either by subjective account or observations by others.	1. Centrally administered CRF in infant rhesus monkeys mimics the behavioral despair syndrome observed after maternal separation.
2. Markedly diminished interest or pleasure in all or almost all activities most of the day, nearly every day.	2. Centrally administered CRF decreases the incidence of sexual behavior in male and female rats.
3. Significant weight loss or weight gain when not dieting or decrease or increase in appetite nearly every day.	3. Centrally administered CRF decreases food consumption in rats.

4. Insomnia or hyposomnia nearly every day.	4. Centrally administered CRF disrupts normal sleep, with concomitant EEG changes.
5. Psychomotor agitation or retardation nearly every day.	5. Centrally administered CRF increases locomotor activity in a familiar environment but produces "stresslike" alterations in locomotion in a novel environment.
6. Fatigue or loss of energy nearly every day.	6. No data.
7. Feelings of worthlessness or excessive or unappropriate guilt nearly every day.	7. No data.
8. Diminished ability to think or concentrate, or indecisiveness, nearly every day.	8. No data.
9. Recurrent thoughts of death, recurrent suicidal ideation, or a suicide attempt.	9. No data.

axis. Gold and his associates (Gold and Chrousos 1985; Gold et al. 1984) and Holsboer and his colleagues (1984) administered CRF to depressed patients and control subjects, and reported that the depressed patients exhibited blunted ACTH but normal cortisol responses. This finding has been replicated by others (Amsterdam et al. 1987, 1988) and by our group in dexamethasone suppression test (DST) nonsuppressor subjects (C. B. Nemeroff, K. R. R. Krishnan, and B. J. Carroll, unpublished observations). These blunted ACTH responses to CRF are believed to be secondary to the normal negative feedback of cortisol on the anterior pituitary corticotrophs and/or to chronic CRF hypersecretion that plausibly might down-regulate the CRF receptors on the corticotrophs.

To directly test the hypothesis that CRF is hypersecreted in depression, we measured the concentration of CRF in cerebrospinal fluid (CSF) using a sensitive and specific radioimmunoassay. A further impetus for these experiments, as noted above (see Table 5-1), was the striking similarities between the signs and symptoms of major depression and the effects of centrally administered CRF in laboratory animals (e.g., decreased libido, disturbed sleep, diminished appetite). In the first study (Nemeroff et al. 1984), conducted in collaboration with Widerlöv and his colleagues in Sweden, the CSF concentration of CRF was found to be elevated in drug-free depressed patients compared with healthy control subjects and patients with schizophrenia or senile dementia (Figure 5-2). In fact 11 of the 23 depressed patients had CSF CRF concentrations that were greater than the highest control value. In a second study (Bánki et al. 1987), conducted in collaboration with Bánki in Hungary, we measured the concentration of CRF in CSF of 138 neurological control subjects with peripheral neurological disorders, 54 depressed patients, 23 schizophrenic patients, and 4 manic patients (see Figure 5-3). The depressed patients exhibited a marked, almost twofold elevation in CSF CRF concentrations. The schizophrenic patients showed a small but significant increase in CSF CRF concentrations, largely because of three patients with high values. In subsequent studies we have confirmed the finding of increased CSF CRF concentrations in depressed patients. Recently we reported (France et al. 1988) that patients with chronic pain, with or without concomitant major depression, do not exhibit this increase in CSF CRF concentrations, whereas a comparison group of patients with major depression again were shown to exhibit this abnormality. In a study (Arató et al. 1989) conducted in collaboration with Arató in Hungary, we obtained cisternal CSF samples from completed suicide victims and sudden-death control subjects and observed marked elevations in CSF CRF

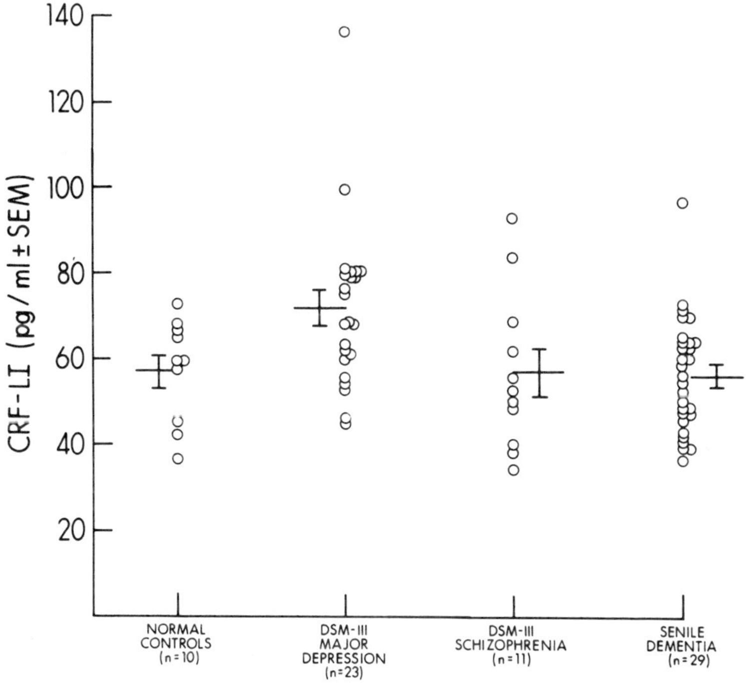

Figure 5-2. Concentration of CRF-like immunoreactivity (CRF-LI) in CSF of normal control subjects (5 males and 5 females) and in CSF of patients with DSM-III major depression (13 males and 10 females), DSM-III schizophrenia (8 females and 3 males), or senile dementia (DSM-III primary degenerative dementia or multi-infarct dementia, or both; 20 females and 9 males). Because the data distribution in the depressed patients was slightly skewed, the data were analyzed by both parametric (ANOVA and Student-Newman-Keuls test) and nonparametric (Mann-Whitney U test) methods. By both methods the CSF CRF-LI concentrations were significantly elevated in the depressed patients when compared with the other diagnostic groups and the control subjects ($P < .05$, ANOVA and Student-Newman-Keuls test; $P < .025$, Mann-Whitney U test). Reprinted from Nemeroff et al. 1984, with permission of the American Association for the Advancement of Science. Copyright 1984, AAAS.

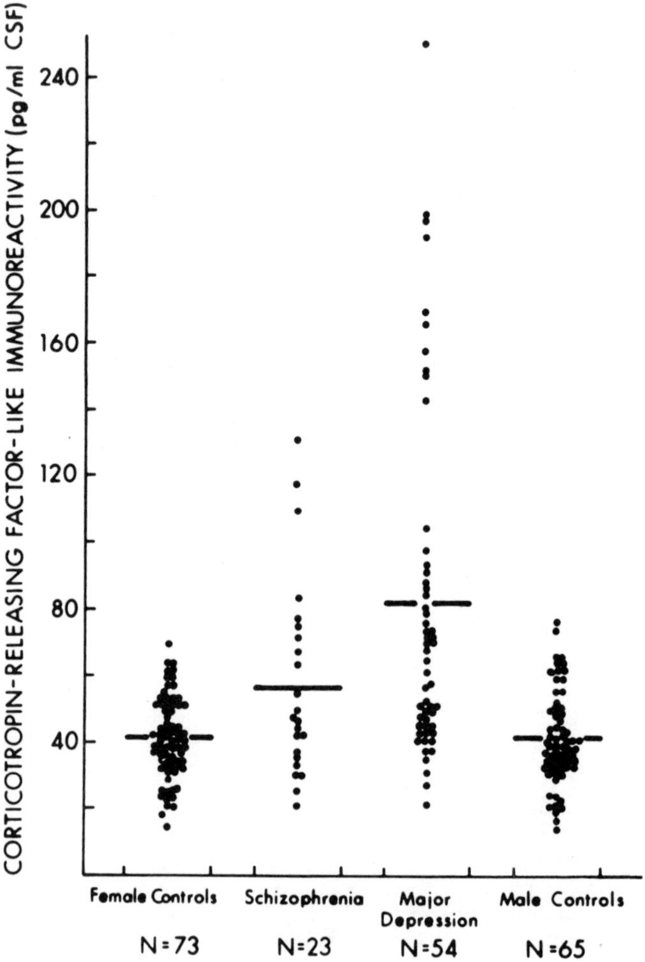

Figure 5-3. CSF CRF-like immunoreactivity in patients with DSM-III schizophrenia, patients with DSM-III major depression, and control subjects with various peripheral neurological diseases. Reprinted from Bánki et al. 1987, with permission of the American Psychiatric Association. Copyright 1987, APA.

concentrations in the former group. By obtaining CSF samples from both cisternal and lumbar samples, we also demonstrated in these experiments a rostral-caudal gradient for CRF in CSF, indicating a supraspinal source for the peptide. We also confirmed the elevation in CSF CRF concentrations in a group of depressed patients compared with control subjects (Arató et al. 1986). Finally, in collaboration with Fink, we measured CSF CRF concentrations in drug-free depressed patients at baseline and after a series of electroconvulsive shock treatments. At baseline the depressed patients had elevated CSF CRF concentrations, but after ECT and concomitant improvement, CSF CRF concentrations were significantly reduced—to normal levels. This biological abnormality, like both the blunted ACTH responses to CRF and dexamethasone nonsuppression, is a state-dependent marker, that is, associated with the state of being depressed.

In contrast to the studies described above, Roy et al. (1987) found no difference in CSF CRF concentrations between depressed patients and control subjects. However, the depressed DST nonsuppressors had significantly higher CSF CRF concentrations than the DST suppressors.

No published studies have appeared in which either CRF concentrations or CRF mRNA levels have been measured in postmortem brain tissue from depressed patients. However, in order to determine whether chronic CRF hypersecretion results in down-regulation of CRF receptors in depression, we measured the number (B_{max}) and affinity (K_d) of CRF receptor binding in the frontal cortex of suicide victims and age- and sex-matched sudden-death control subjects (Nemeroff et al. 1988). The suicide victims had a significantly reduced number (down 23%) of frontal cortical CRF receptors, which is consistent with the hypothesis that CRF hypersecretion in depression results in CRF receptor down-regulation (Figure 5-4).

ALZHEIMER'S DISEASE

Our group (Bissette et al. 1985) was the first to report reductions in CRF concentrations in the frontal and temporal cortex as well as in the caudate nucleus of patients with histologically verified Alzheimer's disease when compared to age- and sex-matched control subjects (Figure 5-5). This finding was confirmed and extended by De Souza and his colleagues (1986), who found marked reductions in cerebrocortical CRF concentrations in Alzheimer's disease and a concomitant increase in CRF receptor number.

Based on these findings of CRF neuronal involvement in Alzheimer's disease, several investigators have measured the concentration of the peptide in CSF of patients with this neurodegenerative disorder. Mouradian et al. (1986) and May et al. (1987) both reported reductions in CSF CRF concentrations in Alzheimer's disease patients. In a group of 15 patients with mild to moderate Alzheimer's disease, we observed a significant correlation between CSF CRF concentrations and global neurological impairment ratings. Greater cognitive impairment was associated with lower CSF CRF concentrations (Pomara et al. 1989).

OTHER NEUROPSYCHIATRIC DISORDERS

The CSF concentration of CRF in anorexia nervosa patients is elevated when compared with control subjects, and the severity of depression correlates significantly with CSF CRF levels (Kaye et al. 1987). When the anorexia nervosa patients attained normal body weight, the CSF CRF concentrations returned to normal. In

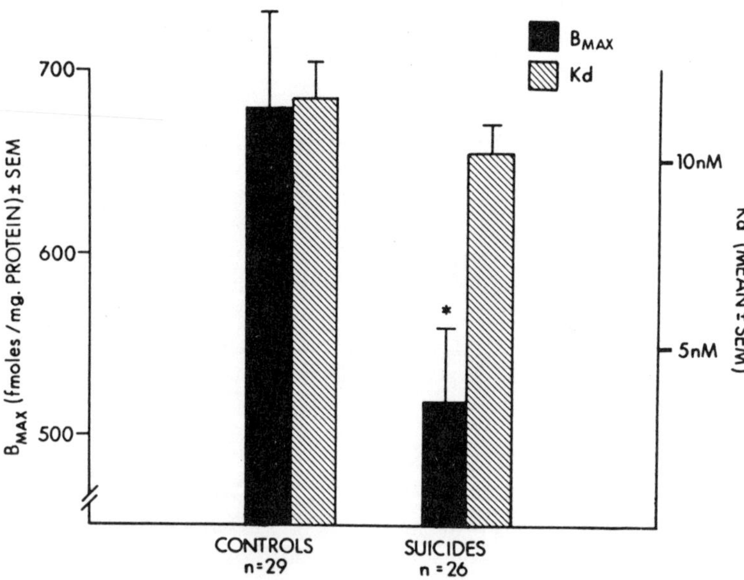

Figure 5-4. Maximum binding (B_{max}) and dissociation affinity constant (K_d) of ^{125}I-labeled Tyr^0-ovine CRF binding sites in frontal cortex in suicide victims and control subjects. Values are mean ± SEM. There was a 23% decrease in the B_{max} in suicide victims compared with control subjects (P = .020 by Student's t test). Analysis of individual B_{max} values showed normal distributions in both suicide and control populations. Adapted from Nemeroff et al. 1988.

Huntington's disease, CSF CRF concentrations are, as in the anorexia nervosa patients, positively correlated with depression severity (Kurlan et al. 1988). Finally, in a study of 5 patients with amyotrophic lateral sclerosis (ALS) and 10 control subjects, the ALS patients had significantly reduced CSF CRF concentrations (Klimek et al. 1986).

In view of the anxiogenic effects of CRF injected intracerebroventricularly or directly into the locus coeruleus (Butler et al. 1990), it would be of interest to measure CRF in CSF of patients with anxiety disorders. We are not aware of any data in this regard. However, Uhde and colleagues at NIMH have observed blunted ACTH responses to CRF in panic disorder patients. This is of particular interest because such patients exhibit DST suppression and may, therefore, have a very subtle form of HPA axis dysregulation.

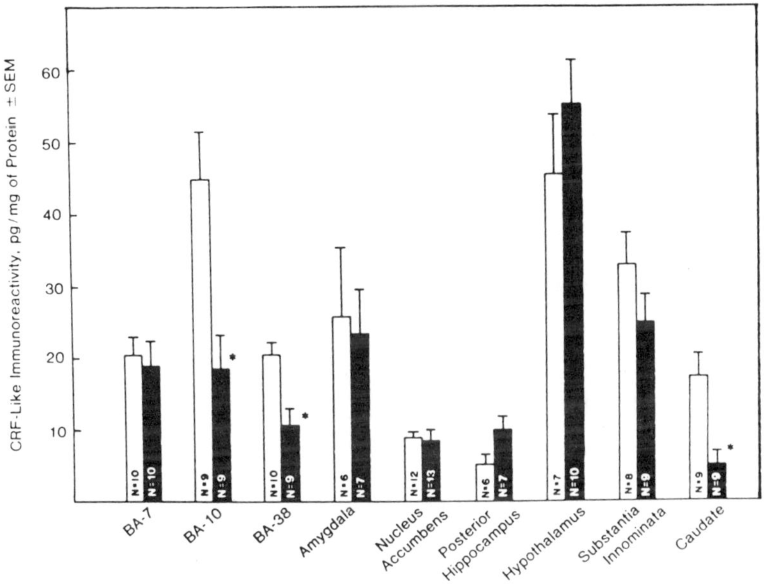

Figure 5-5. Regional brain concentration of CRF-like immunoreactivity (CRF-LI) in patients with senile dementia of Alzheimer's type (solid bars) and in control subjects (open bars). Number of samples from each brain region is shown inside respective bars. Concentration of CRF-LI is shown as mean ± SEM and is reported as picograms per milligram of protein. Statistical significance was sought by Student's t test and is represented by asterisk, which indicates $P < .01$. Reprinted from Bissette et al. 1985, with permission of the American Medical Association. Copyright 1985, AMA.

CONCLUSIONS

It seems clear from the studies described above that CRF-containing neurons are related in several neuropsychiatric disorders, including major depression and Alzheimer's disease. However, the exact nature of the alterations remains obscure. In major depression, CRF is apparently hypersecreted, which results in increased CSF CRF concentrations and down-regulation of CRF receptors in the frontal cortex. This increased CRF secretion may plausibly be responsible for, at least in part, the hyperactivity of the HPA axis commonly observed in depressed patients. It is unclear, however, which CRF-containing neurons are hyperactive in depression. No data have yet been generated in which CRF biosynthesis rates have been evaluated in postmortem brain tissue by, for example, in situ hybridization techniques.

It is now well documented that the concentration of CRF in cerebrocortical tissue is reduced in Alzheimer's disease. However, direct demonstration of degeneration of CRF-containing neurons in this disorder has not been provided. It is also unclear which, if any, symptoms of Alzheimer's disease are secondary to the pathological involvement of CRF neurons in this disease.

Similarly, we remain ignorant of the exact CNS source of CRF in CSF and, moreover, of the CNS contribution, if any, to plasma concentrations of this peptide. Finally, virtually nothing is known about the regulation of the processing of CRF and its liberation from its prohormone nor of the peptidases that degrade the peptide. Nevertheless, the progress made in the last 8 years is impressive, and there is little doubt that it shall continue. The development of CRF receptor antagonists that can cross the blood-brain barrier may lead to novel antidepressant and anxiolytic agents.

REFERENCES

Amsterdam JD, Maeslin G, Winokur A, et al: Pituitary and adrenocortical responses to ovine corticotropin-releasing hormone stimulation test. Arch Gen Psychiatry 44:775–781, 1987

Amsterdam JD, Maeslin G, Winokur A, et al: The oCRH stimulation test before and after clinical recovery from depression. J Affective Disord 14:213–222, 1988

Arató M, Bánki CM, Nemeroff CB, et al: Hypothalamic-pituitary-adrenal axis and suicide. Ann NY Acad Sci 487:263–270, 1986

Arató M, Bánki CM, Bissette G, et al: Elevated CSF CRF in suicide victims. Biol Psychiatry 25:355–359, 1989

Bánki CM, Bissette G, Arató M, et al: Cerebrospinal fluid corticotropin-releasing factor–like immunoreactivity in depression and schizophrenia. Am J Psychiatry 144:873–877, 1987

Bilezikjian LM, Vale WW: Glucocorticoids inhibit corticotropin-releasing factor–induced production of adenosine 3′,5′-monophosphate in cultured anterior pituitary cells. Endocrinology 113:657–662, 1983

Bissette G, Reynolds GP, Kilts CD, et al: Corticotropin-releasing factor–like immunoreactivity in senile dementia of the Alzheimer type: reduced cortical and striatal concentrations. JAMA 254:3067–3069, 1985

Britton KT, Lee G, Dana R, et al: Activating and "anxiogenic" effects of corticotropin releasing factor are not inhibited by blockade of the pituitary-adrenal system with dexamethasone. Life Sci 39:1281–1286, 1986

Butler PD, Weiss JM, Stout JC, et al: Corticotropin-releasing factor produces fear-enhancing and behavioral activating effects following infusion into the locus coeruleus. J Neurosci 10:176–183, 1990

De Souza EB, Perrin MH, Insel TR, et al: Corticotropin-releasing factor receptors in rat forebrain: autoradiographic localization. Science 224:1449–1451, 1984

De Souza EB, Whitehouse PJ, Kuhar MJ, et al: Reciprocal changes in corticotropin-releasing factor (CRF)–like immunoreactivity and CRF receptors in cerebral cortex of Alzheimer's disease. Nature 319:593–595, 1986

Dunn AJ, Berridge CW: Corticotropin-releasing factor administration elicits a stress-like activation of cerebral catecholaminergic systems. Pharmacol Biochem Behav 27:685–691, 1987

Ehlers C, Henriksen S, Wang M, et al: Corticotropin-releasing factor produces increases in brain excitability and convulsive seizures in rats. Brain Res 278:332–336, 1983

Evans DL, Nemeroff CB: The clinical use of the dexamethasone suppression test in DSM-III affective disorders: correlation with the severe depressive subtypes of melancholia and psychosis. J Psychiatr Res 21:185–194, 1987

France RD, Urban B, Krishnan KRR, et al: CSF corticotropin-releasing factor–like immunoreactivity in chronic pain patients with and without major depression. Biol Psychiatry 23:86–88, 1988

Furutani Y, Morimoto Y, Shibahara S, et al: Cloning and sequence analysis of cDNA for ovine corticotropin-releasing factor precursor. Nature 301:537–540, 1983

Gold PW, Chrousos G, Kellner C, et al: Psychiatric implications of basic and clinical studies with corticotropin-releasing factor. Am J Psychiatry 141:619–627, 1984

Gold PW, Chrousos G: Clinical studies with corticotropin-releasing factor: implications for the diagnosis and pathophysiology of depression, Cushing's disease and adrenal insufficiency. Psychoneuroendocrinology 10:401–419, 1985

Holsboer F, Bardeleben U, Gerken A, et al: Blunted corticotropin and normal cortisol response to human corticotropin-releasing factor in depression. N Engl J Med 311:1127, 1984

Kaye WH, Gwirtsman HE, George GT, et al: Elevated cerebrospinal fluid levels of immunoreactive corticotropin-releasing hormone in anorexia nervosa: relation to state of nutrition, adrenal function, and intensity of depression. J Clin Endocrinol Metab 64:203–208, 1987

Kilts CD, Bissette G, Krishnan KRR, et al: The preclinical and clinical neurobiology of corticotropin-releasing factor (CRF), in Hormones and Depression. Edited by Halbreich U. New York, Raven, 1987, pp 297–312

Klimek A, Cieslak D, Kuberska JS, et al: Reduced lumbar cerebrospinal fluid corticotropin-releasing factor (CRF) levels in amyotrophic lateral sclerosis. Acta Neurol Scand 74:72–74, 1986

Kurlan R, Caine E, Rubin A, et al: Cerebrospinal fluid correlates of depression in Huntington's disease. Arch Neurol 45:881–883, 1988

Levine AS, Rogers B, Kneup J, et al: Effects of centrally administered corticotropin-releasing factor (CRF) on multiple feeding paradigms. Life Sci 22:337–339, 1983

May C, Rapoport SI, Tomai TP, et al: Cerebrospinal fluid concentrations of corticotropin-releasing hormone (CRH) and corticotropin (ACTH) are reduced in patients with Alzheimer's disease. Neurology 37:535–538, 1987

Mouradian MM, Farah JM, Mohr E, et al: Spinal fluid CRF reduction in Alzheimer's disease. Neuropeptides 8:393–400, 1986

Nemeroff CB, Widerlöv E, Bissette G, et al: Elevated concentrations of CSF corticotropin-releasing factor–like immunoreactivity in depressed patients. Science 226:1342–1344, 1984

Nemeroff CB, Owens MJ, Bissette G, et al: Reduced corticotropin-releasing factor (CRF) binding sites in the frontal cortex of suicides. Arch Gen Psychiatry 45:577–579, 1988

Pomara N, Singh RR, Deptula D, et al: Corticotropin-releasing factor (CRF) in Alzheimer's disease: relationship to severity of dementia and monoamine metabolites. Biol Psychiatry 26:500–504, 1989

Rivier C, Rivier J, Vale W: Inhibition of adrenocorticotropic hormone secretion in the rat by immunoneutralization of corticotropin-releasing factor. Science 218:377–378, 1982

Roy A, Pickar D, Paul S, et al: CSF corticotropin-releasing hormone in depressed patients and normal control subjects. Am J Psychiatry 144:641–645, 1987

Saffran M, Schally AV: Release of corticotropin by anterior pituitary tissue in vitro. Canadian Journal of Biochemistry and Physiology 33:408–415, 1955

Sawchenko PE, Swanson LW: Localization, colocalization and plasticity of corticotropin-releasing factor immunoreactivity in rat brain. Federation Proceedings 44:221–227, 1985

Sirinathsinghji DJS, Rees LH, Rivier J, et al: Corticotropin-releasing factor is a potent inhibitor of sexual receptivity in the female rat. Nature 305:232–235, 1983

Smith MA, Bissette G, Slotkin TA, et al: Release of corticotropin-releasing factor from rat brain regions in vitro. Endocrinology 118:1997–2001, 1986

Vale W, Speiss J, Rivier C, et al: Characterization of a 41-residue ovine hypothalamic peptide that stimulates secretion of corticotropin and β-endorphin. Science 213:1394–1397, 1981

Young WS III, Mezey E, Siegel RE: Quantitative in situ hybridization histochemistry reveals increased levels of corticotropin-releasing factor mRNA after adrenalectomy in rats. Neurosci Lett 70:198–203, 1986

Chapter 6

Growth Hormone–Releasing Factor and Growth Hormone

S. Craig Risch, M.D.

Chapter 6

Growth Hormone–Releasing Factor and Growth Hormone

In this chapter I briefly summarize the extensive literature of studies of the anterior pituitary hormone growth hormone (GH) in various psychiatric disease states and then focus on more recent studies of the role of the 44–amino-acid hypothalamic peptide human growth hormone–releasing factor (GHRF) in the pathophysiology of GH disturbances in psychiatric illness.

Stress paradigms and various provocative psychopharmacological "challenges" of pituitary GH secretion have been studied in an attempt to understand the pathophysiology of psychiatric illnesses and to provide a laboratory basis aiding in diagnosis and predicting efficacy of psychopharmacological treatments. These studies have been conceptually based on the precis that studies of GH may provide a "window to the brain" because 1) many psychiatric disease states are accompanied by various hormonal dysregulations, and 2) many of the limbic-hypothalamic neurotransmitter systems involved in anterior pituitary GH regulation have been hypothesized to be dysfunctional and underlie the pathogenesis of specific psychiatric illnesses. Classic examples include the dopamine hypothesis of schizophrenia and the catecholamine and indolelamine hypotheses of affective disorders. Extensive literature has implicated aberrant "up-regulated" dopamine neurotransmission (D_2 receptors) in the pathophysiology of hallucinations and delusions in schizophrenia and other psychoses. Likewise, extensive literature has implicated aberrant catecholamine (i.e., dopamine, norepinephrine, serotonin) neurotransmission in depression and mania. These same CNS neurotransmitters regulate anterior pituitary GH secretion, and there have been numerous provocative challenges of GH secretion in schizophrenia and affective disorders.

Unfortunately, as reviewed in more detail elsewhere (Risch and Judd 1987) and summarized below, the literature on psychopharmacological provocative challenges of GH in specific psychiatric nosological states has been both inconsistent and, to date, of limited clinical utility. These conflicting results presumably reflect such issues as diagnostic heterogeneity and lack of sufficient age, sex, diet, activity, menstrual cycle, menopausal status, medication status, and duration of illness controls.

However, the isolation and sequencing of the 44–amino-acid hypothalamic peptide GHRF (Guillemin et al. 1982; Rivier et al. 1982) has allowed new generations of more refined studies of GH physiology and pathophysiology in specific psychiatric disease states.

GROWTH HORMONE PHYSIOLOGY

Growth hormone is a 191–amino-acid peptide secreted by the anterior pituitary. Basal GH secretion tends to have spontaneous bursts during the day, averaging 6 to 7 bursts per 24 hours and decreasing in frequency with age (van Praag 1982). Pituitary GH secretion is markedly augmented by circulating estrogen, and plasma GH concentrations may vary markedly with the menstrual cycle and menopausal status. GH secretion is stimulated by stress, exercise, hypoglycemia, certain hormones (insulin), and a variety of medications, such as amphetamine, L-dopa, apomorphine, morphine, and clonidine. Regarding neurotransmitter regulation, GH secretion is stimulated by dopamine, norepinephrine, and serotonin and inhibited by acetylcholine. It increases during slow-wave sleep, usually early after onset of sleep in the first non-REM phase (Brown et al. 1978).

Hypothalamic GHRF is the major regulatory stimulus for pituitary growth secretion. Hypothalamic GHRF stimulates both GH synthesis and release. Plasma GH, in turn, stimulates liver production of somatomedins, somatomedin C, a 63–amino-acid peptide, being the best characterized and studied somatomedin to date. Somatomedins stimulate glucose production and cartilage growth and development. Circulating somatomedins also stimulate production and release of central somatostatin (see Rubinow et al., Chapter 3, this volume), which in turn is the major inhibitor of the stimulatory hypothalamic GHRF effects on pituitary GH synthesis and release, completing a complex feedback regulatory loop. Circulating adrenal glucocorticoids and triiodothyronine (T_3) enhance the pituitary GH response to hypothalamic GHRF, adding further complexity to GH regulation.

PROVOCATIVE CHALLENGES OF GROWTH HORMONE IN THE AFFECTIVE DISORDERS

As noted above, interpretation of basal GH plasma concentrations is confounded by stress, activity, diet, obesity, sex, menopausal status, stage of menstrual cycle, medication status, and many other factors. When these factors have been controlled for, basal plasma concentrations of GH have been reported to be significantly elevated, particularly during the daytime, in depressed patients as compared with healthy control subjects (Mendlewicz et al. 1985).

One of the most extensively studied provocative challenges of GH in affective disorders has been insulin-induced hypoglycemia. After controlling for the above variables, the clinically minimal adequate response is usually defined as a change in plasma GH response greater than 5 ng/ml after at least a 50% drop in blood glucose level (Gruen 1978; Sachar 1976). Although early studies were sometimes marred by a lack of the above described controls, the literature suggests that an inadequate or "blunted" GH response to insulin-induced hypoglycemia occurs commonly in endogenous depression (Casper et al. 1977; Grof et al. 1982; Gruen et al. 1975; Kathol et al. 1983; Mueller et al. 1969; Sachar et al. 1971, 1973; Winokur et al. 1982). This abnormality appears to be more common in unipolar depressed patients than in bipolar depressed patients (Kathol et al. 1983; Sachar et al. 1973). This GH resistance to insulin challenge also may occur in prepubertal children with major depression, perhaps with a greater frequency than in adults (Puig-Antich and Weston 1983; Puig-Antich et al. 1981, 1984a). These depressed children also secrete significantly more GH during sleep, but there is little overlap between this abnormality and insulin resistance (Puig-Antich and Weston 1983). Both these abnormalities tend to persist for long periods after clinical recovery (Puig-Antich et al. 1984b, 1984c).

In contrast, challenge studies to GH secretion with the dopamine agonists apomorphine, L-dopa, and amphetamine have been unrewarding in differentiating depressed patients from control subjects (Casper et al. 1977; Checkley 1979, 1980; Gruen 1978; Halbreich et al. 1982; Insel and Siever 1981; Linkowski et al. 1983; Maany et al. 1979; Meltzer et al. 1984; Mendlewicz et al. 1979; Sachar et al. 1975).

Unlike these unrewarding results in differentiating depressed patients from control subjects with GH responses to apomorphine, L-dopa, and amphetamine, a reduced GH response to clonidine (an α_2-receptor agonist) has emerged as one of the most powerful and substantive markers for neuroendocrine dysfunction in depression (Charney et al. 1982; Checkley et al. 1981; Matussek et al. 1980; Siever et al. 1981).

Desipramine stimulates GH secretion. A reduced GH response to desipramine has also been observed in depressed patients as compared with controls (Glass et al. 1982; Laakmann and Benkert 1980; Laakmann et al. 1978). These observations, like those with clonidine, support the hypothesis that this abnormality may be selectively noradrenergically, rather than dopaminergically, mediated.

From the above review, it would appear that GH secretion responsivity to insulin, and more specifically and substantively to clonidine and desipramine, is reduced in depressed patients as compared with control subjects. These observations suggest that noradrenergic systems, as least in part, may mediate the pathogenesis of this neuroendocrine abnormality.

PROVOCATIVE CHALLENGES OF GROWTH HORMONE IN SCHIZOPHRENIA

Basal plasma GH concentrations in patients with schizophrenia do not differ from those in healthy control subjects (Loosen and Prange 1980; Prange et al. 1979).

A number of investigators have utilized dopamine agonists (i.e., L-dopa and apomorphine) to pharmacologically challenge anterior pituitary GH secretion in patients with schizophrenia and in control subjects. Because the pathogenesis of schizophrenia may involve increased CNS dopamine activity, it has been hypothesized that patients with schizophrenia might have an augmented response to dopaminergic agonists. In fact, many investigators have reported a significantly augmented response to apomorphine in acute schizophrenic patients with positive symptoms of psychosis as compared with chronic schizophrenic patients or control subjects (Cleghorn et al. 1983; Ettigi et al. 1976; Ferrier et al. 1984; Pandey et al. 1977; Rotrosen et al. 1979; Tamminga et al. 1977).

In general, GH responses to apomorphine in chronic schizophrenia with negative symptoms of psychosis tend to be blunted (Ferrier et al. 1984; Pandey et al. 1977; Rotrosen et al. 1979). An exaggerated GH response to apomorphine in acute schizophrenic patients may predict a favorable response to treatment (Hollister et al. 1980), whereas an exaggerated response in chronic schizophrenic patients may predict relapse (Cleghorn et al. 1983). Tamminga et al. (1977) report that while schizophrenic patients, in general, may demonstrate a blunted GH response to apomorphine, there is no significant difference in GH response to apomorphine in schizophrenic patients with or without tardive dyskinesia. Meltzer et al. (1984) studied GH responses to apomorphine in a large group of unmedicated hospitalized patients with functional psychoses and found no differences in GH among the various diagnostic groups. However, the apomorphine-induced GH response correlated significantly with psychosis ratings and negative symptom-scale scores. Growth hormone response was inversely related to duration of illness, but the correlation was independent of age effect only in patients with major depression. A blunted GH response to intravenously administered methylphenidate in schizophrenia has also been reported (Janowsky et al. 1978). This effect appeared to be independent of medication status.

These various studies may be integrated to suggest that in schizophrenia, although there is some variability, apomorphine-induced GH response may be 1) elevated from normal in acute schizophrenic patients with positive symptoms of psychosis or in chronic schizophrenic patients about to relapse, with an exaggerated response possibly predicting a favorable response to treatment; and 2) blunted in chronic schizophrenic patients with negative symptoms. A blunted GH response to apomorphine is not specific to schizophrenia and, therefore, is of no diagnostic utility, but the test may be useful in predicting and monitoring pharmacotherapy.

Thus, it appears manifest that abnormalities in GH secretion occur in both schizophrenia and affective illness, and may be elicited and studied by a variety of provocative challenge tests.

HYPOTHALAMIC GHRF STUDIES IN PSYCHIATRIC ILLNESS

As noted above, the isolation and sequencing of the hypothalamic peptide GHRF has allowed the initiation of more mechanistically oriented studies of GH physiology and pathophysiology. To date, almost all of the published psychiatric literature using intravenously administered GHRF as a probe of pituitary GH pathophysiology has been on patients with major depressive disorders and matched control subjects. In all the studies reviewed below, carefully diagnosed depressed patients have been matched by age, weight, sex, and menopausal status with healthy control subjects. In most studies patients were medication free for at least 1 week prior to study.

Klaus-Peter Lesch and colleagues in the Departments of Psychiatry and Endocrinology at the University of Würzburg in the Federal Republic of Germany have reported an elegant series of studies of GH response to GHRF in depressed patients and matched control subjects. In their first report (Lesch et al. 1987a), nine patients with either major depression or bipolar depression were compared with control subjects matched for age, sex, menopausal status, and body weight. After an overnight fast, subjects at bed rest received 50 μg of synthetic human GHRH-44amide as an intravenous bolus. Blood was drawn at 15-minute intervals immediately before and after the GHRF infusions. The subjects were drug free for a minimum of 3 days to more than 14 days prior to study. The authors reported that the depressed patients had a "markedly blunted" GH response to GHRF infusion as measured both by the "delta-max" (peak postinfusion GH response minus baseline) and by the "integrated net area under the response curve." In this report the blunted GH responses occurred in the presence of normal baseline plasma GH concentrations.

In a second study, Lesch et al. (1987b) reported the effects of intravenous hypothalamic GHRF on 11 drug-free patients with major depression or bipolar depression and 11 matched control subjects using the methodology described above (Lesch et al. 1987a), except that the dosage of GHRF was 1 μg/kg. In this report they also found a significantly blunted GH response to GHRF in the depressed patients. However, in contrast to their earlier report, the basal serum GH levels were significantly decreased in the depressed patients as compared with matched control subjects. In addition, they also reported increased plasma somatomedin C levels in the depressed patients as compared with the control subjects. The findings of increased somatomedin C in the depressed patients is of particular interest because somatomedin C feeds back negatively on pituitary GH release at the level of both the pituitary and the hypothalamus. The authors also noted in this study that "no relationship was found between GH responses to GHRH and the number of previous affective episodes, total duration of illness, length of present depressive episodes or severity of depressive symptoms in the patient group" (p. 1280).

Finally Lesch et al. (1988a) reported on 20 subjects, 10 patients with major depressive disorder and 10 control subjects matched for age, gender, and ovarian status, receiving 1 μg/kg of synthetic human GHRF in the manner described above. Two days later subjects received the α_2-receptor agonist clonidine (2 μg/kg) intravenously over 10 minutes. The GH response in the clonidine infusion protocol (previously reported by many other investigators to be diminished in depressed patients [see above]) was compared within the same subjects with their GH response to the GHRF infusions. The investigators reported a significant positive correlation ($r_s = .76$, $P<.001$) between GH response to GHRF and GH response to the α_2 agonist clonidine. As reviewed above, clonidine infusions represent a central nervous system (CNS) probe of GH physiology, while intravenously administered GHRF acts directly at the level of the pituitary and does not cross the blood-brain barrier. Thus, this study assesses both the central and peripheral pituitary components of the GH axis dysregulation in depression.

Our own studies (Risch et al. 1988) have replicated in a small group of depressed subjects a significantly attenuated GH response to intravenous hypothalamic GHRF. In our study five patients with major depression and 11 age- and sex-matched healthy control subjects received intravenous GHRF (1 µg/kg) infused over 5 minutes and, on a separate occasion, placebo (saline) infusions performed in an identical manner. Blood samples were obtained every 15 minutes for 30 minutes prior to and for 2 hours subsequent to the intravenous infusions of GHRF and placebo. The five depressed patients as compared with the 11 matched healthy control subjects had a significantly attenuated (diagnostic group x drug x time, $P < .03$) GH response to GHRF, paralleling the previously reported studies of Lesch and colleagues reviewed above. In our ongoing studies (unpublished observations) we have extended our pilot observations in a larger group of patients; these observations suggest that, as reported by Lesch and colleagues (1987a, 1987b, 1988a, 1988b), depressed patients have a significantly attenuated GH response to GHRF as compared with matched control subjects. Of particular note, our current ongoing studies suggest that this attenuated GH response in depression may persist for long periods after clinical remission much like the attenuated GH response to insulin-induced hypoglycemia reviewed above. Lesch et al. (1988b) previously reported no relationship between postdexamethasone plasma cortisol concentrations and GH response to GHRF. In our own studies, to date, we have found no effect of hypothalamic GHRF infusions on plasma cortisol concentrations and no relationship between basal plasma cortisol concentrations and GH response to intravenous GHRF. Our observations, together with those of Lesch and colleagues, suggest that basal hypothalamo-pituitary-adrenal activity may not be a major influence on GH response to intravenous GHRF.

As suggested by Lesch et al. (1988a), the above studies may be integrated to provide a hypothesis of GH pathophysiology in major depression. Despite the reports by Lesch and colleagues of either normal or low basal plasma GH values at the time of the GHRF infusions in depressed subjects, Mendlewicz et al. (1985), by obtaining frequent serial plasma samples over a 24-hour period, have previously demonstrated an episodic *hyper*secretion of GH during the daytime in depressed patients. This could result in the elevated somatomedin C plasma concentrations observed in the studies of

Lesch and colleagues and, via negative feedback by somatomedin C, in attenuated pituitary GH responses to GHRH infusions.

More centrally, as reviewed by Rubinow et al. (Chapter 3, this volume), considerable evidence has accumulated implicating low cerebrospinal fluid (CSF) concentrations of somatostatin in depressed patients. Because somatostatin inhibits hypothalamic GHRF stimulation of pituitary GH secretion, low CNS somatostatin could result in "disinhibition" or hyperactivity of hypothalamic GHRF neurons, which, in time, could "down-regulate" pituitary GHRF receptors. Thus, low CNS somatostatin, causing hypothalamic GHRF hypersecretion, could produce 1) down-regulated pituitary GHRF receptors, and 2) episodic pituitary GH hypersecretion and elevated plasma somatomedin C concentrations. Both mechanisms, not mutually exclusive, could contribute to diminished pituitary GH secretion in response to exogenously administered GHRF.

Because in the studies of Lesch and colleagues the attenuated GH response to GHRF observed in depressed patients was highly correlated within the same patients with an attenuated GH response to the α_2 agonist clonidine, it is conceivable that this hypothesized endogenous hypothalamic GHRF hypersecretion and low CNS somatostatin may in turn reflect altered CNS α_2-adrenergic activity.

Despite the above reviewed findings, both the clinical sensitivity and the specificity of the reported attenuated GH response to GHRF in depression are in doubt. In an elegant study using identical patient control methodology and identical infusion design parameters, Krishnan and colleagues (1988) failed to demonstrate an attenuated GH response to GHRF in depressed patients. In their study, 19 patients with major depression and 19 age- and sex-matched control subjects each received intravenous bolus GHRF 1 μg/kg. All subjects were drug free for at least 1 week prior to testing. Patients with major depression were matched by age, sex, weight, and menopausal status with healthy volunteers who had no history of psychiatric disorders. Blood was collected at 15-minute intervals for 1 hour prior to and 3 hours subsequent to GHRF infusions. In this study there was a significantly *augmented* GH response to GHRF infusion in the depressed patients as compared with the matched healthy control subjects. However, the authors note that this "group difference was mainly attributable to 3 of the 19 depressed patients who exhibited markedly high GH responses to GHRF" (p. 90). Thus, this study suggests an essentially normal, or in a few cases augmented, GH response to hypothalamic GHRF in depressed patients, contrasting with the above noted studies of Lesch and colleagues (1987a, 1987b, 1988a, 1988b) and Risch et al. (1988), who reported a significantly attenuated GH response to GHRF.

Because all these studies used essentially identical GHRF dosages, infusion paradigms, and patient control matching, the current literature suggests a significant heterogeneity among depressed patients in GH responsivity to GHRF infusion. Furthermore, Rapaport et al. (1989) have recently reported a significantly blunted GH response to GHRF infusions in patients with panic disorder as compared with matched control subjects. Thus, the current literature suggests a lack of both sensitivity and specificity of abnormalities of pituitary GH response to GHRF in depression. Unfortunately, to date, there have been no other published studies of the effects of hypothalamic GHRF infusions on plasma GH in other psychiatric illnesses. Of particular note, there have been no reported studies of the effects of GHRF on plasma GH in schizophrenia despite the above reviewed studies of GH abnormalities in schizophrenia, although such studies are clearly needed.

Finally, to date, there has been only one report of CSF concentrations of GHRF in psychiatric patients. Berrettini et al. (1987) reported on CSF concentrations of GHRF in 37 unmedicated healthy volunteers and 24 lithium-treated euthymic bipolar patients. Thirteen of the 24 lithium-treated euthymic bipolar patients provided a second CSF sample during an unmedicated state. In this study there were no group differences or effects of lithium observed. This finding, if replicated and extended to show no differences in CSF GHRF between *actively ill* depressed patients and matched healthy control subjects, suggests that major alterations in CSF concentrations of GHRF may not occur and may not be of mechanistic significance in the pathogenesis of depression, as have alterations in other CSF peptides such as corticotropin-releasing factor (see Nemeroff, Chapter 5, this volume) and somatostatin (see Rubinow et al., Chapter 3, this volume).

CONCLUSIONS

The use of hypothalamic GHRF as an intravenous probe of GH pathophysiology has not yet suggested any utility as a diagnostic marker in affective disorders or other psychiatric illnesses. In part, this may be due to the paucity of studies in the existing literature, and clearly many more studies are necessary before more definitive statements can be made. However, the elegant studies of Lesch and colleagues (reviewed above) have provided a model for the systematic use of GHRF as a physiologic probe to facilitate the understanding of underlying CNS, hypothalamic, and pituitary mechanisms in the pathophysiology of GH secretion in depression and potentially in other psychiatric disease states.

REFERENCES

Berrettini WH, Nurnberger JI, Simmons-Alling S: Growth hormone releasing factor in human cerebrospinal fluid. Psychiatry Res 22:141–147, 1987

Brown GM, Seggie JA, Chambers JW, et al: Psychoendocrinology and growth hormone: a review. Psychoneuroendocrinology 3:131–153, 1978

Casper RC, Davis JM, Pandey GN, et al: Neuroendocrine and amine studies in affective illness. Psychoneuroendocrinology 2:105–113, 1977

Charney DS, Heninger GR, Sternberg DE: Failure of chronic antidepressants, desmethylimipramine and amitriptyline, on the growth hormone response to clonidine. Psychiatry Res 7:135–138, 1982

Checkley SA: Corticosteroid and growth hormone responses to methylamphetamine in depressive illness. Psychol Med 9:107–115, 1979

Checkley SA: A neuroendocrine study of adrenoceptor function in endogenous depression. Acta Psychiatr Scand [Suppl] 280:211–217, 1980

Checkley SA, Slade AP, Shur E: Growth hormone and other responses to clonidine in patients with endogenous depression. Br J Psychiatry 138:51–55, 1981

Cleghorn JM, Brown GM, Brown PJ, et al: Growth hormone responses to graded doses of apomorphine HCl in schizophrenia. Biol Psychiatry 18:875–885, 1983

Ettigi P, Nair NP, Lal S, et al: Effects of apomorphine on growth hormone and prolactin secretion in schizophrenic patients with or without oral dyskinesia, withdrawn from chronic neuroleptic therapy. Neurol Neurosurg Psychiatry 39:870–876, 1976

Ferrier IN, Johnstone EC, Crow TJ: Hormonal effects of apomorphine in schizophrenia. Br J Psychiatry 144:349–357, 1984

Glass IB, Checkley SA, Shur E, et al: The effect of desipramine upon central adrenergic function in depressed patients. Br J Psychiatry 141:372–376, 1982

Grof E, Brown GM, Grof P: Neuroendocrine responses as an indicator of recurrence liability in primary affective illness. Br J Psychiatry 140:320–322, 1982

Gruen PH: Endocrine changes in psychiatric diseases. Med Clin North Am 62:285–296, 1978

Gruen PH, Sachar E, Altman N, et al: Growth hormone responses to hypoglycemia in post-menopausal depressed women. Arch Gen Psychiatry 32:31–33, 1975

Guillemin R, Brazeau P, Bohlen P, et al: Growth hormone–releasing factor from a human pancreatic tumor that caused acromegaly. Science 218:585, 1982

Halbreich U, Sachar EJ, Asnis GM, et al: Growth hormone response to dextramphetamine in depressed patients and normal subjects. Arch Gen Psychiatry 39:189–192, 1982

Hollister L, Davis K, Berger P: Apomorphine in schizophrenia. Communications in Psychopharmacology 4:277–281, 1980

Insel TR, Siever LJ: The dopamine system challenge in affective disorders: a review of behavioral and neuroendocrine responses. J Clin Psychopharmacology 1:207–213, 1981

Janowsky DS, Leichner P, Parker D, et al: The effect of methylphenidate on serum growth hormone: influence of antipsychotic drugs and diagnosis. Arch Gen Psychiatry 35:1384–1389, 1978

Kathol RG, Sherman BM, Winokur G, et al: Dexamethasone suppression, protirelin stimulation, and insulin infusion in subtypes of recovered depressive patients. Psychiatry Res 9:99–106, 1983

Krishnan KRR, Manepalli AN, Ritchie JC, et al: Growth hormone–releasing factor stimulation test in depression. Am J Psychiatry 145:90–92, 1988

Laakman G, Benkert O: Neuroendokrinologie und Psychopharmaka. Arzneim Forsch 28:1277–1280, 1980

Laakman G, Benkert O, Neurlinger E, et al: Beeinflussung der Hypophysen-Vorderlappen-hormon-Sekretion nach akuter und chroniscker Gabe von Desipramin. Arzneim Forsch 28:1292–1294, 1978

Lesch KP, Laux G, Erb A, et al: Attenuated growth hormone response to growth hormone-releasing hormone in major depressive disorder. Biol Psychiatry 22:1491–1495, 1987a

Lesch KP, Laux G, Pfuller H, et al: Growth hormone (GH) response to GH-releasing hormone in depression. J Clin Endocrinol Metab 65:1278–1281, 1987b

Lesch KP, Laux G, Erb A, et al: Growth hormone (GH) and prolactin responses after GH-releasing hormone in major depressive disorder: relationship to somatomedin C levels and dexamethasone suppressibility of cortisol. Psychoneuroendocrinology 13:255–263, 1988a

Lesch KP, Laux G, Erb A, et al: Growth hormone (GH) responses to GH-releasing hormone in depression: correlation with GH release following clonidine. Psychiatry Res 25:301–310, 1988b

Linowski P, Brauman H, Mendlewicz J: Prolactin and growth hormone response to levodopa in affective illness. Neuropsychobiology 9:108–112, 1983

Loosen PT, Prange AJ Jr: Thyrotropin releasing hormone (TRH): a useful tool for psychoneuroendocrine investigation. Psychoneuroendocrinology 5:63–80, 1980

Maany I, Mendels J, Frazer A, et al: A study of growth hormone release in depression. Neuropsychobiology 5:282–289, 1979

Matussek N, Ackenheil M, Hippius H, et al: Effect of clonidine on growth hormone release in psychiatric patients and controls. Psychiatry Res 2:25–36, 1980

Meltzer HY, Kolakowska T, Fang VS, et al: Growth hormone and prolactin response to apomorphine in schizophrenia and the major affective disorders: relation to duration of illness and depressive symptoms. Arch Gen Psychiatry 41:512–519, 1984

Mendlewicz J, Linkowski P, Van Cauter E: Some neuroendocrine parameters in bipolar and unipolar depression. J Affective Disord 1:25–32, 1979

Mendlewicz J, Linkowski P, Kerkhofs M, et al: Diurnal hypersecretion of growth hormone in depression. J Clin Endocrinol Metab 60:505, 1985

Mueller PS, Heninger GR, McDonald RK: Insulin tolerance test in depression. Arch Gen Psychiatry 21:587–594, 1969

Pandey GM, Garver DL, Tamminga C, et al: Postsynaptic supersensitivity in schizophrenia. Am J Psychiatry 134:518–522, 1977

Prange AJ Jr, Loosen PT, Wilson IC, et al: Behavioral and endocrine responses of schizophrenic patients to TRH (protirelin). Arch Gen Psychiatry 36:1086–1093, 1979

Puig-Antich J, Weston B: The diagnosis and treatment of major depressive disorder in childhood. Annu Rev Med 34:231–245, 1983

Puig-Antich J, Tabrizi MA, Davies M, et al: Prepubertal endogenous major depressives hyposecrete growth hormone in response to insulin-induced hypoglycemia. Biol Psychiatry 16:801–818, 1981

Puig-Antich J, Novacenko H, Davies M, et al: Growth hormone secretion in prepubertal children with major depression, I: final report on response to insulin-induced hypoglycemia during a depressive episode. Arch Gen Psychiatry 41:455–460, 1984a

Puig-Antich J, Novacenko H, Davies M, et al: Growth hormone secretion in prepubertal children with major depression, III: response to insulin-induced hypoglycemia after recovery from a depressive episode and in a drug-free state. Arch Gen Psychiatry 41:471–475, 1984b

Puig-Antich J, Goetz R, Davies M, et al: Growth hormone secretion in prepubertal children with major depression, IV: sleep related plasma concentrations in a drug-free fully recovered clinical state. Arch Gen Psychiatry 41:479–483, 1984c

Rapaport MH, Risch SC, Gillin JC, et al: Blunted growth hormone response to peripheral infusion of human growth hormone–releasing factor in patients with panic disorder. Am J Psychiatry 146:92–95, 1989

Risch SC, Judd LL: Provocative challenges of growth hormone and prolactin in schizophrenia and affective disorders, in Handbook of Clinical Psychoneuroendocrinology. Edited by Nemeroff CB, Loosen PT. New York, Guilford, 1987, pp 361–368

Risch SC, Ehlers C, Janowsky DS, et al: Human growth hormone–releasing factor infusion effects on plasma growth hormone in affective disorder patients and normal controls. Peptides 9 (suppl 1):45–48, 1988

Rivier J, Spiess J, Thorner M, et al: Characterization of a growth hormone–releasing factor from a human pancreatic islet tumor. Nature 300:276, 1982

Rotrosen J, Angrist B, Gershon S, et al: Neuroendocrine effects of apomorphine: characterization of response patterns and application to schizophrenia research. Br J Psychiatry 135:444–456, 1979

Sachar EJ: Neuroendocrine dysfunction in depressive illness. Annu Rev Med 27:389–396, 1976

Sachar EJ, Finkelstein J, Hellman L: Growth hormone response in depressive illness. Arch Gen Psychiatry 25:263–269, 1971

Sachar EJ, Frantz AG, Altman N, et al: Growth hormone and prolactin in unipolar and bipolar patients: responses to hypoglycemia and L-dopa. Am J Psychiatry 130:1362–1367, 1973

Sachar EJ, Altman N, Gruen PH, et al: Human growth hormone response to levodopa: relation to menopause, depression, and plasma dopa concentration. Arch Gen Psychiatry 32:502–503, 1975

Siever L, Insel T, Uhde T: Noradrenergic challenges in the affective disorders. J Clin Psychopharmacol 1:193–206, 1981

Tamminga CA, Smith RC, Pandey G, et al: A neuroendocrine study of supersensitivity in tardive dyskinesia. Arch Gen Psychiatry 34:1199–1203, 1977

van Praag HM: The significance of biological factors in the diagnosis of depression, II: hormonal variables. Compr Psychiatry 23:216–226, 1982

Winokur A, Amsterdam J, Caroff S, et al: Variability of hormonal responses to a series of neuroendocrine challenges in depressed patients. Am J Psychiatry 139:39–44, 1982

Chapter 7

Vasopressin

William M. McDonald, M.D.
K. Ranga Rama Krishnan, M.D.

Chapter 7

Vasopressin

Vasopressin is a nonapeptide that is widely distributed in the central nervous system (CNS) and has a number of diverse effects in the brain and peripheral autonomic system. Certain physiological functions of vasopressin, such as the regulation of fluid and electrolyte balance, have been well characterized and are responsible for vasopressin's pseudonym, antidiuretic hormone (ADH). More recent evidence has elucidated vasopressin's role not only as a hormone but also as a potential neuromodulator and neurotransmitter in the CNS. In this chapter we address the neurophysiological effects of vasopressin and the potential implications of this unique neuropeptide for human behavior.

ANATOMY

The primary site of synthesis of vasopressin is the magnocellular (cell bodies 20–30 μm in diameter) neurons in the supraoptic nucleus (SON) and paraventricular nucleus (PVN) of the hypothalamus. After synthesis, vasopressin is packaged with the protein neurophysin into neurosecretory granules. The granules are transported in axons that connect the SON and PVN with the third ventricle, the median eminence, and the posterior lobe of the pituitary.

The major pathway of vasopressin secretion connects the magnocellular PVN and SON of the hypothalamus with the posterior lobe, or neurohypophysis, of the pituitary. This pathway releases vasopressin directly into the systemic circulation forming the hypothalamo-neurohypophyseal system. Although the SON is almost entirely magnocellular, the PVN is a mix of magnocellular and parvocellular cell bodies. The SON, which contains approximately two to four times as many magnocellular neurons as the PVN, is therefore responsible for a majority of the vasopressin secreted into the systemic circulation by the hypothalamo-neurohypophyseal system (Morris et al. 1987).

The parvocellular neurons of the PVN terminate in the portal capillaries of the median eminence of the neurohypophysis and form the second pathway connecting the hypothalamus and the pituitary (Swanson and Sawchenko 1983). Vasopressin from the PVN stimulates secretion of adrenocorticotropin (ACTH) from the anterior lobe of the pituitary (Swanson and Sawchenko 1980) and therefore makes up a part of the hypothalamo-pituitary axis that is distinct from the magnocellular neurons of the neurohypophyseal system.

A third pathway connects the parvocellular nuclei of the PVN to the autonomic centers in the spinal cord and dorsal medulla (primarily the dorsal motor nucleus of the vagus nerve and the nucleus of the tractus solitarius) (Swanson and Sawchenko 1980).

Some researchers have described evidence for a fourth pathway composed of a tract from the hypothalamus to free nerve endings on the floor of the third ventricle particularly at the level of the median eminence and anteriorally near the organum vasculosum of the lamina terminalis (Robinson and Zimmerman 1973; Scott et al. 1974). This pathway accounts for vasopressin being directly secreted into the cerebrospinal fluid (CSF).

The magnocellular neurons receive a number of afferents from the brain stem, and the release of vasopressin is controlled by the action of several neurotransmitters on the hypothalamus and the neurohypophysis. Acetylcholine was one of the first neurotransmitters shown to affect the system. In 1939, Pickford demonstrated the antidiuretic effect of acetylcholine in dogs. Subsequent research has demonstrated that an area dorsolateral to the SON contained cholinergic neurons (De Vries and Buijs 1983; Meyer and Brownstein 1980). The vasopressin neurons also receive afferents from cardiovascular regulatory inputs in the carotid sinus, aortic receptors, and baroreceptors (Swanson and Sawchenko 1983). In addition, noradrenergic fibers project to these neurons from the nucleus tractus solitarius, locus coeruleus, and ventrolateral medulla (Swanson and Sawchenko 1983). Gamma-aminobutyric acid (GABA) appears to act as an inhibitory neurotransmitter via high-affinity chloride channel-associated GABA receptors in the SON (Palacios et al. 1981). Serotinergic fibers project from the midbrain nucleus of the raphe to the PVN and SON, but these fibers appear to be more important in oxytocin regulation than in vasopressin regulation (Swanson and Sawchenko 1983). Dopaminergic fibers have also been shown to innervate the PVN and SON, but their role is unclear (Buijs et al. 1984). In 1975, Zaborszky and his colleagues defined connections from the limbic system to the SON. These inputs include fibers from the hypothalamus, septum, amygdala, and hippocampus. Sladek and Armstrong (1987) reviewed evidence for the effects of other neurotransmitters on the vasopressin system, including histamine, substance P, angiotensin II, and the opioid peptides, including dynorphin, enkephalin, and beta-endorphin.

Recent studies have also shown that vasopressin has an extensive distribution in other areas of the brain. Vasopressin synthesis has also been demonstrated in the suprachiasmatic nucleus (Vandesande et al. 1975), bed nucleus of the stria terminalis (Sofroniew 1983), locus coeruleus, medial amygdala, and parts of the dorsomedial hypothalamus (Caffe and Van Leeuwen 1983; Caffe et al. 1985).

Buijs (1987) has reviewed all the interconnections of vasopressin in the CNS. The vasopressin fibers that originate in the PVN reach the olfactory nucleus, pineal gland, dorsal vagal complex, nucleus ambiguous, dorsal parabrachial nucleus, and lateral reticular nucleus. The vasopressin pathways from the suprachiasmatic nucleus project to the periventricular thalamic nucleus, the dorsomedial hypothalamic nucleus, and the organum vasculosum of the lamina terminalis. The vasopressin pathways that originate in the nucleus of the stria terminalis project to the lateral septum, Broca's diagonal band, area of the anterior amygdala, lateral habenular nucleus, periventricular gray matter, and locus coeruleus. Neurons of the medial amygdala project to the ventral hippocampus and the lateral septum.

Overall, vasopressin neurons have widespread connections in the CNS. Vasopressin is synthesized in hypothalamic and other neurons that project throughout the brain. Hypothalamic projections secrete vasopressin into the systemic circulation via portal capillaries and possibly also directly into the CSF. These interconnections form the basis for considering vasopressin as a neuropeptide influencing human behavior, as well as a hormone influencing distant organs in the body.

ROLE AS A HORMONE

Although vasopressin synthesis occurs in the CNS, the earliest descriptions of vasopressin involved the peptide's role as a hormone in modifying the peripheral autonomic system. Vasopressin receptors have been found not only in the CNS but also in the kidney, heart, liver, and vascular smooth muscle.

In 1895, Oliver and Schafer demonstrated that pituitary gland extracts caused a significant pressor effect in the vascular system. Three years later Howell (1898) determined that the pressor effect was due specifically to posterior pituitary extract. These early observations account for the original description of this peptide as a vaso "pressin."

Vasopressin is one of the most potent vasoconstrictors in the systemic circulation (Altura 1977) and acts directly on vascular smooth muscle, and indirectly through its effect on cardiac baroreceptors, to raise arterial pressure. However, the role of vasopressin in the routine maintenance of blood pressure, or as a cause of essential hypertension, remains controversial (Cowley and Liard 1987). Instead, vasopressin appears to be most clearly involved in the regulation of systemic blood pressure in dehydrated hypovolemic states.

Vasopressin primarily acts on the kidney to conserve water and concentrate urine in an effort to maintain body fluids at a constant osmolality and volume (Valtin 1987). Conditions such as water deprivation or infusions of hypertonic saline that increase plasma osmolality stimulate the osmoreceptors located in the SON and lead to an increase in the synthesis and release of vasopressin into the systemic circulation. Water deprivation and the subsequent decrease in plasma volume are sensed by the volume receptors in the left atrium and the baroreceptors in the carotid arteries. A decrease in plasma volume leads to a diminution of the tonic inhibitory impulse of these baroreceptors and a release of vasopressin. Vasopressin then acts on the kidney to conserve free water, so that serum osmolality is decreased and plasma volume increased.

Destruction of the SON or neurohypophysis leads to diabetes insipidus. Patients with diabetes insipidus excrete large amounts of dilute urine. Patients with the clinical condition of SIADH (or secretion of inappropriate ADH) have the opposite condition. This condition is often induced by medications (including phenothiazines and tricyclic antidepressants) or head injury and is seen in patients who secrete a highly concentrated urine despite low plasma osmolality. Other drugs, such as ethanol, inhibit ADH secretion and lead to the loss of large amounts of free water.

Unlike the effects of vasopressin on the cardiovascular system, its effect on the renal system is more constant. Vasopressin's pressor effects are present mainly at times of hemorrhage or severe volume loss, whereas vasopressin's effect on the kidney constantly acts to maintain serum osmolality within a very narrow range.

Besides having a role in the regulation of fluid and electrolyte balance, vasopressin also acts to regulate the hypothalamo-pituitary-adrenal (HPA) axis. In fact, vasopressin was originally thought to be the endogenous corticotropin-releasing factor (CRF). The effects of vasopressin on the HPA axis may be at several different levels. Although its primary effect is at the level of the pituitary in stimulating the release of ACTH, vasopressin may also act at the hypothalamic level by potentiating the release of CRF (Hedge and Huffman 1987). Vasopressin releases ACTH in a dose-dependent fashion, although this effect is less potent than that of CRF. But the most important role of vasopressin appears to be in potentiating the effect of CRF on ACTH secretion.

The importance of vasopressin in the regulation of the HPA system has also been shown by studies in the Brattleboro rat. The Brattleboro rat has a congenital lack of vasopressin. In this rat, the response of the HPA system to stress is blunted because of multiple physiological changes. These changes include a reduction in the adrenocortical sensitivity to ACTH (Wiley et al. 1974) and an overall reduction in the activity of the HPA system as evidenced by reduced plasma corticosterone concentrations (Mohrin et al. 1978) and reduced plasma and pituitary ACTH concentrations (Buckingham and Leach 1980).

Negative feedback from glucocorticoid secretion by the adrenal glands also appears to regulate vasopressin and CRF secretion. Wolfson et al. (1985) showed that vasopressin and CRF synthesis were both increased in the parvocellular hypothalamic neurons in adrenalectomized animals. Humans with adrenocortical insufficiency have also been shown to have increased plasma levels of vasopressin (Ahmed et al. 1967), indicating that corticosteroids may exert a negative feedback effect on vasopressin release. The release of vasopressin under certain physiological conditions (e.g., stress secondary to hypoxia) is also attenuated by negative feedback from circulating corticosteroids (Raff et al. 1984).

The other major effect of vasopressin upon the endocrine system is to mobilize energy reserves. Vasopressin increases glucagon release (Spruce et al. 1985) and also acts directly on the liver to promote glycogenolysis and gluconeogenesis (Hems 1977).

Vasopressin receptors have been classified into V_1 and V_2 subtypes (Michell et al. 1979). The V_2 receptors are linked to cyclic AMP and are responsible for the renal antidiuretic effects of vasopressin (Jard 1983). The V_1 receptors are found on vascular smooth muscle (Penit et al. 1983) and hepatocytes (Keppens and De Wulf 1979) and may mediate the pressor and glycogenolytic effects of vasopressin. The V_1 receptors also appear to be more prominent in the brain (Van Leeuwen 1987). The V_1 receptors mediate their effects through calcium-dependent channels that facilitate vasopressin release by potassium depolarization (Michell et al. 1979).

ROLE OF VASOPRESSIN AS A NEUROPEPTIDE

Thus far, we have described the hormonal effects of vasopressin released by the pituitary neurohypophysis. These effects are well documented and involve primarily the peripheral autonomic system. More recently, attention has been paid to the CNS effects of vasopressin when acting as a neuromodulator and neurotransmitter.

The pool of vasopressin in the CSF is insulated from the vasopressin in the systemic circulation by the blood-brain barrier (Ang and

Jenkins 1982). The diurnal variation in CSF vasopressin is not affected by the concentration of vasopressin in plasma. The CSF vasopressin appears to be secreted by a different population of neurons and, unlike plasma vasopressin, is not controlled by osmoregulation (Coleman and Reppert 1985).

Vasopressin fibers that project from the PVN, stria terminalis, medial amygdala, and suprachiasmatic nucleus have already been described. Vasopressin has been found in nuclei outside the SON and PVN, specifically in the locus coeruleus, dorsomedial hypothalamus, suprachiasmatic nuclei, medial amygdaloid, and bed nucleus of the stria terminalis. Vasopressin has been posited to act as a neurotransmitter in the sympathetic nervous system rather than by transport through the CSF or systemic circulation (Hanley et al. 1984). In addition, vasopressin increases the firing rate of hippocampal neurons (Muhlethaler and Dreifuss 1982) and may hence act as a neuromodulator in the hippocampus.

Evidence of the influence of vasopressin on behavior comes from the examination of the effects of vasopressin on passive-avoidance behavior in laboratory animals. Learning in this experimental paradigm is assessed by determining the number of trials needed to acquire a conditioned-avoidance behavior. Memory is measured as the length of time to extinction of the conditioned avoidance.

DeWied and his colleagues were the first to demonstrate that vasopressin improved the performance of rats in learning and memory tasks. In 1965, DeWied reported that neurohypophysectomy in a rat increased the rate of extinction of avoidance behavior but not the learning of an active-avoidance task. DeWied also showed that rats deficient in vasopressin due to a genetic defect (e.g., Brattleboro rat) were less proficient in learning to avoid an aversive stimulus. In the Brattleboro rat, DeWied demonstrated that the acquisition of avoidance-response behavior is impaired (DeWied et al. 1975). The extinction of avoidance-response behavior is also more rapid in Brattleboro rats, and this extinction rate can be lowered by replacing or administering vasopressin to the animal.

Memory consolidation of passive-avoidance behavior has also been shown to be facilitated by microinjections of vasopressin into certain limbic midbrain structures, including the hippocampal dentate gyrus, dorsal raphe nucleus, and dorsal septal nucleus (Kovacs et al. 1977). Injections of vasopressin antiserum into the anterior dorsal hippocampus (Kovacs et al. 1982), dorsal raphe nucleus (Kovacs et al. 1980), and lateral ventricles (van Wimersma Greidanus and DeWied 1976) prevented the memory consolidation and retrieval, but not learning, of passive-avoidance behavior.

Since DeWied's initial experiments a number of investigators have attempted to assess the effects of vasopressin on human cognition. Jolles (1987) has reviewed the studies of the effects of vasopressin on human cognition. He points out that there are a number of differences in experimental design that make comparisons across studies difficult. These differences include varying patient populations and variations in the dose, route, frequency, and duration of the vasopressin administered.

When attempting to draw conclusions about the human research studies, several considerations regarding experimental technique need to be kept in mind. First, most investigators would agree that the blood levels of vasopressin found under physiologic conditions do not cross the blood-brain barrier. However, when given in large doses experimentally, vasopressin may pass from the plasma to the CNS in minute but physiologically significant quantities.

Second, vasopressin fragments have been shown to have central activity, and some researchers believe that brain vasopressin may be the precursor for these active fragments. The different experimental designs utilize vasopressin fragments that are assumed to have typical central behavioral effects and differ primarily in their peripheral side effects (e.g., antidiuretic and vasopressor activities). For instance, digestion of the parent compound lysine vasopressin with trypsin destroys pressor, antidiuretic, and CRF activity while maintaining the effects of vasopressin on memory.

Third, the human studies draw conclusions on the effects of vasopressin on cognition and behavior using very different patient populations. These populations have included patients with head trauma, chronic alcoholism, senile dementia, depression, schizophrenia, and anorexia.

Finally, most of the animal studies that examine the effects of vasopressin on memory have focused on aversive paradigms. The few that have examined nonaversively motivated paradigms have reported inconsistent results (Laczi et al. 1983a, 1983b).

Jolles (1987) notes that several diverse patient populations have been utilized. Several investigators have observed patients with head trauma and have generally noted that the therapeutic efficacy of vasopressin on memory was more significant when the trauma was less severe. Patients with an amnestic syndrome associated with chronic alcoholism also appeared to respond preferentially depending upon the severity of their pretreatment amnesia. For example, Laczi and his coworkers (1983a) noted no effect of intranasal dGAVP (a vasopressin congener with no peripheral effects) on attention, spatial orientation, and memory in alcoholic patients with Korsakoff 's syndrome. Yet Blake et al. (1978) did find an effect on memory using lysine vasopressin (which has significant effects on blood pressure and electrolytes) in patients with less severe alcoholism. These results typify the confusion in this field of research, since the different researchers have utilized different vasopressin congeners and patient populations. Some senile patients (Delwaide et al. 1980; Weingartner et al. 1981a, 1981b) showed improvement in memory tasks when administered vasopressin, whereas patients with Alzheimer's disease (Durso et al. 1982; Jennekens-Schinkel et al. 1985) and Parkinson's disease (Jensen 1980) showed no treatment effect.

Many studies of healthy volunteers show that most subjects improve on memory tasks when administered vasopressin (Laczi et al. 1982, 1983a, 1983b; Nebes et al. 1984; Weingartner et al. 1981a, 1981b). However, some studies show no effect of vasopressin on either a mixed gender population (Fehm-Wolfsdorf et al. 1985; Jenkins et al. 1982) or a group of healthy young men (Snel et al. 1987). An additional study (Beckwith et al. 1984) demonstrated a positive effect of vasopressin on memory in males but not females. Jolles (1987) points out that the recent studies are more precise in their methodology and have elucidated certain subgroups of memory that are preferentially affected by vasopressin. The differences in experimental results may be due to the fact that different experimental designs test different memory functions and therefore obtain conflicting results.

Jolles (1987) conceptualizes vasopressin as exerting its effect on cognition by an increase in CNS activation perhaps by modulating the synaptic efficacy of the ascending catecholaminergic systems. Vasopressin may act by increasing the rate at which information is processed and by facilitating attention and concentration. Nebes and his coworkers (1984) refute this hypothesis and show that short-term and long-term memory are improved by vasopressin without an increase in the subject's general level of arousal or response time.

Vasopressin has already been shown to have a number of connections with the deep limbic structures associated with memory, including the hippocampus, amygdala, and hypothalamic nuclei. Jolles (1987) points out that experimental evidence from the animal literature showing that vasopressin's effects on avoidance behavior are blocked by destruction of limbic structures may explain why patients with marked neuronal degeneration (e.g., Korsakoff's syndrome and severe head trauma) may not respond to vasopressin. The experimental design may also be a crucial factor. Data from the animal literature show that only memory tasks involving avoidance behavior yield consistent results. None of the study designs in humans have utilized this experimental paradigm. Interestingly, patients with Lesch-Nyhan syndrome, an X-linked recessive disorder in which there is a presumed defect in passive-avoidance learning, have been tested after having been administered vasopressin (Anderson et al. 1979). In three such children, there was consistent improvement in learning a passive-avoidance task (i.e., punishment to decrease self-mutilation) when vasopressin was administered prior to this task.

VASOPRESSIN IN PSYCHIATRY

Vasopressin was first used in the treatment of schizophrenia in 1952, when Forizs gave Pitressin injections to chronic schizophrenic patients. About one-third of the patients showed improvement, with a decrease in psychomotor activity, autism, and ward problems. In a study of 19 patients suffering from chronic anergic schizophrenia, Korsgaard and his colleagues (1981) found a significant decrease in the thinking disorder scale of the Brief Psychiatric Rating Scale (BPRS) with no change in total BPRS score. Six of the patients became quite agitated, and there was no change noted in anergia.

After pretreatment with vasopressin, dopamine turnover has been shown to be increased in the terminal areas of the nigrostriatum and tuberoinfundibular dopamine systems (Kovacs et al. 1977). Projections of dopamine fibers have also been shown to enervate the PVN and SON; however, their purpose has yet to be defined (Buijs et al. 1984). Researchers who have compared vasopressin concentrations in the CSF of schizophrenic patients with those in healthy control subjects have obtained conflicting results, with some finding no difference (Beckmann et al. 1985; Sorensen et al. 1985) and others showing a decrease in CSF vasopressin in schizophrenia (van Kammen et al. 1981).

A role for vasopressin in affective illness has been proposed by Gold and Goodwin (1978). They describe a number of physiological factors that appear to be influenced by vasopressin and that are also disturbed in mood disorders. They point to evidence that vasopressin may influence memory, pain sensitivity, biological rhythms, REM sleep, and fluid and electrolyte balance.

Two studies have shown an improvement in memory in subjects with major affective disorders and at least some amelioration of affective symptoms (Gold et al. 1979; Weingartner et al. 1981a). Gold et al. demonstrated that CSF vasopressin was significantly lower in depressed patients than in manic patients and healthy control subjects (Gold et al. 1981). However, a later study found CSF vasopressin to be lower only in nonpsychotically depressed bipolar patients compared with control subjects and patients with unipolar depression and mania, and highest in bipolar patients with psychotic depression (Gold et al. 1983b). Gold et al. (1983b) also showed that the secretion of plasma vasopressin in response to a hypertonic saline infusion was generally decreased in depressed bipolar patients compared with manic bipolar patients.

Gold and his colleagues emphasized that vasopressin may play a role in the pathophysiology of affective illness, possibly via the catecholamine system that was previously linked to mood disorders. They further support their hypothesis by pointing out that drugs with an antimanic effect, such as lithium, also decrease sensitivity to peripheral vasopressin receptors (e.g., nephrogenic diabetes insipidus). Conversely, tricyclic antidepressants can increase central vasopressin release and lead to the clinical condition of the secretion of inappropriate ADH (Gold and Goodwin 1978).

Vasopressin has also been shown to influence the release of ACTH in the HPA axis. Carroll has demonstrated that malfunctioning of the HPA with hypersecretion of cortisol in response to a dexamethasone challenge is a reliable test for depression (Carroll et al. 1981). Vasopressin has an additive effect with CRF in releasing ACTH (Gillies et al. 1982). Although neither CRF nor vasopressin alone can cause a significant release of ACTH in the presence of dexamethasone, when the two are added together they produce a considerable increase in ACTH. This indicates not just an additive effect but an overall enhancement of ACTH-releasing activity (Hedge and Smelik 1969).

Gold's hypothesis indicates that in depression there is an overall hypofunctioning of the vasopressin tone. Yet, hypercortisolemia results from a hyperfunctioning of the HPA axis and (an as yet unproven) possible increase in vasopressin tone potentiating ACTH release. These apparently disparate theories are reconciled by the fact that the vasopressin-secreting cells in the HPA axis are part of the parvocellular neurons in the PVN. These cells form a distinct subgroup from the magnocellular nuclei controlling the vasopressin response to osmotic stimuli such as isotonic saline and the cells secreting vasopressin into the CSF. The vasopressin nuclei that form a part of the HPA axis secrete vasopressin into the systemic circulation via the portal capillaries. As previously discussed, the blood-brain barrier does not allow vasopressin in the systemic circulation to enter the CSF at physiologic concentrations. Measurements of CSF, vasopressin, and systemic vasopressin in response to hypertonic saline challenges probably measure the function of a different subset of vasopressin nuclei distinct from the nuclei that control ACTH secretion in the HPA axis.

The role of vasopressin in patients with anorexia nervosa has also been investigated. Gold et al. (1983a) hypothesized that anorexic patients had abnormalities in vasopressin secretion as demonstrated clinically by the patients' inability to maintain urinary concentration. These patients showed abnormalities in the HPA axis, with abnormal secretions of gonadatropins, thyroid-stimulating hormone, and growth hormone. Gold et al. demonstrated markedly abnormal responses in vasopressin secretion in the plasma and CSF following challenge with hypertonic saline solution. These defects persisted for several months. Nishita and his colleagues (1989) have extended these findings to include patients with bulimia nervosa.

In summary, vasopressin appears to have a number of possible implications for further study in psychiatric disorders. Vasopressin's function as a hormone, neuropeptide, and putative neurotransmitter is reason to postulate a significant role for this peptide in human behavior.

REFERENCES

Ahmed ABJ, George BC, Gonzalez-Auvert C, et al: Increased plasma arginine vasopressin in clinical adrenocortical insufficiency and its inhibition by glucosteroids. J Clin Invest 46:111–123, 1967

Altura BM: Comparative cellular and pharmacologic actions of neurohypophyseal hormones on smooth muscle. Federation Proceedings 36:1840–1841, 1977

Anderson LT, David R, Bonnet K, et al: Passive avoidance learning in Lesch-Nyhan disease: effect of 1-desamino-8-arginine-vasopressin1. Life Sci 24:905–910, 1979

Ang VTY, Jenkins JS: Blood-cerebrospinal fluid barrier to arginine-vasopressin, desmopressin and desglycinamide arginine-vasopressin in the dog. J Endocrinol 93:319–325, 1982

Beckmann H, Lang RE, Gattaz WF: Vasopressin-oxytocin in cerebrospinal fluid of schizophrenic patients and normal controls. Psychoneuroendocrinology 10:187–191, 1985

Beckwith BE, Robert ET, Schneider V: Vasopressin analog (DDAVP) improves memory in human males. Peptides 5:819–822, 1984

Blake DR, Dodd MJ, Grimley Evans J: Vasopressin in amnesia. Lancet 1:608, 1978

Buckingham JC, Leach JH: Hypothalamo pituitary-adrenocortical function in rats with inherited diabetes insipidus. J Physiol 305;397–404, 1980

Buijs RM: Vasopressin localization and putative functions in the brain, in Vasopressin: Principles and Properties. Edited by Gash DM, Boer GJ. New York, Plenum, 1987, pp 91–116

Buijs RM, Geffard M, Pool CW, et al: The dopaminergic innervation of the supraoptic and paraventricular nucleus: a light and electron microscopical study. Brain Res 323:65–72, 1984

Caffe AR, Van Leeuwen FW: Vasopressin-immunoreactive cells in the dorsomedial hypothalamic region, medial amygdaloid nucleus and locus coeruleus of the rat. Cell Tissue Res 233:23–33, 1983

Caffe AR, Van Leeuwen FW, Buijs RM, et al: Coexistence of vasopressin, neurophysin and noradrenaline immunoreactivity in medium-sized cells of the locus coeruleus and subcoeruleus in the rat. Brain Res 338:160–164, 1985

Carroll BJ, Feinberg M, Greden JF, et al: A specific laboratory test for the diagnosis of melancholia. Arch Gen Psychiatry 38:15–22, 1981

Coleman RJ, Reppert SM: CSF vasopressin rhythm is effectively insulated from osmotic regulation of plasma vasopressin. Am J Physiol 248:346–352, 1985

Cowley AW, Liard JF: Cardiovascular actions of vasopressin, in Vasopressin: Principles and Properties. Edited by Gash DM, Boer GJ. New York, Plenum, 1987, pp 389–434

Delwaide PJ, Devoitille JM, Ylieff M: Acute effects of drugs upon memory of patients with senile dementia. Acta Psychiatr Belg 80:748–754, 1980

De Vries GJ, Buijs RM: The origin of the vasopressinergic and oxytocinergic innervation of the rat brain, with special reference to the lateral septum. Brain Res 273:307–317, 1983

DeWied D: The influence of the posterior and intermediate lobe of the pituitary and pituitary peptides on the maintenance of a conditioned avoidance response in rats. Int J Neuropharmacol 4:157–167, 1965

DeWied D, Bohus B, van Wimersma Greidanus TB: Memory deficit in rats with hereditary diabetes insipidus. Brain Res 85:152–156, 1975

Durso R, Fedio P, Brouwers P, et al: Lysine vasopressin in Alzheimer's disease. Neurology 32:674–677, 1982

Fehm-Wolfsdorf G, Born J, Elbert T, et al: Vasopressin does not enhance memory processes: a study in human twins. Peptides 6:297–300, 1985

Forizs L: Treatment of mental patients with antidiuretic hormone of the posterior pituitary. Diseases of the Nervous System 13:44–47, 1952

Gash DM, Boer GJ (eds): Vasopressin: Principles and Properties. New York, Plenum, 1987

Gillies GE, Linton EA, Lowry PJ: Corticotropin releasing activity of the new CRF is potentiated several times by vasopressin. Nature 299:355–357, 1982

Gold PW, Goodwin FK: Vasopressin in affective illness. Lancet 1:1233–1235, 1978

Gold PW, Weingartner H, Ballenger JC, et al: Effects of 1 desamino-8-D-arginine vasopressin on behaviour and cognition in primary affective disorder. Lancet 2:992–994, 1979

Gold PW, Goodwin FK, Post RM, et al: Vasopressin function in depression and mania. Psychopharmacol Bull 17:7–9, 1981

Gold PW, Kaye W, Robertson GL, et al: Abnormalities in plasma and cerebrospinal-fluid arginine vasopressin in patients with anorexia nervosa. N Engl J Med 308:1117–1123, 1983a

Gold PW, Robertson GL, Ballenger JC, et al: Neurohypophyseal function in affective illness. Psychopharmacol Bull 19:426–431, 1983b

Hanley MR, Benton HP, Lightman SL, et al: A vasopressin-like peptide in the mammalian sympathetic nervous system. Nature 309:257–261, 1984

Hedge GA, Huffman LJ: Vasopressin and endocrine function, in Vasopressin: Principles and Properties. Edited by Gash DM, Goer GJ. New York, Plenum, 1987, pp 435–476

Hedge GA, Smelik PG: The action of dexamethasone and vasopressin on hypothalamic CRF production and release. Neuroendocrinology 4:242–253, 1969

Hems DA: Short-term hormonal control of hepatic carbohydrate and lipid catabolism. FEBS Lett 80:237–245, 1977

Howell WH: The physiological effects of extracts of the hypophysis cerebri and infundibular body. J Exp Med 5:245–253, 1899

Jard S: Vasopressin isoreceptors in mammals: relation to cyclic AMP–independent transduction mechanisms, in Current Topics in Membranes and Transport. Edited by Kleinzeller A. New York, Academic, 1983, pp 255–285

Jenkins JS, Mather HM, Coughlan AK: Effect of desmopressin on normal and impaired memory. J Neurol Neurosurg Psychiatry 45:830–831, 1982

Jennekens-Schinkel A, Wintzen AR, Lanser JBK: A clinical trial with desglycinamide arginine vasopressin for the treatment of memory disorders in man. Prog Neuropsychopharmacol Biol Psychiatry 9:273–284, 1985

Jensen JPA: Vasopressin therapy in Parkinson's disease. Acta Neurol Scand 62:197–199, 1980

Jolles J: Vasopressin and human behavior, in Vasopressin: Principles and Properties. Edited by Gash DM, Boer GJ. New York, Plenum, 1987, pp 549–578

Keppens S, De Wulf: The nature of the hepatic receptors involved in vasopressin-induced glycogenolysis. Biochim Biophys Acta 588:63–69, 1979

Korsgaard S, Casey DE, Pedersen NED, et al: Vasopressin in anergic schizophrenia. Psychopharmacology (Berlin) 74:379–381, 1981

Kovacs GL, Vecsei L, Szabo G, et al: The involvement of catecholaminergic mechanisms in the behavioural action of vasopressin. Neurosci Lett 5:337–344, 1977

Kovacs GL, Bohus B, Versteeg DHG, et al: Effect of oxytocin and vasopressin on memory consolidation: sites of action and catecholaminergic correlates after local microinjection into limbic-midbrain structures. Brain Res 175:303–314, 1979

Kovacs GL, Vecsei L, Medve L, et al: Effect on memory processes of anti-vasopressin serum microinjected into the dorsal raphe nucleus: the role of catecholaminergic neurotransmission. Exp Brain Res 38:357–361, 1980

Kovacs GL, Buijs RM, Bohus B, et al: Microinjection of arginine^{8}-vasopressin antiserum into the dorsal hippocampus attenuates passive avoidance behavior in rats. Physiol Behav 28:45–48, 1982

Laczi F, Valkuz Z, Laszlo FA, et al: Effects of lysine-vasopressin and 1-desamino-8-D-arginine-vasopressin on memory in healthy individuals and diabetes insipidus patients. Psychoneuroendocrinology 7:185–193, 1982

Laczi F, Van Ree JM, Balogh L, et al: Lack of effect of DGAVP on memory in patients with Korsakoff syndrome. Acta Endocrinol 104:177–182, 1983a

Laczi F, Van Ree JM, Wagner A, et al: Effects of desglycinamide-arginine-vasopressin (DGAVP) on memory processes in diabetes insipidus patients and in non-diabetic subjects. Acta Endocrinol 102:205–212, 1983b

Meyer DK, Brownstein MJ: Effect of surgical deafferentation of the supraoptic nucleus on its choline acetyltransferase content. Brain Res 193:566–569, 1980

Michell RH, Kirk CJ, Billah MM: Hormonal stimulation of phosphatidylinositol breakdown, with particular reference to the hepatic effects of vasopressin. Biochemical Society Transaction, 83rd Meeting, Cambridge, UK, 1979

Mohrin J, Kohrs G, Mohring B, et al: Effects of prolonged vasopressin treatment in Brattleboro rats with diabetes insipidus. Am J Physiol 234:106–111, 1978

Morris JF, Chapman DB, Sokol HW: Anatomy and function of the classic vasopressin-secreting hypothalamus-neurohypophysial system, in Vasopressin: Principles and Properties. Edited by Gash DM, Boer GJ. New York, Plenum, 1987, pp 1–90

Muhlethaler M, Dreifuss JJ: Vasopressin excites hippocampal neurons. Nature 296:749–751, 1982

Nebes RD, Reynolds CF, Horn LC: The effect of vasopressin on memory in the healthy elderly. Psychiatry Res 11:49–59, 1984

Nishita JK, Ellinwood EH Jr, Rockwell WJK, et al: Abnormalities in the response of plasma arginine vasopressin during hypertonic saline infusion in patients with eating disorders. Biol Psychiatry 26:73–86, 1989

Oliver G, Schafer EA: On the physiological action of extracts of pituitary body and certain other glandular organs. J Physiol (Lond) 18:276–279, 1895

Palacios JM, Wamsley JK, Kuhar MJ: High affinity GABA receptors: autoradiographic localization. Brain Res 222:285–307, 1981

Penit J, Faure M, Jard S: Vasopressin and angiotensin II receptors in rat aortic smooth muscle cells in culture. Am J Physiol 244:72–82, 1983

Pickford M: The inhibitory effect of acetylcholine on water diuresis in the dog and its pituitary transmission. J Physiol (Lond) 95:226–238, 1939

Raff H, Shinsako J, Keil LC, et al: Feedback inhibition of adrenocorticotropin and vasopressin responses to hypoxia by physiological increases in endogenous plasma corticosteroids in dogs. Endocrinology 114:1245–1249, 1984

Robinson AG, Zimmerman EA: Cerebrospinal fluid and ependymal neurophysin. J Clin Invest 52:1260–1267, 1973

Scott DE, Kozlowski GP, Sheridan MN: Scanning electron microscopy in the ultrastructural analysis of the mammalian cerebral ventricular system. Neurosecretory Axon Terminals 37:349–388, 1974

Sladek CD, Armstrong WE: Effect of neurotransmitters and neuropeptides on vasopressin release, in Vasopressin: Principles and Properties. Edited by Gash DM, Boer GJ. New York, Plenum 1987, pp 275–316

Snel J, Taylor J, Wegman M: Does DGAVP influence memory, attention and mood in young healthy men? Psychopharmacology (Berlin) 92:224–229, 1987

Sofroniew MV: Morphology of vasopressin and oxytocin neurons and their central and vascular projections, in The Neurohypophysis: Structure, Function and Control. Progress in Brain Research. Edited by Cross BA, Leng G. Amsterdam, Elsevier, 1983, pp 101–114

Sorensen PS, Gjerris A, Hammer M: Cerebrospinal fluid vasopressin in neurological and psychiatric disorders. J Neurol Neurosurg Psychiatry 48:50–57, 1985

Spruce BA, McCulloch AJ, Burd J, et al: The effect of vasopressin infusion on glucose metabolism in man. Clin Endocrinol 22:463–468, 1985

Swanson LW, Sawchenko PE: Paraventricular nucleus: a site for the integration of neuroendocrine and autonomic mechanisms. Neuroendocrinology 31:410–417, 1980

Swanson LW, Sawchenko PE: Hypothalamic integration: organization of paraventricular and supraoptic nuclei. Annu Rev Neurosci 6:269–324, 1983

Valtin H: Physiological effects of vasopressin on the kidney, in Vasopressin: Principles and Properties. Edited by Gash DM, Boer GJ. New York, Plenum, 1987, pp 369–388

Vandesande R, Dierick K, DeMey J: Identification of the vasopressin-neurophysin producing neurons of the rat suprachiasmatic nuclei. Cell Tissue Res 156:377–380, 1975

van Kammen DP, Waters RN, Gold P, et al: Spinal fluid vasopressin, angiotensin I and II, beta-endorphin, and opioid activity in schizophrenia: a preliminary evaluation, in Biological Psychiatry. Edited by Perris C, Struwe G, Jansson B. Amsterdam, Elsevier North-Holland, 1981, pp 339–344

Van Leeuwen FW: Vasopressin receptors in the brain and pituitary, in Vasopressin: Principles and Properties. Edited by Gash DM, Boer GJ. New York, Plenum, 1987, pp 477–496

Van Wimersma Greidanus TB, DeWied D: Modulation of passive avoidance behavior of rats by intracerebroventricular administration of anti-vasopressin serum. Behav Biol 18:325–333, 1976

Weingartner H, Gold PW, Ballenger JC, et al: Effects of vasopressin on human memory functions. Science 211:601–603, 1981a

Weingartner H, Kaye W, Gold PW, et al: Vasopressin treatment of cognitive dysfunction in progressive dementia. Life Sci 29:2721–2726, 1981b

Wiley MK, Pearlmutter AE, Miller RE: Decreased adrenal sensitivity to ACTH in vasopressin-deficient (Brattleboro) rat. Neuroendocrinology 14:257–270, 1974

Wolfson B, Manning RW, Davis LG, et al: Co-localization of corticotropin releasing factor and vasopressin mRNA in neurones after adrenalectomy. Nature 315:59–61, 1985

Zaborszky L, Leranth C, Makara GB, et al: Quantitative studies on the supraoptic nucleus in the rat, II: afferent fiber connections. Exp Brain Res 22:525–540, 1975

Chapter 8

The Psychiatric Significance of Oxytocin

Cort A. Pedersen, M.D.

Chapter 8

The Psychiatric Significance of Oxytocin

For most of this century oxytocin has been viewed solely as a posterior pituitary hormone that stimulates milk ejection and uterine contraction. Although neural lobe oxytocin was proven 40 years ago to originate from anterior hypothalamic magnocellular nuclei, the widespread distribution of oxytocin pathways and receptors within the central nervous system (CNS) has only recently come to light (Buijs et al. 1985; Tribollet et al. 1988; Van Leeuwen et al. 1985). Central oxytocin has numerous behavioral and physiological effects (Kovacs 1986), and in the past few years oxytocin synthesis and release have been discovered in several peripheral endocrine glands (Nicholson et al. 1984; Wathes 1984).

The goal of this chapter is to review those aspects of this new body of knowledge that suggest that oxytocin affects human behavior and psychopathology. I will begin with an overview of oxytocin systems in the brain, with an emphasis on findings that have psychiatric implications. Behavioral effects of oxytocin in animals that may shed light on human behavior will then be discussed. I will conclude by summarizing the considerable evidence supporting a role for oxytocin in major affective disorders as well as psychiatric disorders associated with changes in female reproductive states. My hope is to stimulate interest and awareness of oxytocin as a potential regulator of normal and pathological human behavior.

CENTRAL OXYTOCIN: GENERAL PSYCHIATRIC CONSIDERATIONS

Oxytocin pathways originating in the anterior hypothalamus project

The author's research is supported by National Institute of Mental Health Grant MH-33127 and National Institutes of Health Grants HD 20640 and HD-24086, and by a grant from the Foundation of Hope for Research and Treatment of Mental Illness. The excellent secretarial assistance of Ms. Betsy Shambley is also appreciated.

to numerous regions within the CNS. Some pathways terminate in the septum, hippocampus, amygdala, and the nucleus accumbens, limbic brain sites that play key roles in mood, affect, and cognition (Buijs et al. 1985). Other oxytocinergic pathways terminate in lower brain-stem and spinal-cord sites involved in central regulation of autonomic function (Hancock and Nicholas 1987; Sofroniew and Schrell 1981; Swanson and McKellar 1979). The adrenal medulla also contains oxytocin (Nicholson et al. 1984). Central oxytocin administration affects cardiovascular function in some species (Tran et al. 1982; Versteeg et al. 1979) and inhibits firing of thoracic sympathetic preganglionic neurons (Gilbey et al. 1982). Oxytocin probably affects autonomically mediated symptoms of anxiety and stress. Within the basal forebrain, oxytocin influences motivated behaviors such as parenting, sex, social behavior, and, very likely, food intake (see following sections for more detail). These considerations suggest that oxytocin regulates emotion, thought, and neurovegetative functions that are often disturbed in psychiatric disorders.

Among the large body of evidence that psychopathology has biological origins are observations that psychiatric populations differ in central neurotransmitter activity, neuroendocrine regulation, and patterns of diurnal change such as sleep and cortisol secretion (Meltzer 1987). It may, therefore, be of psychiatric significance that oxytocinergic brain systems have been implicated in all of these areas.

Oxytocinergic pathways terminate in the substantia nigra and the locus coeruleus; fibers of passage may also synapse in the ventral tegmental area and the raphe nuclei (Buijs et al. 1985). This pattern of distribution suggests that oxytocin may regulate ascending monoamine systems that affect behavior and psychopathology. Indeed, a small number of studies have found that oxytocin has regionally specific effects on brain biogenic amines (Kovacs 1986). Utilization of dopamine is decreased by oxytocin in most brain sites tested; synthesis of dopamine may also be decreased. Behavioral interactions with dopaminergic drugs (amphetamine, apomorphine) indicate that oxytocin selectively increases postsynaptic dopamine receptor sensitivity in the mesolimbic system but decreases presynaptic dopamine receptor sensitivity in the nigrostriatal system. A number of fragments of the oxytocin molecule, especially C-terminal tripeptide fragments, have very potent effects on dopamine utilization and dopamine receptor sensitivity. Cerebrospinal fluid (CSF) levels of oxytocin and oxytocin-associated neurophysin are elevated in schizophrenia (Beckman et al. 1985; Linkowski et al. 1984), a disorder associated with excessive mesolimbic dopamine activity. Oxytocin also appears to alter norepinephrine and serotonin utilization in hypothalamic, limbic, and midbrain sites. The effects of oxytocin on acetylcholine, gamma-aminobutyric acid (GABA), and other neurotransmitters have not yet been studied.

Oxytocin appears to regulate the release of a number of anterior pituitary hormones. Oxytocinergic fibers, originating from the paraventricular nucleus, terminate in the median eminence (Vandesand and Dierickx 1975). High concentrations of oxytocin have been measured in hypophysial portal blood (Gibbs 1984; Plotsky 1987), suggesting that oxytocin is released into this vascular link between the hypothalamus and the anterior pituitary. Oxytocin affects corticotropin-releasing factor (CRF)–induced adrenocorticotropin (ACTH) release (Legros et al. 1984; Page et al. 1990) and stimulates prolactin and luteinizing hormone release (Johnston and Negro-Vilar 1988; Samson et al. 1986).

Oxytocin concentration in CSF cycles diurnally in primates and man (Reppert 1985). Levels rise three to five times from their low point in the early hours of the morning to their high point in the late afternoon. It may be of significance that this pattern is opposite to the diurnal rhythm of cortisol secretion. In subprimate mammals most diurnal rhythms are controlled by oscillations within the suprachiasmatic nucleus. However, in primates the CSF oxytocin cycle and other diurnal cycles, such as cortisol secretion and body temperature, are independent of the suprachiasmatic nucleus. Perhaps the central oxytocin rhythm serves as a diurnal *Zeitgeber* in primates and man.

MAJOR BEHAVIORAL EFFECTS OF OXYTOCIN

Oxytocin and Memory

Studies of oxytocin effects on memory are summarized in Kovacs (1986). Oxytocin treatment facilitated extinction of learned avoidance behavior, an effect opposite to that of vasopressin. Intracerebroventricular administration of oxytocin antiserum increased retention of passive-avoidance behavior. This evidence has been interpreted to suggest that oxytocin endogenous to the brain is a naturally occurring amnestic substance. Oxytocin effects on retention of avoidance behavior have been localized to the dentate gyrus of the hippocampus and the dorsal raphe nucleus

Oxytocin effects on memory may be mediated by fragments produced by two types of specific peptidases: a C-terminal cleaving peptidase (which releases the terminal tripeptide of oxytocin, prolyl-leucyl-glycinamide [PLG]) and an aminopeptidase that opens the N-terminal ring structure and cleaves several amino acids (Kovacs 1986). Administration of PLG increased retention of learned active-avoidance behavior and reversed retrograde amnesia produced by puromycin, CO_2, and electroconvulsive shock. In contrast, oxytocin 4-9 (a product of N-terminal aminopeptidase activity) facilitated extinction of learned passive-avoidance behavior at one hundredth the minimally effective dose of oxytocin itself.

While numerous studies of vasopressin effects on human memory have been published, only three studies of oxytocin effects have appeared in print. Ferrier et al. (1980) and Kennett et al. (1982) found that intravenous infusion or intranasal inhalation of large doses of oxytocin significantly impaired delayed but not immediate recall of words and associations between paired words. Recall of photographs of faces and associations between pairs of photographs was also impaired.

Fehm-Wolfsdorf et al. (1984) compared the effects of intranasally administered oxytocin, lysine-vasopressin, or placebo on recall of newly and previously presented lists of 15 words. Overall, comparisons of results between all treatment groups were not statistically significant, but, compared with subjects treated with vasopressin, subjects treated with oxytocin exhibited significantly impaired recall of old and newly presented lists. While the results of Ferrier et al. (1980) and Kennett et al. (1982) parallel the results of animal studies suggesting that oxytocin interferes with retention but not acquisition of memory, the results of Fehm-Wolfsdorf et al. (1984) imply that oxytocin may impair both retention and acquisition of memory in man.

Animal and human studies summarized above strongly suggest that oxytocin decreases performance on tests of recall of learned material. Investigators may have been too quick to interpret these effects as primary alterations of memory without carefully assessing oxytocin effects on other cognitive dimensions such as attention, motivation, and perception, deficits of which might account for decrements in recall performance.

Despite the lack of clarity concerning the nature of its effects on recall, oxytocin may play a role in real or perceived cognitive deficits accompanying neurological and psychiatric disorders. Some investigators have reported elevated levels of oxytocin in the hippocampus and temporal cortex of brains from patients with dementia of the Alzheimer type (Mazurek et al. 1987), although CSF levels were normal in this disorder (Raskind et al. 1986). Oxytocin may be a factor in the decreased motivation to perform that cognitively underlies the pseudodementia of major depression.

Oxytocin and Addiction

The development of tolerance to addictive substances has been hypothesized to be a form of adaptation similar to learning. Because of the effects of nonapeptides on memory, a number of investigators have tested the effects of these peptides on the development of tolerance and physical dependence. The results of these experiments suggest that oxytocin does not alter the acute effects of addictive substances (narcotics, ethanol) but does alter changes in response that develop with repeated exposure (Kovacs 1986). Administration of oxytocin to rats prior to acute or chronic morphine treatment significantly inhibited the development of tolerance to morphine analgesia. These effects of oxytocin were localized to the hippocampus and the nucleus accumbens. Central administration of oxytocin antiserum facilitated the development of tolerance. In addition, subcutaneous administration of oxytocin prior to implantation of a morphine pellet prolonged the latency of onset of withdrawal and diminished withdrawal symptoms occurring after naloxone treatment. C-Terminal fragments of oxytocin (PLG, cyclo-Leu-Gly, Pro-Leu) have all been reported to affect narcotic tolerance and dependence. It remains to be determined whether oxytocin effects on tolerance, dependence, or narcotic self-administration (see below) depend on proteolytic cleavage of the nonapeptide molecule. Some investigators have also reported that oxytocin administration decreased tolerance and withdrawal symptoms in ethanol-dependent mice.

Oxytocin may also diminish the reinforcing properties of addictive substances (Kovacs 1986). While oxytocin did not affect the acquisition of heroin self-administration, oxytocin decreased the amount of heroin intake in tolerant rats exhibiting a stable level of heroin self-administration. Antagonism of tolerance and physical dependence may contribute to the decline in heroin self-administration following oxytocin injection. However, oxytocin may also influence brain mechanisms mediating reward. In support of this view, Schwarzberg et al. (1976) found that oxytocin significantly increased electrical self-stimulation in rats with electrodes placed in the medial forebrain bundle, a pathway that has been strongly implicated in positive reinforcement. Further investigation will be required, however, to determine how oxytocin can decrease self-administration of heroin but increase electrical self-stimulation. Perhaps oxytocin substitutes for heroin in activating reward-mediating pathways. On the other hand, oxytocin may increase the potency of heroin in activating those pathways.

Given the compelling animal findings summarized above it is critical that studies of oxytocin effects on drug tolerance, dependence, and self-administration be conducted in man. Deficits in oxytocin release or sensitivity may increase vulnerability to drug dependency. Comparisons of oxytocin effects and oxytocin release between healthy subjects and drug-free addicts would be useful in testing this hypothesis. Oxytocin may also have potential as a treatment for addiction and craving.

Oxytocin and Maternal and Sexual Behavior

Oxytocinergic neurons project to almost every brain site that has been implicated in maternal behavior as well as female and male sexual behavior. Gonadal steroids, which regulate these reproductive behaviors, have powerful effects on oxytocin neurons and receptors in the brain (Pedersen et al. 1988). Behavioral pharmacological studies that are summarized below suggest that central oxytocin regulates maternal and sexual behaviors.

Oxytocin appears to be a physiologically critical trigger for the activation of mothering behavior (Pedersen et al. 1988). Intracerebroventricular administration of oxytocin rapidly induced maternal behavior in virgin rats. This effect of oxytocin was dependent upon estrogen. Intracerebroventricular administration of oxytocin antiserum or a potent oxytocin antagonist blocked the onset of maternal behavior in parturient and ovarian steroid-treated nulliparous rats. Recently, oxytocin has been reported to stimulate maternal behavior in mice and sheep, suggesting that oxytocin may activate mothering in a number of mammalian species.

Central oxytocin systems change markedly near parturition (i.e., the time period during which maternal behavior appears). Between late pregnancy and the morning after parturition in rats, oxytocin content decreases in anterior hypothalamic sites where the peptide is synthesized, while content increases in extrahypothalamic projection sites, some of which (e.g., the ventral septum) are involved in maternal behavioral regulation (Caldwell et al. 1987). These shifts in regional content may reflect transport to and/or release within behaviorally relevant brain sites near the time of parturition. The topography of oxytocin immunostaining in the basal forebrain also undergoes dramatic and complex changes before and after parturition (Jirikowski et al. 1989). Increased numbers of dendrites and an expansion of the dendritic zone occur within the supraoptic nucleus (which contains a large number of oxytocin neurons) during experimental induction of maternal behavior (Salm et al. 1988). The observation of Kendrick et al. (1986) that oxytocin concentration rises in CSF in sheep during labor, parturition, and nursing suggests that oxytocin is released centrally at those times. Oxytocin binding is located in the amygdala, a brain site that has been implicated in the regulation of maternal behavior (Numan 1988; Tribollet et al. 1988; Van Leeuwen et al. 1985). Estrogen, which is critical to the postpartum activation of mothering in animals, increases oxytocin binding in several brain areas, including the amygdala (de Kloet et al. 1986). Postpartum increases in oxytocin binding occur in the bed nucleus of the stria terminalis (Insel 1986).

Intracerebroventricular infusion of oxytocin in rats increases lordosis behavior, the principal component of female sexual receptivity (Pedersen et al. 1988). This effect of oxytocin, like the induction of maternal behavior, was dependent upon estrogen. Oxytocin facilitation of lordosis has been localized to the medial preoptic area and ventromedial nucleus of the hypothalamus. Intromission may release oxytocin within these brain sites. Mating of sexually receptive rats increased oxytocin content and decreased oxytocin immunostaining in the medial preoptic area.

Changes in estrogen and progesterone levels during the ovarian cycle, which regulate female sexual behavior in rodents, also affect oxytocinergic neurons. The oxytocin content of the paraventricular nucleus cycles significantly across the estrous cycle (Greer et al. 1986). Ovarian steroid treatments that stimulate sexual receptivity alter oxytocin content and immunostaining pattern in the basal forebrain (Caldwell et al. 1988). In rats oxytocin concentrations in hypophysial portal blood rise dramatically on the afternoon of proestrus concomitant with the surge in progesterone that stimulates the heightened sexual receptivity appearing on the evening of proestrus (Sarkar and Gibbs 1984).

Long before central effects were investigated, peripheral administration of oxytocin was reported to decrease latency to ejaculate and increase ejaculate size in male rabbits (Fjellstrom et al. 1968). Recently, central administration of oxytocin in rats has been observed to increase the frequency of penile erections (Argiolas et al. 1986) and to alter various dimensions of male sexual behavior (Arletti et al. 1985; Stoneham et al. 1985). In rabbits oxytocin levels in plasma were elevated at the time of ejaculation (Stoneham et al. 1985), while in rats CSF concentrations of oxytocin rose after ejaculation (Hughes et al. 1987). Carmichael et al. (1987) and Murphy et al. (1987) measured significant increases in blood levels of oxytocin during genital self-stimulation and orgasm in men and women. While oxytocin has been reported to be an effective treatment for impotence (Lidberg 1972), its effects on sexual arousal in healthy men and women have yet to be tested.

The parent-infant relationship and sexuality have long been considered critical factors in the development of human personality

(Shapiro and Hertzig 1988). Sexual interest and the protective, nurturing instincts of parents are among the most powerful of motivations in men and women. These fundamental drives are often impaired or distorted by psychiatric disorders. Despite the great importance of these drives, the biological origins of human parental and sexual motivation remain almost unexplored. Studies focusing on neuroendocrine factors, such as oxytocin, that have been implicated by animal studies in the activation of reproductive behaviors may expand our understanding of the physiological basis of parental attachment and sexual interest in man. This, in turn, may provide powerful tools with which to investigate disturbances of relationship formation seen in developmental and personality disorders.

OXYTOCIN AS A FACTOR IN AFFECTIVE DISORDERS

Several lines of evidence suggest that a deficiency of or an insensitivity to oxytocin may contribute to depression. To begin with, oxytocin has potent effects in animal screening tests for antidepressant efficacy. Oxytocin treatment antagonized immobility in the Porsolt swim test and reversed learned helplessness (Arletti and Bertolini 1987; Meisenberg 1981). These effects of oxytocin depended upon proteolytic degradation of the nonapeptide (Arletti and Bertolini 1987). It is of interest that Ehrensing and Kastin (1974, 1978) observed a significant improvement in patients with major depression following administration of PLG, the C-terminal tripeptide of the oxytocin molecule. However, PLG was ineffective in animal screening tests for antidepressant efficacy (Arletti and Bertolini 1987). Treatment with oxytocin itself has not been tested in major depression. In a recent case report (Ansseau et al. 1987), oxytocin improved symptoms of obsessive-compulsive disorder, an illness that often responds to antidepressants.

Oxytocin is a stress hormone (Gibbs 1986) and is released most vigorously under aversive conditions in which test animals are helpless and have no available coping strategy (e.g., immobilization, cold water swim, hanging by the tail). Other stressful situations in which animals can adjust behaviorally (e.g., introduction into a novel cage) are not accompanied by oxytocin release. Oxytocin plays a physiological role in ACTH release under the former but not the latter conditions. These observations, taken together with antidepressant effects, suggest that oxytocin may be an endogenous coping factor. Repeated exposure to uncontrollable stress decreased blood levels of oxytocin in monkeys (Kalin et al 1985). Prolonged exposure to unmanageable stressors may produce depression in humans and depression-like behavioral effects in animals by exhausting oxytocin systems in the brain.

Oxytocin appears to regulate some appetitive, hedonic behaviors that decline in depression. Evidence is summarized above that CNS oxytocin facilitates female and male sexual behavior. Loss of sexual interest is a classic symptom of depression. Oxytocin stimulates maternal behavior in rodents and sheep. As suggested above oxytocin may play a broader role in relationship formation. Depression is often characterized by a loss of interest, confidence, and pleasure in relationships (Hirschfeld and Goodwin 1988). Studies demonstrating release associated with food intake and satiety suggest that oxytocin may mediate some of the rewarding aspects of eating (Verbalis et al. 1986). Loss of appetite or overeating are, of course, other classic symptoms of depression.

Major affective disorders have been associated with a number of hormonal abnormalities. The most common and widely studied neuroendocrine finding in major depression and bipolar disorder is hyperactivity of the hypothalamo-pituitary-adrenal (HPA) axis as indicated by increased levels of cortisol in blood and urine, loss of diurnal variation in blood cortisol levels, and failure to suppress cortisol after dexamethasone (Evans 1988). Decreased stimulated release of prolactin has also been reported in patients with major depression (Grof et al. 1983). Oxytocin may be a physiologically relevant brake on the HPA axis in primates and man. In monkeys oxytocin blood levels rise considerably after treatment with large doses of dexamethasone, implying that oxytocin may be involved in negative feedback on the HPA axis (Kalin et al. 1985). This hypothesis is strengthened by reports that CSF oxytocin levels rise during daylight hours when cortisol levels decline (Reppert 1985). In human subjects oxytocin infusion suppresses ACTH and cortisol levels (Legros et al. 1984). Animal studies have proven oxytocin to be a physiologically significant stimulus for prolactin release (Johnston and Negro-Vilar 1988; Samson et al. 1986). These observations suggest that diminished oxytocin release or insensitivity to oxytocin may account for two of the more prominent neuroendocrine abnormalities associated with major affective disorders, especially HPA axis hyperactivity. CSF oxytocin levels in manic patients are low (Demitrack et al. 1990) but have not been measured in depressive patients.

OXYTOCIN AND PSYCHIATRIC DISORDERS ASSOCIATED WITH FEMALE REPRODUCTIVE STATES

Ovarian steroids potently affect oxytocin content, synthesis, binding, and probably release within the brain (Caldwell et al. 1988, 1989; de

Kloet et al. 1986; Greer et al. 1986; Insel 1986). Central and peripheral oxytocin also regulates ovarian cycling, ovulation, and menstruation, as well as parturition and nursing (Wathes 1984). Reproductive states involving changes in gonadal hormones are often associated with or affected by specific psychiatric disturbances in women. For reasons summarized below, oxytocin may play a role in these psychiatric disorders.

Anorexia Nervosa

CSF oxytocin levels have been reported to be quite low in anorexic patients. Insufficient central oxytocin may produce several of the prominent symptoms of anorexia nervosa, including amenorrhea, preoccupation with and avoidance of food, and poor adjustment to feminine sexual and maternal roles (Halmi et al. 1987). Deficiencies in CNS oxytocin may also contribute to the neuroendocrine abnormalities observed in anorexic patients. Luteinizing hormone (LH) release, which is necessary for ovulation, depends upon oxytocin (Johnston and Negro-Vilar 1988). In preovulatory women oxytocin levels rise in parallel with LH levels (Mitchell et al. 1981; Wathes 1984). Inadequate release of oxytocin into the hypophyseal portal system may result in anovulation and amenorrhea as well as the low blood levels of gonadotropins and decreased estrogen-stimulated LH release found in anorexic patients (Halmi et al. 1987). Release of oxytocin occurs during eating and has been linked to the sensation of satiety (Verbalis et al. 1986). Oxytocin also facilitates sexual and maternal behavior in female animals (Pedersen et al. 1988). Perhaps low central oxytocin activity results in the altered perception of hunger and fullness as well as the diminished sexual and maternal interest exhibited by many anorexic patients. Underweight anorexic individuals usually hypersecrete cortisol and are dexamethasone suppression test nonsuppressors (Halmi et al. 1987). As discussed above, oxytocin probably acts in man as a brake on the HPA axis. Diminished central oxytocin may disinhibit the HPA axis in acutely ill, emaciated anorexic patients.

Premenstrual Syndrome (Late Luteal-Phase Dysphoria)

In addition to ovulation, oxytocin facilitates luteolysis, that is, the regression of the corpus luteum in the midluteal phase of the ovarian cycle, resulting in cessation of progesterone synthesis and subsequently, in primates, menstruation (Wathes 1984). While most experiments on the luteolytic effects of oxytocin have been conducted in farm animals, recent reports suggest that oxytocin has a similar effect in primates and man. Oxytocin is synthesized within the corpus luteum. Under the influence of the midluteal rise in estrogen, oxytocin receptor binding increases in the endometrium. After release from the corpus luteum, oxytocin acts at endometrial receptors to release prostaglandin F2α, which exerts a direct luteolytic effect. Subsequently, oxytocin receptor concentrations diminish as estrogen levels decline. Thus, oxytocin may initiate the late luteal-phase decline in progesterone that corresponds with the onset of symptoms of the premenstrual syndrome (PMS) (Gold 1985).

Central changes in oxytocin release and binding may parallel peripheral changes occurring during the late luteal phase of the menstrual cycle. The observation that breast stimulation releases oxytocin in the luteal phase, but not the follicular phase, suggests that central mechanisms controlling oxytocin also change across the menstrual cycle (Leake and Fisher 1985). Abnormal shifts in central oxytocin systems in the late luteal phase may contribute to the affective lability, anxiety, depression, decreased interest, and altered appetite that are symptoms of PMS.

Postpartum Psychiatric Disorders

Women are at the greatest psychiatric risk of their lives in the first few months of the postpartum period. Oxytocin systems within the brain undergo considerable alteration near parturition and in the postpartum period (Jirikowski et al. 1989). Central release of oxytocin normally increases at parturition and during nursing in animals (Kendrick et al. 1986; Pedersen et al. 1988) and probably in women. Oxytocin may play a role in coping with the stress of the peripartum period and may help stabilize neurotransmitter systems in the midst of the enormous changes in hormone levels occurring at parturition. Aberrant evolution of CNS oxytocin systems in the puerperium may increase vulnerability to postpartum psychiatric disorders.

Three discrete postpartum psychiatric disorders have been described (Inwood 1985): the relatively rare but dramatic postpartum psychosis; the very common, mild, and transient postpartum adjustment disorder with depressed mood ("postpartum blues"); and postpartum major depression. Postpartum psychosis, which usually appears within the first 10 days after the infant is delivered, shares some clinical features with mania. Bipolar women are at considerable risk of developing this psychiatric disorder (Campbell and Winokur 1985). Depressed CSF levels of oxytocin have been reported in mania (Strupp et al. 1986). Perhaps women that develop puerperal psychosis release insufficient oxytocin centrally in the postpartum period. Symptoms of postpartum blues are akin to symptoms of PMS, and, indeed, a prior history of PMS has been related to postpartum mood instability (O'Hara et al. 1984). Changes in central oxytocin release or binding may contribute to the postpartum blues just as we have hypothesized such a mechanism may contribute to PMS.

Postpartum major depression occurs in approximately 10% of new mothers (Inwood 1985). The risk of postpartum major depression is considerably higher in women with a family history of depression (O'Hara 1986). Marital discord is also correlated with postpartum depression (O'Hara 1986). As emphasized above CNS oxytocin systems undergo enormous changes near parturition. Many of the events that are specific to the puerperium (e.g., large changes in ovarian steroid levels, labor and delivery, nursing, attachment to the infant) further tax central oxytocin. In some women, postpartum changes in central oxytocin may be abnormal or CNS oxytocin systems may become depleted. As I have argued in a previous section of this chapter, disturbances of central oxytocin may precipitate major depression.

Inadequate mother-infant bonding may also contribute to depression in the puerperium. Depressed postpartum women often insist that they are failures as mothers and express guilt about not developing warm feelings toward their babies (Brockington and Kumar 1982). While complaints of this sort can be seen as typical depressive self-deprecation, they may also reflect a failure of biological mechanisms, such as CNS oxytocin, that promote emotional attachment to the infant. Indeed, depressed mothers are often significantly impaired in their ability to meet the emotional and physical needs of their children (Zuckerman and Beardslee 1987). Failure of biological attachment mechanisms may leave some women with all of the stressors of new motherhood and none of the rewarding feelings of love toward their newborns. This difficult situation may lead to depression especially in those who are genetically predisposed and have no compensatory support from the father of the child.

CONCLUSIONS

Animal studies reviewed in this chapter have firmly established that CNS oxytocin activates some rewarding behaviors (e.g., maternal and sexual behaviors) and influences aspects of adaptation (e.g., recall of learned avoidance behavior, tolerance to addictive substances, ACTH release under specific stressful conditions). Oxytocin very likely affects other rewarding and adaptive behaviors as well (e.g., eating). The network of oxytocinergic projections within the brain may allow this nonapeptide to coordinate appropriate neurotransmitter, endocrine, and autonomic responses with each of these behavioral states. Dysregulation of CNS oxytocin systems may contribute to the disturbances of thought, mood, and behavior, as well as the neurochemical and neuroendocrine abnormalities that characterize specific psychiatric syndromes. In this chapter I have emphasized the role of oxytocin in mood disorders, psychiatric disorders associated with changes in female reproductive states, and addiction. However, its full spectrum of effects suggests that oxytocin may be a determinant of a broader range of psychopathology, including personality disorders, dementias, sleep disorders, primary sexual disorders, and psychotic disorders. Clearly the time has come for an increased focus on oxytocin in studies of normal and pathological human behavior.

REFERENCES

Ansseau M, Legros JJ, Mormont C, et al: Intranasal oxytocin in obsessive-compulsive disorder. Psychoneuroendocrinology 12:231–236, 1987

Argiolas A, Melis MR, Gessa GL: Oxytocin: an extremely potent inducer of penile erection and yawning in male rats. Eur J Pharmacol 130:265–272, 1986

Arletti R, Bertolini A: Oxytocin acts as an antidepressant in two animal models of depression. Life Sci 41:1725–1730, 1987

Arletti R, Bazzani C, Castelli M, et al: Oxytocin improves male copulatory performance in rats. Horm Behav 19:14–20, 1985

Beckmann H, Lang RE, Gattza WF: Vasopressin-oxytocin in cerebrospinal fluid of schizophrenic patients and normal controls. Psychoneuroendocrinology 10:187–191, 1985

Brockington JD, Kumar R (eds): Motherhood and Mental Illness. New York, Grune & Stratton, 1982

Buijs RM, De Vries GJ, Van Leeuwen FW: The distribution and synaptic release of oxytocin in the central nervous system, in Oxytocin: Clinical and Laboratory Studies. Edited by Amico JA, Robinson AG. Amsterdam, Elsevier, 1985, pp 77–86

Caldwell JD, Greer ER, Johnson MF, et al: Oxytocin and vasopressin immunoreactivity in hypothalamic and extrahypothalamic sites in late pregnant and postpartum rats. Neuroendocrinology 46:39–47, 1987

Caldwell JD, Jirikowski GF, Greer ER, et al: Ovarian steroids and sexual interaction alter oxytocinergic content and distribution in the basal forebrain. Brain Res 446:236–244, 1988

Caldwell JD, Brooks PJ, Jirikowski GF, et al: Estrogen alters oxytocin mRNA levels in the preoptic area. J Neuroendocrinol 1:273–278, 1989

Campbell JL, Winokur G. Postpartum affective disorders: selected biological aspects, in Recent Advances in Postpartum Psychiatric Disorders. Edited by Inwood DG. Washington DC, American Psychiatric Press, 1985, pp 19–39

Carmichael MS, Humbert R, Dixen J, et al: Plasma oxytocin increases in the human sexual response. J Clin Endocrinol Metab 64:27–31, 1987

de Kloet ER, Voorhuis DAM, Boschma Y, et al: Estradiol modulates density of putative "oxytocin receptors" in discrete rat brain regions. Neuroendocrinology 44:415–421, 1986

Demitrack MA, Lesem MD, Listwak SJ, et al: CSF oxytocin in anorexia nervosa and bulimia nervosa: clinical and pathophysiologic considerations. Am J Psychiatry 147:882–886, 1990

Ehrensing RH, Kastin AJ: Melanocyte-stimulating hormone-release inhibiting hormone as an antidepressant. Arch Gen Psychiatry 30:63–65, 1974

Ehrensing RH, Kastin AJ: Dose-related biphasic effect of prolyl-leucylglycinamide (MIF-I) in depression. Am J Psychiatry 135:562–566, 1978

Evans DL: Use of the dexamethasone suppression test in clinical psychiatry, in Recent Advances in Hypothalamic-Pituitary-Adrenal Axis: Physiology and Pathophysiology. Edited by Nemeroff CB, Schatzburg AS. New York, Raven, 1988, pp 133–155

Fehm-Wolfsdorf G, Born J, Voight K, et al: Human memory and neurohypophyseal hormones: opposite effects of vasopressin and oxytocin. Psychoneuroendocrinology 9:285–292, 1984

Ferrier BM, Kennett DJ, Devlin MC: Influence of oxytocin on human memory processes. Life Sci 27:2311–2317, 1980

Fjellstrom D, Kihlstrom JE, Melin P: The effect of synthetic oxytocin upon seminal characteristics and sexual behavior in male rabbits. J Reprod Fertil 17:207–209, 1968

Gibbs DM: High concentrations of oxytocin in hypophyseal portal plasma. Endocrinology 124:1216–1218, 1984

Gibbs DM: Vasopressin and oxytocin: hypothalamic modulators of the stress response: a review. Psychoneuroendocrinology 22:131–140, 1986

Gilbey MP, Coote JH, Fleetwood-Walker S, et al: The influence of the paraventriculo-spinal pathway, and oxytocin and vasopressin on sympathetic preganglionic neurones. Brain Res 252:283–290, 1982

Gold JH (ed): The Psychiatric Implications of Menstruation. Washington DC, American Psychiatric Press, 1985

Greer ER, Caldwell JD, Johnson MF, et al: Variations in concentration of oxytocin and vasopressin in the paraventricular nucleus of the hypothalamus during the estrous cycle in rats. Life Sci 38:2311–2318, 1986

Grof E, Brown GM, Grof P: Neuroendocrine strategies in affective disorders. Prog Neuropharmacol Biol Psychiatry 7:557–562, 1983

Halmi KA, Ackerman S, Gibbs J, et al: Basic biological overview of the eating disorders, in Psychopharmacology: The Third Generation of Progress. Edited by Meltzer HY. New York, Raven, 1987, pp 1255–1266

Hancock MB, Nicholas AP: Oxytocin-immunoreactive projections onto medullary adrenaline neurons. Brain Res Bull 18:213–219, 1987

Hirschfeld RMA, Goodwin FK: Mood disorders, in The American Psychiatric Press Textbook of Psychiatry. Edited by Talbott JA, Hales RE, Yudofsky SC. Washington, DC, American Psychiatric Press, 1988, pp 403–441

Hughes AM, Everitt BJ, Lightman SL, et al: Oxytocin in the central nervous system and sexual behavior in male rats. Brain Res 414:133–137, 1987

Insel TR: Postpartum increases in brain oxytocin binding. Neuroendocrinology 44:515–518, 1986

Inwood DG: The spectrum of postpartum psychiatric disorders, in Recent Advances in Postpartum Psychiatric Disorders. Edited by Inwood DG. Washington DC, American Psychiatric Press, 1985, pp 1–18

Jirikowski GF, Caldwell JD, Pilgrim CH, et al: Changes in oxytocin immunostaining in the female rat forebrain during late pregnancy, parturition and early lactation. Cell Tissue Res 256:411–417, 1989

Johnston CA, Negro-Vilar A: Role of oxytocin in prolactin secretion during proestrus and in different physiological or pharmacological paradigms. Endocrinology 122:341–350, 1988

Kalin NH, Gibbs DM, Barksdale CM, et al: Behavioral stress decreases plasma oxytocin concentrations in primates. Life Sci 36:1275–1280, 1985

Kendrick KM, Keverne EB, Baldwin BA, et al: Cerebrospinal fluid levels of acetylcholinesterase, monoamines and oxytocin during labour, parturition, vaginocervical stimulation, lamb separation and suckling in sheep. Neuroendocrinology 44:149–156, 1986

Kennett DJ, Devlin MC, Ferrier BM: Influence of oxytocin on human memory processes: validation by a control study. Life Sci 31:273–275, 1982

Kovacs GL: Oxytocin and behavior, in Neurobiology of Oxytocin. Edited by Ganten D, Pfaff D. Heidelberg, Springer-Verlag, 1986, pp 91–120

Leake RD, Fisher DA: Oxytocin secretion and milk ejection in the human, in Oxytocin: Clinical and Laboratory Studies. Edited by Amico JA, Robinson AG. Amsterdam, Elsevier, 1985, pp 200–206

Legros JJ, Chiodera P, Geenen V, et al: Dose-response relationship between plasma oxytocin and cortisol and adrenocorticotropin concentrations during oxytocin infusion in normal men. J Clin Endocrinol Metab 58:105–109, 1984

Lidberg L: The effect of Syntocinon® on patients suffering from impotence. Pharmacopsychiatry 5:187–190, 1972

Linkowski P, Geenen V, Kerkhofs M, et al: Cerebrospinal fluid neurophysins in affective illness and in schizophrenia. Eur Arch Psychiatry Neurol Sci 234:162–165, 1984

Mazurek MF, Beal MF, Bird ED, et al: Oxytocin in Alzheimer's disease: postmortem brain levels. Neurology 37:1001–1003, 1987

Meisenberg G: Short-term behavioral effects of posterior pituitary peptides in mice. Peptides 2:1–8, 1981

Meltzer HY (ed): Psychopharmacology: The Third Generation of Progress. New York, Raven, 1987

Mitchell MD, Haynes PJ, Anderson ABM, et al: Plasma oxytocin concentrations during the menstrual cycle. Eur J Obstet Gynecol Reprod Biol 12:195–200, 1981

Murphy MR, Seckl JR, Burton SA, et al: Changes in oxytocin and vasopressin secretion during sexual activity in men. J Clin Endocrinol Metab 65:738–741, 1987

Nicholson HD, Swann RW, Burford GD, et al: Identification of oxytocin and vasopressin in the testis and in adrenal tissue. Regul Pept 8:141–146, 1984

Numan M: Maternal behavior, in The Physiology of Reproduction. Edited by Knobil E, Neill J. New York, Raven, 1988, pp 1569–1645

O'Hara MW: Social support, life events, and depression during pregnancy and the puerperium. Arch Gen Psychiatry 43:569–573, 1986

O'Hara MW, Neubaer DJ, Zekoski EM: A prospective study of postpartum depression: prevalence, course and predictive factors. J Abnorm Psychol 93:158–171, 1984

Page SR, Ang VTY, Jackson R, et al: The effect of oxytocin infusion on adenohypophyseal function in man. Clin Endocrinol 32:307–313, 1990

Pedersen CA, Caldwell JD, Jirikowski GF: Oxytocin and reproductive behaviors, in Recent Progress in Posterior Pituitary Hormones. Edited by Yoshida S, Share L. Amsterdam, Elsevier, 1988, pp 141–149

Plotsky PM: Regulation of hypophysiotropic factors mediating ACTH secretion. Ann N Y Acad Sci 512:205–217, 1987

Raskind MA, Peskind ER, Lampe TH, et al: Cerebrospinal fluid vasopressin, oxytocin, somatostatin, and β-endorphin in Alzheimer's disease. Arch Gen Psychiatry 43:382–388, 1986

Reppert SM: Circadian rhythm of oxytocin in primate cerebrospinal fluid, in Oxytocin: Clinical and Laboratory Studies. Edited by Amico JA, Robinson AG. Amsterdam, Elsevier, 1985, pp 133–142

Salm AK, Modney BK, Hatton GI: Alterations in supraoptic nucleus ultrastructure of maternally behaving virgin rats. Brain Res Bull 231:685–691, 1988

Samson WK, Lumpkin MD, McCann SM: Evidence for a physiological role for oxytocin in the control of prolactin secretion. Endocrinology 119:554–560, 1986

Sarkar SK, Gibbs DM: Cyclic variation of oxytocin in the blood of pituitary portal vessels of rats. Neuroendocrinology 39:481–483, 1984

Schwarzberg H, Hartmann G, Kovacs GL, et al: The effect of intraventricular administration of oxytocin and vasopressin on self-stimulation of rats. Acta Physiol Hung 47:127–131, 1976

Shapiro T, Hertzig ME: Normal growth and development, in The American Psychiatric Press Textbook of Psychiatry. Edited by Talbott JA, Hales RE, Yudofsky SC. Washington, DC, American Psychiatric Press, 1988, pp 91–122

Sofroniew MB, Schrell U: Evidence for a direct projection from oxytocin and vasopressin neurons in the hypothalamic paraventricular nucleus to the medulla oblongata: immunohistochemical visualization of both the horseradish peroxidase transported and the peptide produced by the same neurons. Neurosci Lett 22:211–217, 1981

Stoneham MD, Everitt BJ, Hansen S, et al: Oxytocin and sexual behaviour in the male rat and rabbit. J Endocrinol 107:97–106, 1985

Swanson LW, McKellar S: The distribution of oxytocin- and neurophysin-sustained fibers in the spinal cord of the rat and monkey. J Comp Neurol 188:87–106, 1979

Tran LD, Montastruc JL, Montastruc P: Effects of lysine-vasopressin and oxytocin on central cardiovascular control. Br J Pharmacol 77:69–73, 1982

Tribollet E, Barberis C, Jard S, et al: Localization and pharmacological characterization of high affinity sites for vasopressin and oxytocin in the rat brain by light microscopic autoradiography. Brain Res 442:105–118, 1988

Vandesand F, Dierickx K: Identification of the vasopressin-producing and of the oxytocin-producing neurons in the hypothalamic magnocellular neurosecretory system of the rat. Cell Tissue Res 164:153–162, 1975

Van Leeuwen FW, Van Heerikhuize J, Van der Meulen G, et al: Light microscopic autoradiographic localization of ^{3}H-oxytocin binding sites in the rat brain, pituitary and mammary glands. Brain Res 359:320–325, 1985

Verbalis JG, McCann MJ, McHale CM, et al: Oxytocin secretion in response to cholecystokinin and food: differentiation of nausea from satiety. Science 232:1417–1419, 1986

Versteeg CA, Bohus B, DeJong W: Inhibitory effects of neuropeptides on centrally evoked pressor responses, in Prophylactic Approach to Hypertensive Diseases. Edited by Yamori Y. New York, Raven, 1979, pp 329–335

Wathes DC: Possible actions of gonadal oxytocin and vasopressin. J Reprod Fertil 71:315–345, 1984

Zuckerman BS, Beardslee WR: Maternal depression: a concern for pediatricians. Pediatrics 79:110–117, 1987

Chapter 9

Neurotensin

Beth Levant, Ph.D.
Garth Bissette, Ph.D.
Charles B. Nemeroff, M.D., Ph.D.

Chapter 9

Neurotensin

One of the most exciting recent developments in biological psychiatry has been the discovery of the involvement of neuromodulatory peptides in the action of classical neurotransmitters in the central nervous system (CNS). Since the isolation and characterization of neurotensin by Carraway and Leeman (1973, 1975), considerable progress has been made toward elucidating the role of this neuropeptide in the CNS. The interaction between this endogenous tridecapeptide and the classical catecholamine neurotransmitter dopamine has been of particular interest, for these two systems may be integrally involved in the pathogenesis of schizophrenia as well as in the mechanism of action of antipsychotic drugs. In this chapter we focus on interactions of neurotensin and dopamine in the CNS and the clinical implications of these interactions. Recent findings from our laboratory are highlighted.

Neurotensin (pyro-Glu-Leu-Tyr-Glu-Asn-Lys-Pro-Arg-Arg-Pro-Tyr-Ile-Leu-OH), first identified in bovine hypothalamic extracts, has been found to exist in all classes of vertebrates. In the CNS of humans and other mammals, neurotensin is heterogeneously distributed, with relatively high concentrations in the substantia nigra, periaqueductal gray matter, amygdala, nucleus accumbens, and certain hypothalamic nuclei; moderate concentrations in the caudate nucleus, globus pallidus, and hippocampus; low concentrations in the cerebral cortex and cerebellum (Manberg et al. 1982). The neuroanatomic localization of neurotensin-containing cell bodies has been achieved, and certain of the putative projections of these cell bodies have also been identified. Among these putative pathways, and of particular interest, is a neurotensin projection from the ventral tegmental area (VTA) (A_{10}) to the nucleus accumbens (Kalivas and Miller 1984).

Neurotensin receptors appear to be composed of two different subunits (each molecular weight 50,000) linked by a noncovalent

Supported by National Institute of Mental Health Grant MH-39415 and the Schizophrenia Research Foundation. We are grateful to Sheila Walker for preparation of this manuscript.

bond (Mazella et al. 1985). These receptors have been found to be coupled to G-proteins that modulate intracellular levels of cyclic nucleotides and inositol phosphates in cultured neuroblastoma cells (Mazella et al. 1987). Saturable, reversible, high-affinity binding of $[^{125}I]$neurotensin and $[^{3}H]$neurotensin has been observed in membrane preparations from rat and human brain (Kanba et al. 1986). Recently, two neurotensin receptor subtypes with different subcellular localizations and affinities for neurotensin and other drugs have been detected (Schotte et al. 1988). Autoradiographic studies have revealed a heterogeneous distribution of neurotensin receptors that parallels the distribution of this tridecapeptide in many brain regions, with notable exceptions being in the cortex, where neurotensin is low and receptor density is high (Lazarus et al. 1977), and in the striatum, where the converse is true (Goedert et al. 1983). The areas of highest receptor density include the zona compactae of the substantia nigra (A_9) and the VTA (A_{10}) dopamine cell body regions, and dopamine terminal fields such as the frontal cortex and the olfactory tubercles (Young and Kuhar 1981). A similar distribution of neurotensin receptors has been found in the human brain (Sarrieu et al. 1985).

In addition to the aforementioned findings that describe a heterogeneous CNS distribution of neurotensin, the projection of known neurotensin neuronal pathways, and the location and characteristics of saturable and specific binding of this neuropeptide to neurotensin receptors, neurotensin has satisfied several other criteria for recognition as a neurotransmitter. Although the biosynthetic pathway for neurotensin has yet to be thoroughly described, the rat gene encoding this tridecapeptide has been isolated and sequenced, and the tissue-specific expression determined (Kislauskis et al. 1988). Synaptic localization of neurotensin (Kataoka et al. 1979), release upon neuronal depolarization (Iversen et al. 1978), and degradation by peptidases (Dupont and Merand 1978) have been demonstrated. Neurotensin-containing vesicles in nerve terminals have also been observed in electron micrographs (Uhl and Snyder 1977).

NEUROTENSIN-DOPAMINE INTERACTIONS

Neurotensin appears to interact with a number of classical neurotransmitter systems including certain dopaminergic, cholinergic, serotonergic, and noradrenergic neurons, and produces a variety of pharmacological effects that are beyond the scope of this chapter (for extensive review see Levant and Nemeroff 1988). The interactions between neurotensin and the CNS dopaminergic systems are of particular interest because of their potential involvement in schizophrenia and antipsychotic drug action (see below). Consequently, neurotensin's effects on dopaminergic neurons have been evaluated more extensively than the interactions with other neurotransmitters. It is also important to note that the doses of centrally administered neurotensin that alter dopaminergic neuronal activity are, in general, considerably lower than those affecting other neurotransmitter systems.

Anatomical Evidence

Neurotensin and dopamine have been shown to have a largely overlapping distribution in the CNS (Anderson et al. 1984) and are colocalized with dopamine in a number of brain nuclei, such as the arcuate (A_{12}) and periventricular (A_{14}) nuclei of the hypothalamus and in some mesencephalic dopaminergic neurons, particularly the retrorubral area (A_8), substantia nigra (A_9), and VTA (A_{10}) (Hökfelt et al. 1984). Accordingly, 6-hydroxydopamine (6-OHDA) lesions of dopaminergic neurons in the VTA were found to produce an increase in neurotensin binding sites in the prefrontal cortex (Tassin et al. 1988), indicating a potential decrease in neurotensin release in this region. A decrease in neurotensin concentration was also found in that brain region by these investigators but not in the striatum or nucleus accumbens (Studler et al. 1988). In contrast, our group has found that destruction of dopaminergic neurons with 6-OHDA fails to produce decreases in neurotensin concentration in the frontal cortex, nucleus accumbens, or caudate nucleus (Bissette et al. 1983); nor are neurotensin concentrations altered in Parkinson's disease where nigroneostriatal and mesolimbic dopaminergic pathways degenerate, except in the hippocampus (Bissette et al. 1985). However, treatment with 1-methyl-4-phenyl-1,2,3,6-tetrahydropyridine (MPTP) does decrease neurotensin concentration in several dopaminergic terminal regions in the mouse (Levant et al. 1988b). While these findings appear to be discrepant, it is likely that the subpopulation of neurons in which neurotensin and dopamine are colocalized are either not susceptible to the neuronal degeneration observed after 6-OHDA or in Parkinson's disease, or they represent only a small percentage of these dopaminergic cells. Alternatively, the neurotensin immunoreactivity in the VTA is mostly contained in nerve terminals and not in perikarya, making it impossible to detect a decrease in the concentration of the peptide after lesions of dopaminergic cell bodies in this region.

Neurotensin binding sites have been found in high density on dopaminergic perikarya in such areas as the substantia nigra (A_9) and the VTA (A_{10}) (Palacios and Kuhar 1981) and on some dopaminergic terminals and terminal fields (Quirion et al. 1985). The density of neurotensin binding sites in these dopaminergic terminal areas appears to be regulated by dopaminergic neurotransmission (Herve et al. 1986).

Electrophysiological and Neurochemical Evidence

Neurotensin appears to have a stimulatory effect on dopaminergic neurons. In electrophysiological studies, iontophoretically applied neurotensin produced excitation of midbrain dopaminergic neurons (Andrade and Aghajanian 1981). The peptide has also been shown to increase tyrosine hydroxylase activity (Reches et al. 1982) and to increase dopamine release from a variety of in vitro brain slice preparations (Myers and Lee 1984a, 1984b; Starr 1982). Likewise, neurotensin has been found to potentiate the release of endogenous dopamine from striatal synaptosomes (Jiang et al. 1988). In vivo intracisternal or intracerebroventricular administration of neurotensin increases dopamine turnover as determined by increased concentrations of the dopamine metabolites 3,4-dihydroxyphenylacetic acid (DOPAC) and homovanillic acid (HVA), especially in the mesolimbic dopaminergic terminal fields, and by increased accumulation of dopa after treatment with the L-aromatic amino acid decarboxylase inhibitor NSD 1015 (Widerlöv et al. 1982a). While intracisternal neurotensin increases dopamine turnover in the nucleus accumbens, the olfactory tubercles, and the striatum (Nemeroff et al. 1983a), microinjection of neurotensin into the VTA (A_{10}) results in a selective increase in dopamine turnover only in the nucleus accumbens and olfactory tubercles, terminal regions of the mesolimbic dopaminergic projection (Kalivas and Taylor 1985).

Pharmacological Evidence

Central administration of pharmacological doses of neurotensin produces a variety of behavioral effects that require the integrity of CNS dopaminergic systems. The effects of neurotensin on locomotor behavior depend on whether neurotensin is applied to dopaminergic perikarya or dopaminergic terminal fields. Microinjection of neurotensin into the VTA, the site of origin of the dopaminergic perikarya that comprise the mesolimbicocortical dopaminergic system, produces a dose-related increase in exploratory behaviors such as locomotion, sniffing, and rearing (Kalivas et al. 1981). This increase in motor activity is associated with an increase in dopamine utilization in the nucleus accumbens, a major terminal field of the mesolimbic dopaminergic projection (Kalivas et al. 1983). Conversely, when administered intracerebroventricularly (Nemeroff et al. 1977) or microinjected directly into the nucleus accumbens, neurotensin produces a dose-dependent antagonism of dopamine-induced locomotion and rearing. Moreover, bilateral injection of neurotensin into the nucleus accumbens blocks the stimulatory effects of this tridecapeptide applied to the VTA (Kalivas et al. 1982).

As would be predicted from the data described above, neurotensin antagonizes many of the behavioral effects induced by the indirect dopamine agonist dextroamphetamine. Bilateral injections of neurotensin into the nucleus accumbens antagonize the increases in locomotor activity observed after parenteral dextroamphetamine administration. In contrast, intracaudate injection of neurotensin fails to block amphetamine-induced stereotypy (Ervin et al. 1981). Intracisternally administered neurotensin also blocks methylphenidate- and cocaine-induced hyperactivity in both mice and rats (Nemeroff et al. 1983a); however, neurotensin has no effect on scopolamine- or caffeine-induced increases in locomotion (Skoog et al. 1986). Thus, the antagonism of drug-induced locomotor hyperactivity appears to be limited to those pharmacological agents that activate the mesolimbic dopaminergic system. Furthermore, we have recently shown that L-dopa–induced locomotor activity in rats with dopaminergic neurons destroyed by 6-OHDA is blocked by intra-accumbens injection of neurotensin (Ervin and Nemeroff 1988). This is conclusive evidence that the action of neurotensin is on neurons postsynaptic to the dopaminergic neurons.

In addition to altering locomotor behavior, centrally administered neurotensin alters a number of other dopamine-mediated behaviors. Neurotensin injection into the VTA has been shown to produce aphagia (Luttinger et al. 1982a), to have a rewarding effect (Glimcher et al. 1987), and to alter learning and memory performance in several conditioned avoidance paradigms (Luttinger et al. 1982b; van Wimersma Greidanus et al. 1982).

SIMILARITY OF NEUROTENSIN TO ANTIPSYCHOTIC DRUGS

In addition to altering behaviors that are clearly dopamine-mediated, centrally administered neurotensin produces a number of other pharmacological effects (see Levant and Nemeroff 1988). There is a remarkable similarity between these pharmacological actions of neurotensin and those of clinically efficacious antipsychotic drugs. Briefly, both centrally administered neurotensin and neuroleptics increase dopamine turnover in the nucleus accumbens, the olfactory tubercles, and, to a lesser extent, the caudate nucleus. Likewise, neurotensin and neuroleptics both potentiate barbiturate- and ethanol-induced sedation, produce hypothermia, decrease locomotor activity, produce catalepsy and muscle relaxation, and inhibit avoidance (but not escape) behavior in a conditioned-avoidance behavioral paradigm. Furthermore, as noted above, neurotensin, like antipsychotic drugs, blocks the hyperactivity produced by dextroamphetamine and other psychostimulants.

Although neurotensin shares several pharmacological properties with antipsychotic drugs, some differences exist. While classical neuroleptics inhibit the binding of radiolabeled dopamine agonists and antagonists to CNS membrane receptors, neurotensin fails to alter the binding of the dopamine antagonist [^{3}H]spiperone in the rat CNS in vitro and ex vivo (Nemeroff et al. 1983a). Furthermore, while haloperidol blocks dextroamphetamine-induced hyperactivity and stereotypy, neurotensin blocks only the former. In this way, neurotensin is similar to the atypical antipsychotic drugs such as clozapine that also fail to antagonize dextroamphetamine-induced stereotypy. Finally, intracerebroventricular neurotensin produces antinociception, whereas neuroleptics do not.

EFFECT OF DOPAMINERGIC NEURONAL MANIPULATIONS ON ENDOGENOUS NEUROTENSIN

Chronic treatment with antipsychotic drugs increases neurotensin concentrations in certain brain areas in the rat, particularly the nucleus accumbens and the striatum, terminal fields of the mesolimbic and nigroneostriatal dopaminergic projections, respectively. Increases in neurotensin concentration in the nucleus accumbens were seen 16 hours after a single dose of haloperidol and persisted for at least 8 hours. Maximal increases were seen after 14 days of daily injections. Similar increases in neurotensin concentration in the nucleus accumbens were also observed after chronic treatment with other clinically effective antipsychotic drugs, including chlorpromazine, trifluoperazine, and pimozide. Two clinically ineffective phenothiazines, promazine and promethazine, failed to produce any increase in neurotensin concentration in this brain area (Govoni et al. 1980). Interestingly, withdrawal from long-term (8-month) haloperidol administration decreases neurotensin concentration in the caudate nucleus and nucleus accumbens to below control levels (Radke et al. 1989). This rebound decrease may result from the renewed stimulation of dopamine receptors rendered supersensitive by haloperidol, thus leading to a decrease in neurotensin synthesis. A less likely alternative is that long-term haloperidol treatment may have a toxic effect on neurotensin-containing neurons.

Our group has studied the increase in neurotensin concentration after treatment with other dopamine receptor antagonists. We treated rats chronically with the dopamine antagonist (+)-butaclamol, or (−)-butaclamol, which possesses all of the properties of the (+)-enantiomer except dopamine receptor blockade–mediated antipsychotic activity. The (+)-butaclamol produced an increase in neurotensin concentration in the nucleus accumbens and caudate nucleus, whereas the (−)-isomer did not (Bissette et al. 1988a). D_2 receptors appear to be the principal dopamine receptor subtype involved in the neurotensin alterations observed after chronic dopaminergic blockade (Letter et al. 1987). Furthermore, recent evidence suggests that the number of neurotensin-immunoreactive neurons in the striatum increases after treatment with haloperidol (Eggerman and Zahm 1988), and this increase may be responsible for the observed increase in neurotensin concentration.

The atypical antipsychotic drug clozapine, which purportedly produces no acute extrapyramidal side effects or tardive dyskinesia (Rupniak et al. 1984), has been observed by our group to increase neurotensin concentration in the nucleus accumbens but not in the caudate nucleus (Kilts et al. 1988). This increase in neurotensin concentration in the nucleus accumbens, produced by both haloperidol and clozapine, may be a function of their actions at limbic and cortical dopaminergic terminal fields, reflecting their shared properties as effective antipsychotic agents. Because haloperidol increased neurotensin concentration in the caudate nucleus while clozapine did not, it was hypothesized that the lack of untoward extrapyramidal effects of clozapine may be related to its inability to increase neurotensin concentration in the caudate nucleus. One possibility, of course, is that this phenomenon might be mediated by the drug's intrinsic anticholinergic activity; however, recent findings in our laboratory have shown that anticholinergic drugs, such as atropine, administered concomitantly with antidopaminergic drugs do not modulate the regional specificity of the neurotensin alterations produced by dopamine receptor blockade, nor do anticholinergic drugs increase neurotensin concentration when administered alone (Levant et al. 1988a). Thus, the data accumulated to date are concordant with the hypothesis that the increase in neurotensin concentrations in the nucleus accumbens after antipsychotic drug treatment is predictive of antipsychotic drug efficacy, whereas the increase in neurotensin in the caudate nucleus is indicative of a liability toward extrapyramidal effects and/or tardive dyskinesia.

The increases in regional neurotensin concentration observed after treatment with antipsychotic drugs do not require the integrity of mesolimbic and nigrostriatal dopaminergic projections. Haloperidol produced increases in neurotensin concentrations in the nucleus accumbens and caudate of rats after destruction of dopaminergic neurons by 6-OHDA (Bissette et al. 1988b). Thus, while the postsynaptic dopamine receptor seems to be required for antipsychotic drug-induced increases in neurotensin concentration in these brain regions, the presynaptic dopaminergic neuron does not.

The effects of several direct and indirect dopamine agonists on regional brain neurotensin concentrations have also been evaluated. Interestingly, chronic treatment with the direct dopamine agonist bromocriptine increases the concentration of neurotensin in the substantia nigra, whereas treatment with L-dopa decreases neurotensin concentration in this region (DeCeballos et al. 1986). Drugs that purportedly increase dopamine availability in the synapse, such as methamphetamine and its derivatives, have been shown to increase neurotensin concentration in the striatum, the nucleus accumbens, and the substantia nigra (Merchant et al. 1987). It should be noted, however, that the doses of methamphetamine and its derivatives used in these studies were quite large. The effects on regional neurotensin concentration may therefore be the result of neurotoxic effects of the psychostimulants or depolarization block of the dopaminergic neurons rather than dopamine receptor activation.

In addition to alterations in the concentrations of neurotensin in certain brain areas, chronic treatment with neuroleptic drugs produces an increase in the number of neurotensin receptors in the rat substantia nigra (Uhl and Kuhar 1984). Finally, it should be noted that stress, which is known to activate the mesolimbic dopaminergic system, also increases the concentration of neurotensin in the VTA (Deutch et al. 1987).

CLINICAL STUDIES

Neurotensin concentrations have been measured in cerebrospinal fluid (CSF) and in various postmortem brain regions of patients with a variety of neuropsychiatric disorders. Our group has measured the concentration of neurotensin in CSF of drug-free schizophrenic patients and healthy control subjects. Schizophrenic patients were found to have lower mean CSF neurotensin concentrations than did age- and sex-matched control subjects, as shown in Figure 9-1 (Lindström et al. 1988; Nemeroff et al. 1989). Moreover, in a group of schizophrenic patients who were found to have low CSF neurotensin concentrations, these concentrations were observed to increase to normal levels after treatment with neuroleptic drugs for 1 month (Widerlöv et al. 1982b). In a study of postmortem brain samples from

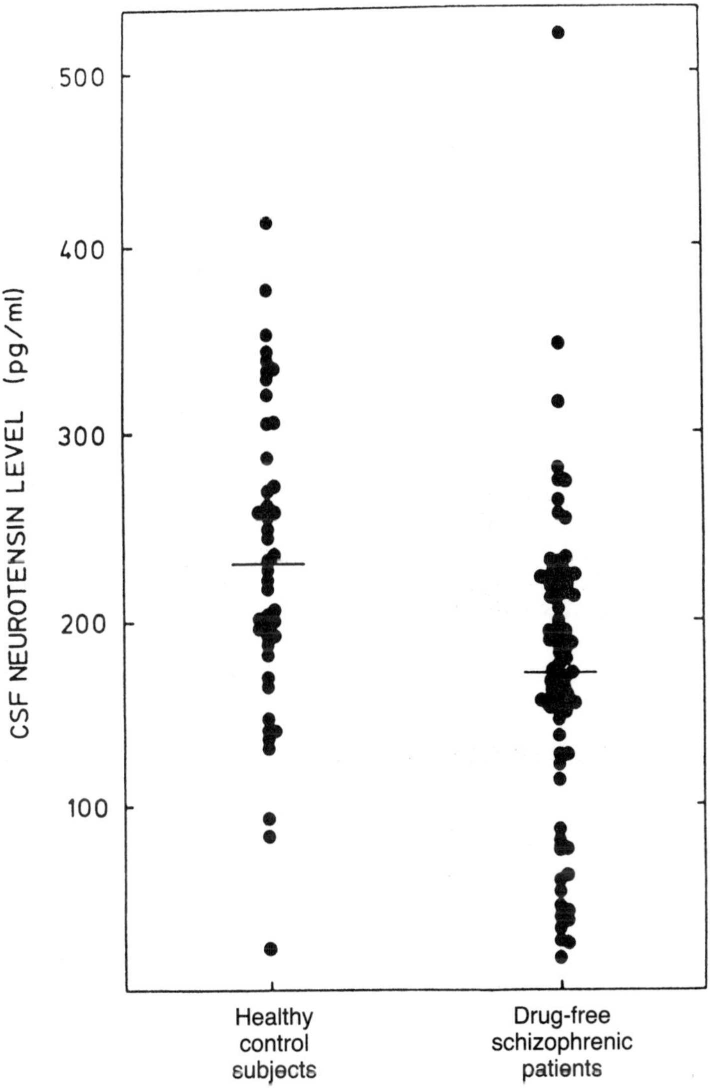

Figure 9-1. CSF concentrations of neurotensin in healthy control subjects (left) and drug-free schizophrenic patients (right). As a group, the schizophrenic patients have a lower CSF neurotensin concentration than do healthy volunteers. The horizontal bars indicate the means. Reprinted, with permission, from Lindström et al. 1988. Copyright 1988, Elsevier Science Publishers.

schizophrenic patients, neurotensin concentration was found to be increased in Brodmann's area 32 of the frontal cortex (Nemeroff et al. 1983b). Several alterations in neurotensin neurons have been reported in patients with Parkinson's disease. The concentration of neurotensin has been reported to be decreased in the hippocampus, but not in the substantia nigra, VTA, striatum, nucleus accumbens, or frontal cortex, in postmortem samples from patients with Parkinson's disease (Bissette et al. 1985). In addition, decreased neurotensin binding has been observed in the substantia nigra of patients with Parkinson's disease, indicating a depletion of nigral neurotensin receptors (Sadoul et al. 1984), as would be expected in view of the well-documented loss of nigral dopaminergic neurons.

While diseases affecting the dopaminergic systems have been of principal interest, alterations in neurotensin concentration in CSF, brain tissue, or plasma have been observed in several other neuropsychiatric disorders, including Huntington's disease, Down's syndrome, and menopausal hot flashes. Neurotensin concentrations have, to date, been found to be unaltered in depression, anorexia-bulimia, premenstrual syndrome (Nemeroff et al. 1989), and Alzheimer's disease. We have also found no evidence for a rostral-caudal gradient for neurotensin in CSF nor any age or sex effect. However, we have recently reported in infants very high CSF neurotensin concentrations that decline rapidly in childhood (Hedner et al. 1989). Neurotensin alterations in neuropsychiatric disorders are summarized in Table 9-1.

CONCLUSIONS

There is considerable evidence that neurotensin fulfills many of the requisite criteria for neurotransmitter status in the mammalian CNS. Although it is not possible to determine to what degree the pharmacological actions of the peptide adumbrate its normal physiological roles, the neuromodulatory influence of exogenously applied neurotensin on dopaminergic neuronal activity includes several dopamine-mediated behaviors. The changes in endogenous neurotensin concentrations after treatment with dopamine agonists and antagonists are noteworthy. Moreover, alterations in CSF and regional neurotensin concentration and neurotensin receptor density have been observed in neuropsychiatric disorders that purportedly involved the CNS dopaminergic systems. This concatenation of findings strongly suggests that neurotensin plays an important physiological role in the CNS, especially in certain pathological states. The striking similarity between the pharmacological effects of neurotensin and those of clinically effective antipsychotic drugs, particularly when

Table 9-1. Neurotensin alterations in neuropsychiatric disorders

Neuropsychiatric disorder	Tissue	Neurotensin alteration	Reference
Schizophrenia	CSF	Decreased NT concentration	Widerlöv et al. 1982b Nemeroff et al. 1983b Lindström et al. 1988 Nemeroff et al. 1989
	Brain	Increased NT concentration in Brodmann's area 32 (frontal cortex)	Nemeroff et al. 1983b
Parkinson's disease	Brain	Decreased NT concentration in hippocampus Unaltered in substantia nigra, ventral tegmental area, striatum, nucleus accumbens, or frontal cortex	Bissette et al. 1985
		Decreased NT binding in substantia nigra	Sadoul et al. 1984 Uhl et al. 1984
Huntington's chorea	Brain	Increased NT concentration in caudate nucleus	Nemeroff et al. 1983b
		Increased NT concentration in globus pallidus	Emson et al. 1985

Table 9-1. Neurotensin alterations in neuropsychiatric disorders—continued

Neuropsychiatric disorder	Tissue	Neurotensin alteration	Reference
Down's syndrome	Brain	Increased NT concentration in caudate nucleus, temporal cortex, and frontal cortex	Yates et al. 1985
Menopausal hot flashes	Plasma	Increased NT concentration	Kronenberg and Carraway 1985
Alzheimer's disease	Brain	None	Biggins et al. 1983 Yates et al. 1985 Emson et al. 1985
Depression	CSF	None	Nemeroff et al. 1989
	Brain	None	Biggins et al. 1983
Anorexia/Bulimia	CSF	None	Nemeroff et al. 1989
Premenstrual syndrome	CSF	None	Nemeroff et al. 1989
	Plasma	None	Chuong et al. 1985

Note. CSF = cerebrospinal fluid; NT = neurotensin.

taken in light of the observed alterations in neurotensin concentration in schizophrenic patients, suggests that this tridecapeptide may play a major role in the pathogenesis of this disease and/or in the mechanism of action of antipsychotic drugs. Further progress in the study of neurotensin will undoubtedly increase not only our understanding of the role of this peptide in the CNS but our understanding of the pathogenesis of schizophrenia, suggesting a direction for rational development of novel treatment strategies with greater antipsychotic efficacy and fewer side effects.

REFERENCES

Anderson CM, Bissette G, Nemeroff CB, et al: Microtopographic distribution of neurotensin and catecholamine concentrations at the level of individual rat brain nuclei. Society of Neuroscience Abstracts 10:437, 1984

Andrade R, Aghajanian GK: Neurotensin selectively activates dopamine neurons in the substantia nigra. Society of Neuroscience Abstracts 7:573, 1981

Biggins JA, Perry EK, McDermott JR, et al: Post mortem levels of thyrotropin-releasing hormone and neurotensin in the amygdala in Alzheimer disease, schizophrenia and depression. J Neurol Sci 58:117–122, 1983

Bissette G, Jennes L, Prange AJ Jr, et al: Neurotensin and dopamine are not co-localized in rat brain. Society of Neuroscience Abstracts 9:290, 1983

Bissette G, Nemeroff CB, Decker MW, et al: Alterations in regional brain concentrations of neurotensin and bombesin in Parkinson's disease. Ann Neurol 17:324–329, 1985

Bissette G, Dauer WT, Kilts CD, et al: The effect of the stereoisomers of butaclamol on neurotensin content in discrete regions of the rat brain. Neuropsychopharmacology 1:329–335, 1988a

Bissette G, Dole K, Johnson M, et al: Antipsychotic drugs increase neurotensin concentrations after destruction of dopamine neurons by 6-hydroxydopamine. Society of Neuroscience Abstracts 14:1211, 1988b

Carraway RE, Leeman SE: The isolation of a new hypotensive peptide, neurotensin, from bovine hypothalami. J Biol Chem 248:6854–6861, 1973

Carraway RE, Leeman SE: The amino acid sequence of a hypothalamic peptide, neurotensin. J Biol Chem 250:1907–1911, 1975

Chuong CJ, Coulam CB, Kao PC, et al: Neuropeptide levels in premenstrual syndrome. Fertil Steril 44:760–765, 1985

DeCeballos ML, Boyce S, Jenner P, et al: Alterations in [Met^5]- and [Leu^5]enkephalin and neurotensin content in basal ganglia induced by the long-term administration of dopamine agonist and antagonist drugs to rats. Eur J Pharmacol 130:305–309, 1986

Deutch AY, Bean AJ, Bissette G, et al: Stress-induced alterations in neurotensin, somatostatin and corticotropin-releasing factor in mesotelencephalic dopamine system regions. Brain Res 417:350–354, 1987

Dupont A, Merand Y: Enzymic inactivation of neurotensin by hypothalamic and brain extracts of the rat. Life Sci 22:1623–1630, 1978

Eggerman KW, Zahm DS: Numbers of neurotensin-immunoreactive neurons selectively increased in rat ventral striatum following acute haloperidol administration. Neuropeptides 11:125–132, 1988

Emson PC, Horsfield PM, Goedert M, et al: Neurotensin in human brain: regional distribution and effects of neurological illness. Brain Res 347:239–244, 1985

Ervin GN, Nemeroff CB: Antagonization of the behavioral activation produced by direct stimulation of forebrain dopamine receptors caused by intraaccumbens injections of neurotensin. Neuropsychopharmacology 1:243–250, 1988

Ervin GN, Birkemo LS, Nemeroff CB, et al: Neurotensin blocks certain amphetamine behaviors. Nature 291:73–76, 1981

Glimcher PW, Giovino AA, Hoebel BG: Neurotensin self-injection in the ventral tegmental area. Brain Res 403:147–150, 1987

Goedert M, Mantyh PW, Hunt SP, et al: Mosaic distribution of neurotensin-like immunoreactivity in the cat striatum. Brain Res 274:176–179, 1983

Govoni S, Hong JS, Yang H-YT, et al: Increase of neurotensin content elicited by neuroleptics in nucleus accumbens. J Pharmacol Exp Ther 215:413–417, 1980

Hedner J, Hedner T, Lundell KH, et al: Cerebrospinal fluid concentrations of neurotensin and corticotropin-releasing factor in pediatric patients. Biol Neonate 55:260–267, 1989

Herve D, Tassin JP, Studler JM, et al: Dopaminergic control of ^{125}I-labeled neurotensin binding site density in corticolimbic structures of the rat brain. Proc Natl Acad Sci USA 83:6203–6207, 1986

Hökfelt T, Everitt BJ, Theodorsson-Norheim E, et al: Occurrence of neurotensin-like immunoreactivity in subpopulations of hypothalamic, mesencephalic, and medullary catecholamine neurons. J Comp Neurol 222:543–559, 1984

Iversen LL, Iversen SD, Bloom F, et al: Calcium-dependent release of somatostatin and neurotensin from rat brain in vitro. Nature 273:161, 1978

Jiang D, Feng D, Zhu L, et al: Neurotensin potentiates the endogenous dopamine release from striatal synaptosomes of rat. Life Sci 43:27–33, 1988

Kalivas PW, Miller JS: Neurotensin neurons in the ventral tegmental area project to the medial nucleus accumbens. Brain Res 300:157–160, 1984

Kalivas PW, Taylor S: Behavioral and neurochemical effect of daily injections with neurotensin into the ventral tegmental area. Brain Res 358:70–76, 1985

Kalivas PW, Nemeroff CB, Prange AJ Jr: Increase in spontaneous motoractivity following infusion of neurotensin into the ventral tegmental area. Brain Res 229:525–529, 1981

Kalivas PW, Nemeroff CB, Prange AJ Jr: Neuroanatomical site specific modulation of spontaneous motor activity by neurotensin. Eur J Pharmacol 78:471–474, 1982

Kalivas PW, Burgess SK, Nemeroff CB, et al: Behavioral and neurochemical effects of neurotensin microinjection into the ventral tegmental area of the rat. Neuroscience 8:495–505, 1983

Kanba KS, Kanba S, Okazaki H, et al: Binding of [^{3}H]neurotensin in human brain: properties and distribution. J Neurochem 46:946–952, 1986

Kataoka K, Mizumo N, Frohman LA: Regional distribution of immunoreactive neurotensin in monkey brain. Brain Res Bull 4:57–60, 1979

Kilts CD, Anderson CM, Bissette G, et al: Differential effects of antipsychotic drugs on the neurotensin content of discrete rat brain nuclei. Biochem Pharmacol 37:1547–1554, 1988

Kislauskis E, Bullock B, McNeil S, et al: The rat gene encoding neurotensin and neuromedin N. J Biol Chem 263:4963–4968, 1988

Kronenberg F, Carraway RE: Changes in neurotensin-like immunoreactivity during menopausal hot flashes. J Clin Endocrinol Metab 60:1081–1086, 1985

Lazarus LH, Brown MR, Perrin HH: Distribution, localization, and characterization of neurotensin binding sites in the rat brain. Neuropharmacology 16:625–629, 1977

Letter AA, Matsuda LA, Merchant KM, et al: Characterization of dopaminergic influence on striatal-nigral neurotensin systems. Brain Res 422:200–203, 1987

Levant B, Nemeroff CB: The psychobiology of neurotensin, in The Neuroendocrinology of Mood, Vol 8. Edited by Ganten D, Pfaff D. Berlin, Springer-Verlag, 1988, pp 231–262

Levant B, Bissette G, Nemeroff CB: Anticholinergic drugs do not alter neurotensin concentration in the nucleus accumbens or striatum. Society of Neuroscience Abstracts 14:114, 1988a

Levant B, Bissette G, Parker Y-M, et al: Alterations in neurotensin and bombesin-like immunoreactivity in MPTP-treated mice. Ann NY Acad Sci 537:515–517, 1988b

Lindström LH, Widerlöv E, Bissette G, et al: Reduced CSF neurotensin concentration in drug-free schizophrenic patients. Schizophrenia Research 1:55–59, 1988

Luttinger D, King RA, Shepperd D, et al: The effect of neurotensin on food consumption in the rat. Eur J Pharmacol 81:499–504, 1982a

Luttinger D, Nemeroff CB, Prange AJ Jr: The effects of neuropeptides on discrete-trial conditioned avoidance responding. Brain Res 237:183–192, 1982b

Manberg PJ, Youngblood WW, Nemeroff CB, et al: Regional distribution of neurotensin in human brain. J Neurochem 38:1777–1780, 1982

Mazella J, Kitabgi P, Vincent J-P: Molecular properties of neurotensin receptors in rat brain. J Biol Chem 260:508–514, 1985

Mazella J, Amar S, Bozou JC, et al: Functional properties and molecular structure of central and peripheral neurotensin receptors. J Recept Res 7:157–165, 1987

Merchant KM, Letter AA, Johnson M, et al: Effects of amphetamine analogs on neurotensin concentrations in rat brain. Eur J Pharmacol 138:151–154, 1987

Myers RD, Lee TF: In vivo release of dopamine during perfusion of neurotensin in the substantia nigra of the unrestrained rat. Peptides 4:955–961, 1984a

Myers RD, Lee TF: Neurotensin perfusion of rat hypothalamus: dissociation of dopamine release from body temperature change. Neuroscience 12:241–253, 1984b

Nemeroff CB, Bissette G, Prange AJ Jr, et al: Neurotensin: central nervous system effects of a hypothalamic peptide. Brain Res 128:485–496, 1977

Nemeroff CB, Luttinger D, Hernandez DE, et al: Interactions of neurotensin with brain dopamine systems: biochemical and behavioral studies. J Pharmacol Exp Ther 225:337–345, 1983a

Nemeroff CB, Youngblood W, Manberg PJ, et al: Regional brain concentrations of neuropeptides in Huntington's chorea and schizophrenia. Science 221:972–975, 1983b

Nemeroff CB, Bissette G, Widerlöv E, et al: Neurotensin-like immunoreactivity in cerebrospinal fluid of patients with schizophrenia, depression, anorexia nervosa–bulimia and premenstrual syndrome. Journal of Neuropsychiatry and Clinical Neuroscience 1:16–20, 1989

Palacios JM, Kuhar MJ: Neurotensin receptors are located on dopamine-containing neurons in rat midbrain. Nature 294:587–589, 1981

Quirion R, Chiueh CC, Everist HD, et al: Comparative localization of neurotensin receptors on nigrostriatal and mesolimbic dopaminergic terminals. Brain Res 327:385–389, 1985

Radke JM, MacLennan AJ, Beinfeld MC, et al: Effects of short- and long-term haloperidol administration and withdrawal on regional brain cholecystokinin and neurotensin concentrations in the rat. Brain Res 480:178–183, 1989

Reches A, Burke RE, Jiang D, et al: The effect of neurotensin on dopaminergic neurons in rat brain. Ann NY Acad Sci 400:420–421, 1982

Rupniak NMJ, Mann S, Hall MD, et al: Comparison of the effects on striatal DA receptor function of chronic administration of haloperidol, clozapine or sulpiride to rats for up to 23 months, in Catecholamines: Neuropharmacology and CNS—Theorectical Aspects. Edited by Usdin E, Carlsson A, Dahlstrom A, et al. New York, Alan R Liss, 1984, pp 91–98

Sadoul J-L, Checler F, Kitabgi P, et al: Loss of high affinity neurotensin receptors in substantia nigra from parkinsonian subjects. Biochem Biophys Res Commun 125:395–404, 1984

Sarrieu A, Javoy-Agid F, Kitabgi P, et al: Characterization and autoradiographic distribution of neurotensin binding sites in the human brain. Brain Res 348:375–380, 1985

Schotte A, Rostene W, Laduron PM: Different subcellular localization of neurotensin-receptor and neurotensin-acceptor sites in the rat brain dopaminergic system. J Neurochem 50:1026–1031, 1988

Skoog KM, Cain ST, Nemeroff CB: Centrally administered neurotensin suppresses locomotor hyperactivity induced by D-amphetamine but not by scopolamine or caffeine. Neuropharmacology 25:777–782, 1986

Starr MS: Influence of peptides on ^{3}H-dopamine release from superfused rat striatal slices. Neurochemistry International 4:233–240, 1982

Studler J-M, Kitabgi P, Tramu G, et al: Extensive co-localization of neuro tensin with dopamine in rat meso-cortico-frontal dopaminergic neurons. Neuropeptides 11:95–100, 1988

Tassin JP, Kitabgi P, Tramu G, et al: Rat mesocortical dopaminergic neurons are mixed neurotensin/dopamine neurons: immunohistochemical and biochemical evidence. Ann NY Acad Sci 537:531–533, 1988

Uhl GR, Kuhar MJ: Chronic neuroleptic treatment enhances neurotensin receptor binding in human and rat substantia nigra. Nature 309:350–352, 1984

Uhl GR, Snyder SH: Regional and subcellular distribution of brain neurotensin. Life Sci 19:1827–1832, 1977

Uhl GR, Whitehouse PJ, Price DL, et al: Parkinson's disease: depletion of substantia nigra neurotensin receptors. Brain Res 308:186–190, 1984

van Wimersma Greidanus TB, van Praag MCG, Kalmann R, et al: Behavioral effects of neurotensin. Ann NY Acad Sci 400:319–329, 1982

Widerlöv E, Kilts CD, Mailman RB, et al: Increase in dopamine metabolites in rat brain by neurotensin. J Pharmacol Exp Ther 222:1–6, 1982a

Widerlöv E, Lindström LH, Bešev G, et al: Subnormal CSF levels of neurotensin in a subgroup of schizophrenic patients: normalization after neuroleptic treatment. Am J Psychiatry 139:1122–1126, 1982b

Yates CM, Fink G, Bennie JG, et al: Neurotensin immunoreactivity in post-mortem brain is increased in Down's syndrome but not in Alzheimer-type dementia. J Neurol Sci 67:327–335, 1985

Young WS III, Kuhar MJ: Neurotensin receptor localization by light microscopic autoradiography in rat brain. Brain Res 220:273–285, 1981

Chapter 10

The Opioid Model in Psychiatric Research

Ede Frecska, M.D.
Kenneth L. Davis, M.D.

Chapter 10

The Opioid Model in Psychiatric Research

Since their discovery in the early 1970s, endogenous opioid peptides have been implicated as being either causative or curative agents in a variety of mental disorders. A tremendous effort was made to investigate their possible role in psychopathology and use in psychopharmacology, but initial successes gave way to discouraging results. Most of the early work focused on schizophrenia and affective disorders. Recently, other areas, particularly childhood autism and eating disorders, have received increasing attention.

SCHIZOPHRENIA

Evidence for a role of the opioid system in schizophrenia is quite confusing. Two opposing hypotheses were formulated, one suggesting a deficiency and the other an excess of opioid function in this disorder. The roots of the dichotomy go back to the discovery that hypokinesia is induced by beta-endorphin. This same phenomenon was interpreted by Jacquet and Marks (1976) as neuroleptic-like bradykinesia, but by Bloom and colleagues (1976) as catatonia. Thus, on the one hand, neuroleptic-like effects and, on the other, psychotogenic properties have been attributed to opioid peptides. These notions led to various therapeutic approaches: 1) studies of the effects of opioid agonists, particularly beta-endorphin, on the symptomatology of schizophrenia; 2) studies of administration of opioid peptides with neuroleptic-like activity, such as gamma-type endorphins, to schizophrenic patients; 3) attempts to wash out endorphin-like peptides from the circulation of schizophrenic patients with peritoneal dialysis or hemodialysis; and 4) the use of opioid receptor blockers on target symptoms of schizophrenia.

This work was supported in part by a grant from the Veterans Administration, Schizophrenia Biologic Research Center (4125-020). The authors would like to thank Dr. Patricia Warne for her assistance in the preparation of this manuscript.

None of these strategies resulted in any practical or hypothetical advances. While reduction of auditory hallucinations and paranoid ideation was reported in the first uncontrolled study with beta-endorphin intravenously administered to schizophrenic patients (Kline et al. 1977), later use of a double-blind, cross-over design demonstrated only statistically significant but not clinically apparent beneficial effects (Berger et al. 1980). Moreover, deterioration of patients' behavior was described under well-controlled conditions (Gerner et al. 1980). Diverse effects were observed among schizophrenic patients (Pickar et al. 1981), with some improvement in mood and anxiety but no relief in psychotic symptoms (Petho et al. 1982). The initially promising des-tyrosine-gamma-endorphin (Verhoeven et al. 1979), which was observed in animal models to have neuroleptic-like properties without opioid activity (Davis et al. 1981; DeWied et al. 1978), later proved to be disappointingly ineffective in humans (Emrich et al. 1982b; Tamminga et al. 1981).

The strategy of decreasing levels of endorphin-like peptides by hemodialysis was derived from the misconception that abnormal, psychotogenic endorphin (i.e., leucine-5-beta-endorphin) is produced by schizophrenic patients and can be removed by dialysis (Wagemaker and Cade 1977). Subsequent controlled experiments failed to confirm this observation (Wagemaker et al. 1984). Furthermore, no investigator has been able to prove the existence of a leucine form of beta-endorphin.

Experiments using the opiate receptor antagonist naloxone were also inconclusive. In the majority of studies, low doses of naloxone were virtually ineffective, although higher doses reduced auditory hallucinations and unusual thought contents in a subgroup of schizophrenic patients. Furthermore, these effects generally occurred at time points later than would be expected given the pharmacodynamics of the drug. Therefore, any interpretation of opioid mechanisms based on these observations is not straightforward.

The "endorphin excess" theory of schizophrenia is also based on the psychotomimetic properties of opiate agonists. Brain sigma-type receptors are thought to mediate the psychotogenic effects of certain opiates (e.g., benzomorphans) and phencyclidine. Although the classification of the sigma binding sites as opioid receptors is questionable, and phencyclidine is not an opiate drug, it is worthwhile to mention here that this agent surpasses amphetamine in modeling schizophrenia (Hollister 1986). Haloperidol and many other antipsychotic drugs exhibit high affinity for a subclass of sigma receptors, binding with a strength that at least equals their affinity for dopamine receptors. However, these sigma receptors differ from phencyclidine-sensitive binding sites and probably contribute to the extrapyramidal side effects of neuroleptics (Walker et al. 1988).

Measurement of total opioid binding by radioreceptor assay or beta-endorphin–like immunoreactivity by radioimmunoassay in biological samples from schizophrenic patients received considerable attention in a series of studies characterized by inadequate diagnostic evaluations and statistical methods. Different studies of cerebrospinal fluid (CSF) opioid levels in schizophrenic patients reported changes in different directions. Increases in these levels were reported by Terenius et al. (1976), Lindström et al. (1978), and Rimon et al. (1980); but decreases were observed by Dupont et al. (1978) and Naber et al. (1981). Neuroleptic-free schizophrenic patients had no significant differences from healthy control subjects in their CSF and plasma beta-endorphin levels (Emrich et al. 1979b; Gerner and Sharp 1982; Naber et al. 1981; Ross et al. 1979). Studies in human autopsy material could be useful in clearing up the inconsistency of in vivo studies, but they are still in their nascent phase (Kleinman et al. 1983; Reisine et al. 1980).

AFFECTIVE DISORDERS

Opium has been shown to have antidepressant effects. Indeed, before the introduction of electroconvulsive therapy (ECT), it was widely used for this purpose. The so-called "laudanum cure" was a course of 2 months treatment with progressive increases in dosage followed by gradual withdrawal. The classical descriptions (Kraepelin 1905) recommended this treatment especially for agitated depression and considered it not only palliative but curative because the whole depressive syndrome disappeared after 2 months of treatment.

In the 1970s several studies suggested that the endogenous opioid system is deficient in patients with depression, and reported symptom relief following acute intravenous administration of beta-endorphin. Kline et al. (1977) observed that 1.8 to 9.0 mg of intravenous human beta-endorphin improved mood, increased spontaneity, and diminished anxiety of depressed patients; however, the effects disappeared within a few hours. In a study by Angst et al. (1979), four bipolar and two unipolar depressive patients showed improvement in energy, anxiety, and restlessness within 20 to 30 minutes after a 10-mg intravenous injection of beta-endorphin. Four of the six patients showed relapse after 2 hours, two patients' improvement persisted, and three patients became hypomanic during or soon after the trial. Unfortunately, these trials were not adequately controlled to rule out the roles of expectation, experimental stress, or sleep deprivation. No hypomania was in fact noted in subsequent double-blind, placebo-controlled studies (Catlin et al. 1980; Gerner et al. 1980), but patients manifested significant improvement in depressive symptoms as reflected in their animated speech, bright facial expression, increased sociability, and psychomotor activation. Negative results have also been reported with beta-endorphin (Pickar et al. 1981) and Met-enkephalin (Klein et al. 1981). In the few studies on the effect of subchronic opiate administration, relief of depression has been attained with cyclazocine (Fink et al. 1970), buprenorphine (Emrich et al. 1982a), and methadone (Pickar et al. 1982a). Owing to the risk of addiction, these studies did not approach the duration of the "laudanum cure," and relapse was practically immediate. Despite these disappointing results, the majority of studies on opioid agonist administration in depressive illness support the traditional notion that depressed patients experience symptom reduction following this treatment.

However, the opposite strategy, using opiate antagonists, provided no additional support for the hypothesis that endogenous opioids are involved in the pathophysiology of affective disorders. There is little evidence that these drugs have marked effects on mood. No change of mood was documented after a moderate (10-mg) dose of naloxone, neither in depressed subjects (Davis et al. 1977; Emrich et al. 1979a; Terenius et al. 1977) nor in healthy volunteers (Grevert and Goldstein 1978; Hoehn-Saric and Masek 1981). The administration of high doses (20–30 mg) of naloxone was reported to cause an observable reduction in manic symptoms (Janowsky et al. 1978), but subsequent attempts to replicate this finding were unsuccessful (Davis et al. 1979; Emrich et al. 1979a; Pickar et al. 1982c). Using a single-blind design, Cohen and his colleagues (1983) observed increases in anxiety with very high doses of naloxone (1–6 mg/kg) in healthy subjects, and depressive patients manifested a more marked and subjectively more intense worsening compared with control subjects (Cohen et al. 1984a). While the specificity of the antagonist is questionable at this dose, these authors postulate a chronic activation of the opioid system in depression, resulting in a naloxone-sensitive, withdrawal-prone physiological state.

Measurements of CSF opioid levels in manic and depressive patients have also yielded inconclusive results. Initially Terenius et al.'s work (1976) indicated that fraction I opioid activity was elevated in bipolar patients, with a tendency for manic patients to have higher values. However, many of their subjects were not medication free. Two other groups did not report any difference in total opioid activity among manic, depressive, and euthymic individuals (Davis et al. 1982; Pickar et al. 1982b), although four bipolar patients in the latter study showed higher levels during the manic phase than in a depressive episode. CSF beta-endorphin immunoreactivity was not different between patients with affective disorders and healthy volunteers (Black et al. 1986; Pickar et al. 1982b).

Whereas most studies examined levels of endogenous opioid peptides between diagnostic groups and controls, some evidence is available suggesting that the activity of the opioid system may relate to symptoms that run across psychiatric diagnoses. It now appears that CSF opioid activity may be associated more with stress and anxiety than with any other psychiatric condition (Post et al. 1984), with concordance of the finding by Cohen et al. (1983) that anxiety increases following opioid blockade.

Although basal plasma beta-endorphin–like immunoreactivity in depression does not seem to show a consistent abnormality (elevated levels: Brambilla et al. 1981, Risch 1982; no abnormality: Alexopoulos et al. 1983, Cohen et al. 1984b), some observations are noteworthy. Dexamethasone failed to suppress plasma beta-endorphin and/or beta-lipotropin values in 50% to 69% of depressive patients (Gispen-de Wied et al. 1987; Matthews et al. 1986). Moreover, thyrotropin-releasing hormone (TRH), luteinizing-hormone–releasing hormone (LHRH), and physostigmine raised plasma beta-endorphin levels in depressed subjects but had less or no effect in control subjects (Brambilla et al. 1986; Risch et al. 1982). Early escape of cortisol in the dexamethasone suppression test (DST) is a measure of a corticotropin-releasing hormone (CRH)–related hyperactivity of the proopiomelanocortin system (Gold et al. 1986b), and the observed increase in beta-endorphin responsivity may be a proximal sign of the same dysfunction. Convergence is not necessary between cortisol and beta-endorphin nonsuppression because of individual differences in adrenal gland autonomy.

Some studies have been successful in relating opioid activity to hypothalamo-pituitary-adrenal axis dysfunction associated with major depression. Urinary free cortisol was increased significantly and correlated positively with CSF opioid activity in depressed subjects but not in healthy individuals (Rubinow et al. 1981). This finding is consistent with the report of a direct relationship between levels of plasma cortisol and plasma beta-endorphin–like activity only in cases of major depression (Cohen et al. 1984b). Early resumption of morphine-suppressed cortisol secretion was associated with a diagnosis of major depression and with abnormal DST results (Zis et al. 1985a). In the interpretations of these data, the cross-tolerance that can develop between opioids and glucocorticoids (Fekete et al. 1984) is usually overlooked and may shed light on some aspects of these results, for example, the decreased opiate sensitivity of cortisol nonsuppressors in the DST.

There have been attempts to utilize neuroendocrine challenge by narcotic alkaloids to test opioid hyporesponsivity in depression. Early reports indicated that the prolactin response to morphine or methadone might be diminished in depressive patients (Extein et al. 1980; Judd et al. 1982; Robertson et al. 1984), but later studies were less supportive (Bánki and Arato 1987; Frecska et al. 1989; Zis et al. 1985b).

Animal models of depression and the action of antidepressants indicate that opioid mechanisms may be operative. Inescapable shock and forced swimming—both of which cause opioid-dependent analgesia—lead to learned helplessness and behavioral despair, respectively. These models of depression involve opioid hyperactivity at onset followed by tolerance to the endogenously released opioids over time (Christie and Chesher 1982). On the other hand, tricyclic antidepressants and electroconvulsive shock are synergistic with morphine, and some of the resulting behavioral effects are antagonized by naloxone (Devoize et al. 1984; Holaday et al. 1986). However, it would be premature to draw any conclusions about how the opioid system might be involved in the behavioral models of depression and in the mechanisms of action of antidepressant treatment.

CHILDHOOD AUTISM AND SELF-INJURIOUS BEHAVIOR

Autistic children appear less sensitive to pain, seldom cry, and seem to have a low desire for social interaction. They are less emotional, show lability in their affect, fail to express physical affection, have episodes of increased motor activity alternating with quiescence, and evidence an extreme resistance to behavioral extinction (Prior and Werry 1986). A range of autistic-like symptoms such as elevation of pain threshold, reduction of distress vocalization, diminution of the desire for companionship, poor clinging behavior, fluctuating responsiveness to stimuli, and learning abnormalities characterized by prolonged extinction can be elicited by enhancement of endogenous opioid function or by administration of opiate alkaloids in infant animals (Panksepp et al. 1985). In addition, both autistic children and children exposed in utero to opiate drugs often are retarded in height and bone development, have feeding problems, and are prone to epileptic seizures. Based on these observations, excessive brain opioid activity has been postulated in the etiology of infantile autism (Panksepp 1979). If this concept is correct, autistic children would have developed tolerance for and dependence on their endogenous opioids, they would manifest symptoms analogous to the behavior of opiate addicts, and they would be sensitive to opioid receptor blockade.

Habitual self-mutilation is a bizarre, sometimes dramatic stereotypy consisting of repetitious and self-inflicted physical harm and tissue damage. Several kinds of self-injurious behavior, such as banging the head, hitting the body, biting self, and picking sores, are reported to occur among 40% of institutionalized psychotic children (Shodell and Reiter 1968) and between 8% to 14% of mentally retarded individuals (Baumeister and Rollings 1976). In both diagnostic groups, self-injurious behavior and other stereotypies (e.g., rocking, bouncing) are extremely resistant to extinction; mere cessation of the behavior seems to be unpleasant for the patients and leads to more violent self-abuse. Chronic administration of opioid alkaloids to rodents results in stereotyped behavior including self-mutilation, which is enhanced by drug withdrawal (Ahtee 1974). Therefore, it has been suggested that these kinds of behavior, especially self-injury that would result in the pain-induced endorphin release, are attempts of the addicted organism to prevent the symptoms of narcotic withdrawal. Thus, self-injurious behavior in autistic children may be a sign of dependence on endogenous opioids (Sandman et al. 1983).

Most of the research examining the opioid system in autism and self-injurious behavior relates to these notions. The strongest evidence linking opioid dysfunction to these abnormal conditions is found in case reports of trials with naloxone and naltrexone. Despite the fact that relatively low doses of naloxone were administered (usually no more than 1.2 mg), seven of eight reports in the literature (Bernstein et al. 1984; Davidson et al. 1983; Gillman and Sandyk 1985; Richardson and Zaleski 1983; Sandman et al. 1983, 1987; Sandyk 1985) found a palliative effect of these agents. Only Beckwith et al. (1986) reported failure of naloxone to reduce self-mutilation in two developmentally disabled female patients. So far at least 11 patients with self-injurious behavior have been treated with naloxone, and decreased frequency and/or intensity of self-injury was reported in nine of them. However, most of these studies had several weaknesses in design, and the results must be regarded as very preliminary. Most of the patients treated with naloxone were mentally retarded, and the etiologies of retardation were different among them. Subjects exhibited self-mutilation with considerable variation over time and thus did not have stable baselines. In addition, history of other medication was imperfectly documented in these papers.

If autistic children or self-abusive patients are addicts of their endogenous opioids, administration of an antagonist should have precipitated withdrawal-like phenomena. However, only one study reported the transient increase of self-mutilation during naloxone administration (Richardson and Zaleski 1983). Interestingly, this study used the highest dose (6-hour infusion at 1 and 2 mg per hour), and self-mutilation declined below baseline level in the postdrug period, presumably due to the absence of reward. Future studies on opioid antagonist treatment of self-injurious behavior have to address this possible biphasic effect and must entail prolonged observation.

To date, there are three reports of the use of naltrexone in treating autistic children (Campbell et al. 1987; Herman et al. 1986; Szymanski et al. 1987). The finding of Szymanski's group was negative, but the other studies reported improvement in these patients, with increased socialization and reduced self-mutilation. Taken as a whole, 14 children with autism have been treated with naltrexone: 12 had a statistically significant response, and the change in 8 of these 12 was clinically relevant. Finally, in a dose-dependent manner, naltrexone reduced self-injurious behavior in three male adolescents with developmental deficit (Herman et al. 1987) and in three of four mentally retarded adults (Sandman 1988).

Weizman et al. (1984) examined plasma concentrations of an endogenous opioid ligand, designated humoral endorphin (a unique opioid peptide that is not cross-reactive with alpha-, beta-, or gamma-endorphin, dynorphin, or enkephalin), in 10 autistic children and, contrary to expectations, observed lowered levels. This deficiency does not appear to be specific to autism, since a similar decrease was found in untreated schizophrenic youths in the same study. However, in the study of Gillberg and his coworkers (1985), self-injurious autistic children had higher fractions I and II of endorphin in their CSF than did those patients who had not manifested self-mutilation. There was a trend toward a correlation between high fraction II levels and self-destructiveness and decreased pain sensitivity. The major opioid in fraction II of human CSF is Met-enkephalin. Coid et al. (1983) reported elevated Met-enkephalin concentrations in the plasma of habitually self-mutilating patients. In a population of 40 developmentally disabled individuals, stereotypic and self-injurious patients had higher levels of plasma beta-endorphin than did control subjects (Sandman 1988).

Auto-addiction is a tempting explanation for self-abusiveness. However, increased levels of endogenous opioids are not sufficient to prove the presence of auto-addiction in these patients. They may explain elevated pain threshold, but decreased pain sensitivity alone is not enough to perpetuate self-injury. The missing links have yet to be provided. In conclusion, the opioid paradigm of infantile autism is a promising research area, and there are sufficient data to justify well-designed clinical trials of opiate antagonists in autistic children with a profile of self-injurious behavior.

EATING DISORDERS

"Vomunt ut edant, edunt ut vomant." ("They vomit to eat, and eat to vomit.") Thus Seneca bitterly described the self-perpetuating circularity of self-induced purging and binge eating as a practice of ancient Rome. *Bulimia* is not a culturally accepted custom but an ingrained habit that commonly presents with episodic binge eating followed by self-induced vomiting and catharsis (Halmi 1985). It is hypothesized that bulimic individuals develop an addictive behavior that begins with emotional distress, which is relieved by eating. Overwhelmed by a fear of obesity, they then treat themselves by self-induced purging, which brings with it an ultimately rewarding euphoria mediated by endogenous opioids released during the stress of vomiting (Abraham and Joseph 1986–1987). For many patients much of the binge eating behavior becomes chronic, for they tend to binge and vomit without feeling stressed.

Evidence for this theory is not definitive but is quite suggestive. Stress can induce eating in experimental animals, with concomitant activation of the opioid system (Morley et al. 1983). Since the pioneering study of Holtzman in 1974, which showed that naloxone reduced food intake in rats, several subsequent studies have demonstrated that opioid antagonists decrease feeding in a variety of species ranging from the slug to the human (Morley and Blundell 1988). These reports prompted trials of opioid receptor blockers in the treatment of bulimia. In an open trial with 10 antidepressant-resistant bulimic patients, treatment with naltrexone resulted in complete resolution in three patients and proved to be effective in reducing binge eating and purging in five more (Jonas and Gold 1986–1987). This finding is consistent with a double-blind, placebo-controlled study of intravenously administered naloxone, which demonstrated significant decreases in the amount of food and caloric intake during episodes of binge eating of five bulimic individuals (Mitchell et al. 1986). In their recent study, Jonas and Gold (1988b) gave increased support for the potential utility of opioid receptor blockade in treating bulimia, and they emphasized that doses of antagonist greater than those needed to block exogenous opiates may be required for therapeutic efficacy.

Opioid involvement in feeding behavior is complex and appears to be dependent on a variety of pathways. Probably different opioid mechanisms are responsible for food seeking, hoarding, intake, palatability, and gratification. The kappa receptor and its endogenous ligand, dynorphin, is particularly important in appetite stimulation (Morley and Levine 1983). It would be relevant to determine if kappa antagonists with higher specificity and potency than naloxone and naltrexone are more effective in relieving binge eating of bulimic individuals. However, it should be noted that demonstration of the decrease of a symptom after administration of an antagonist does not prove that the symptom is caused by the endogenous compound.

At present, direct investigations concerning the role of opioids in binge eating are inadequate and conflicting. Bulimic patients who purge have significantly higher plasma beta-endorphin levels than do control subjects (Fullerton et al. 1986), and nonvomiting bulimic patients have levels similar to those of healthy individuals (Fullerton et al. 1988), raising the possibility that the observed group differences in plasma beta-endorphin are due to the stress of vomiting. Although increased beta-endorphin could not be a primary factor in this illness, it may perpetuate the pathological behavior, because the purging-associated decrease in depression (and rise in pain tolerance) was blocked by naloxone (Abraham and Joseph 1986–1987). Unfortunately, this study did not measure plasma beta-endorphin. In contrast to these findings and interpretations, Waller and colleagues (1986) reported plasma beta-endorphin levels in bulimic patients that were lower than those in control subjects and that were negatively correlated with vomiting. Clinical condition and interval of fasting prior to blood sampling were not clear in this study.

The abnormal negative attitude toward food consumption and weight gain, which defies life-sustaining biological drives, is the most puzzling symptom of *anorexia nervosa*. In addition to the disturbance of appetite, anorexia nervosa is invariably associated with various forms of endocrine dysfunction, including hypothalamic hypogonadism (Vigersky and Loriaux 1977) and hypercortisolism (Gold et al. 1986a). The discovery that endogenous opioid peptides contribute to the regulation of eating behavior and neuroendocrine function has raised the question of whether a disturbance of the endogenous opioid system is involved in the pathophysiology of anorexia nervosa. Data supporting such suggestions are less consistent, and the evidence for possible endorphin participation in anorexia nervosa is more complex than in the case of bulimia. One may expect from the opioid effect on food consumption that anorexic patients have opioid hypofunction. However, the endocrine and metabolic alterations in this disorder, such as suppressed pulsatile gonadotropin secretion and decreased basal metabolic rate and body temperature, suggest the opposite notion, since opioids inhibit LHRH secretion, reduce energy expenditure, and lower the set point for body temperature (Margules 1979). We describe below how these concepts are not mutually exclusive and can result from differential functions of separate opioid systems.

Kaye and coworkers (1982) have demonstrated a correlation of total CSF opioid activity, measured by radioreceptor assay, with the degree of severity and acuteness of anorexia nervosa. It has been reported that certain anorexic patients may be responsive to naloxone (Moore et al. 1981) or naltrexone (Luby et al. 1987). These findings are somewhat surprising considering that these drugs reduce food intake and body weight. Nevertheless, opioids in particular mediate the palatability of food, and patients with anorexia nervosa are often obsessed with food (e.g., they hoard it) and frequently report fear of being unable to stop eating—that is why they refuse to start. Their fears "may be of excessive high drives rather than excessive fears of normal drives" (Marrazzi and Luby 1986, p. 200). Kaye and colleagues speculate that the increased opioid activity in underweight patients with anorexia nervosa is a consequence of a compensatory mechanism to decrease metabolic rate, which simultaneously stimulates the preoccupation with food. The binge eating and intense craving for food that occur in anorexia nervosa may be due to a periodic breakthrough of the appetite-stimulating properties of endogenous opioid peptides.

However, Gerner and Sharp (1982) found no significant difference in CSF beta-endorphin immunoreactivity between healthy subjects and anorexic patients, and Kaye's group (1987a) reported reduced CSF beta-endorphin and other proopiomelanocortin-related peptides in low-weight anorexic patients that normalized after weight restoration. The discrepancy between these two studies and Kaye et al.'s 1982 study (see above) may be explained by the greater mean weight of patients, who were undergoing refeeding, in the Gerner and Sharp study. In addition, the inconsistency of Kaye's results is virtual and due to the different methodological approach: the radioreceptor assay used in the 1982 study measures total opioid activity, and the radioimmunoassay of the 1987 study targets particular peptides of the opioid family. Thus, detection of opioid peptides other than beta-endorphin itself may explain the difference between the results of the two studies. If Kaye's finding of low equimolar quantities of proopiomelanocortin-derived peptides in CSF is valid, then the reports of elevated baseline beta-endorphin plasma levels (Brambilla et al. 1985) with increased responsiveness to clonidine stimulation (Brambilla et al. 1987), and of high concentrations of CSF CRH (Kaye et al. 1987b) in anorexia nervosa, suggest that the pituitary and the hypothalamic proopiomelanocortin systems may be dissociated in this disorder. It is plausible that in anorexic patients the pituitary adrenocorticotropin–beta-endorphin hyperactivity contributes to the endocrinologic and metabolic changes (conservation of energy), and that the decreased hypothalamic proopiomelanocortin function helps to sustain the behavioral symptoms (food refusal).

The hypothesis that opioid peptides could play a role in inhibition of luteinizing hormone secretion in anorexia nervosa (Baranowska et al. 1984) now appears to be untenable, because two other groups have not found an increase in gonadotropin levels in these patients after naloxone administration (Giusti et al. 1988; Grossman et al. 1982). Hyperactivity is another characteristic sign of anorexia nervosa that does not fit the opioid model. The effect of opioids on locomotion is too complex to make reliable interpretations of the data. Many of these peptides have biphasic effects, first decreasing then increasing activity, and many have opposite actions at different doses and act at different receptors (Olson et al. 1989).

Eating disorders share common features with primary affective disorders (Hudson et al. 1983), but recent phenomenological studies of individuals with bulimia or anorexia nervosa provide a substantial body of evidence relating these conditions to substance abuse as well. Approximately 25% to 30% of persons with a history of eating disorder may manifest drug or alcohol abuse in their lives, and a 34% rate of eating disorders was reported among adult children of alcoholic individuals (Jonas and Gold 1988a).

SUMMARY

Even after more than a decade of intensive research, firm conclusions cannot be drawn regarding the role of opioid neuropeptides in psychiatric disorders. There is no compelling evidence to link endogenous opioids to schizophrenia, and interest is waning. The initial optimism in affective disorders has also faded. Nonetheless, there is accumulating evidence that the endogenous opioid system may contribute to the abnormality of the hypothalamo-pituitary-adrenal axis in depression. Studies of the roles of opioids in self-mutilation and eating disorders are on the upsurge. However, most of these works are currently in their early trial phases. Of the eating disorders, bulimia holds the most promise of yielding straightforward evidence of opioid involvement.

Increasing knowledge of the multiplicity of opioid ligands and receptors highlights the importance of studying each peptide individually and the appropriate receptors of the family. Because monolithic theories are usually short-lived in neurosciences, interactions with other neuroregulators must be also taken into consideration.

REFERENCES

Abraham HD, Joseph AB: Bulimic vomiting alters pain tolerance and mood. Int J Psychiatry Med 16:311–316, 1986–1987

Ahtee L: Catalepsy and stereotypies in rats treated with methadone: relation to striatal dopamine. Eur J Pharmacol 27:221–230, 1974

Alexopoulos GS, Inturrisi CE, Lipman R, et al: Plasma immunoreactive beta-endorphin levels in depression: effect of electroconvulsive therapy. Arch Gen Psychiatry 40:181–183, 1983

Angst J, Autenrieth V, Brem F, et al: Preliminary results of treatment with beta-endorphin in depression, in Endorphins in Mental Health Research. Edited by Usdin E, Bunney WE Jr, Kline NS. New York, Oxford University Press, 1979, pp 518–528

Bánki CM, Arato M: Multiple hormonal responses to morphine: relationship to diagnosis and dexamethasone suppression. Psychoneuroendocrinology 12:3–11, 1987

Baranowska B, Rozbicka G, Jeske W, et al: The role of endogenous opiates in the mechanism of inhibited luteinizing hormone (LH) secretion in women with anorexia nervosa: the effect of naloxone on LH, follicle-stimulating hormone, prolactin, and beta-endorphin secretion. J Clin Endocrinol Metab 59:412–416, 1984

Baumeister AA, Rollings JP: Self-injurious behavior, in International Review of Research in Mental Retardation. Edited by Ellis NR. New York, Academic, 1976, p 8

Beckwith BE, Couk DI, Schumacher K: Failure of naloxone to reduce self-injurious behavior in two developmentally disabled females. Applied Research in Mental Retardation 7:183–188, 1986

Berger PA, Watson SJ, Akil H, et al: Beta-endorphin and schizophrenia. Arch Gen Psychiatry 37:635–640, 1980

Bernstein GA, Hughes JR, Thompson T: Naloxone reduces the self-injurious behavior of a mentally retarded adolescent. Paper presented at the annual meeting of the American Academy of Child Psychiatry, Toronto, October 1984

Black PM, Ballantine HT Jr, Carr DB, et al: Beta-endorphin and somatostatin concentrations in the ventricular cerebrospinal fluid of patients with affective disorder. Biol Psychiatry 21:1077–1081, 1986

Bloom F, Segal D, Ling N, et al: Endorphins: profound behavioral effects in rats suggest new etiological factors in mental illness. Science 194:630–632, 1976

Brambilla F, Genazzani AR, Facchinetti F, et al: Beta-endorphin and beta lipotropin plasma levels in chronic schizophrenia, primary affective disorders and secondary affective disorders. Psychoneuroendocrinology 6:321–330, 1981

Brambilla F, Cavagnini F, Invitti C, et al: Neuroendocrine and psychopathological measures in anorexia nervosa: resemblances to primary affective disorders. Psychiatry Res 16:165–176, 1985

Brambilla F, Petraglia F, Facchinetti F, et al: Abnormal beta-endorphin and beta-lipotropin responses to TRH and LRH administration in primary and secondary affective disorders. Acta Endocrinol 112:481–486, 1986

Brambilla F, Lampertico M, Sali L, et al: Clonidine stimulation in anorexia nervosa: growth hormone, cortisol, and beta-endorphin responses. Psychiatry Res 20:19–31, 1987

Campbell M, Small AM, Sokol MS, et al: Naltrexone in autistic children: an acute dose range tolerance trial. Report to the Stallone Foundation, 1987

Catlin DH, Gorelick DA, Gerner RH, et al: Clinical effects of beta-endorphin infusions, in Advances in Biochemical Psycho-pharmacology, Vol 22: Neural Peptides and Neuronal Communication. Edited by Costa E, Trabucchi EM. New York, Raven, 1980, pp 465–472

Christie MJ, Chesher GB: Physical dependence on physiologically released endogenous opiates. Life Sci 30:1173–1177, 1982

Cohen MR, Cohen RM, Pickar D, et al: High-dose naloxone infusions in normals: dose-dependent behavioral, hormonal, and physiological responses. Arch Gen Psychiatry 40:613–619, 1983

Cohen MR, Cohen RM, Pickar D, et al: High dose naloxone in depression. Biol Psychiatry 19:825–832, 1984a

Cohen MR, Pickar D, Extein I, et al: Plasma cortisol and beta-endorphin immunoreactivity in nonmajor and major depression. Am J Psychiatry 141:628–632, 1984b

Coid J, Allolio B, Rees LH: Raised plasma metenkephalin in patients who habitually mutilate themselves. Lancet 2:545–546, 1983

Davidson PW, Kleene BM, Carroll M, et al: Effects of naloxone on self-injurious behavior: a case study. Applied Research in Mental Retardation 4:1–4, 1983

Davis GC, Bunney WE Jr, de Fraites EG, et al: Intravenous naloxone administration in schizophrenia and affective illness. Science 197:74–77, 1977

Davis GC, Bunney WE Jr, Buchsbaum MS, et al: Use of narcotic antagonists to study the role of endorphins in normal and psychiatric patients, in Endorphins in Mental Health Research. Edited by Usdin E, Bunney WE Jr, Kline NS. New York, Oxford University Press, 1979, pp 393–406

Davis GC, Buchsbaum MS, Naber D, et al: Altered pain perception and cerebrospinal endorphins in psychiatric illness. Ann NY Acad Sci 398:366–373, 1982

Davis KL, Samuel A, Mathe AA, et al: Intracerebral des-tyrosine-gamma-endorphin inhibits methylphenidate induced locomotor activity. Life Sci 28:2421–2424, 1981

Devoize JL, Rigal F, Eschalier A, et al: Influence of naloxone on anti-depressant drug effects in the forced swimming test in mice. Psychopharmacology (Berlin) 84:71–75, 1984

DeWied D, Kovacs GL, Bohus B, et al: Neuroleptic activity of the neuropeptide beta-LPH$_{62}$ $_{77}$([des tyr^1]-gamma-endorphin; DTgammaE). Eur J Pharmacol LPH 62–77, 1978

Dupont A, Villeneuve A, Bouchard JP, et al: Rapid inactivation of enkephalin-like material by CSF in chronic schizophrenia. Lancet 2:1107, 1978

Emrich HM, Cording C, Piree S, et al: Actions of naloxone in different types of psychoses, in Endorphins in Mental Health Research. Edited by Usdin E, Bunney WE Jr, Kline NS. New York, Oxford University Press, 1979a, pp 352–360

Emrich HM, Hollt V, Kissling W, et al: Beta-endorphin-like immunoreactivity in cerebrospinal fluid and plasma of patients with schizophrenia and other neuropsychiatric disorders. Pharmakopsychiatrie, Neuropsychopharmakologie 12:269–276, 1979b

Emrich HM, Vogt P, Herz A: Possible antidepressive effects of opioids: action of buprenorphine. Ann NY Acad Sci 398:108–112, 1982a

Emrich HM, Zaudig M, Kissling W, et al: Clinical trial of des-tyr-gamma-endorphin in mental illness. Ann NY Acad Sci 398:470–477, 1982b

Extein I, Pottash AL, Gold MS, et al: Deficient prolactin response to morphine in depressed patients. Am J Psychiatry 137:845–846, 1980

Fekete MI, Kanyicska B, Szentendrei T, et al: Loss of sensitivity to morphine induced by prolonged ACTH treatment. Pharmacol Biochem Behav 20:879–882, 1984

Fink M, Simeon J, Itil TM, et al: Clinical antidepressant activity of cyclazocine—a narcotic antagonist. Clin Pharmacol Ther 11:41–48, 1970

Frecska E, Arato M, Bánki CM, et al: Prolactin response to fentanyl in depression. Biol Psychiatry 25:692–696, 1989

Fullerton DT, Swift WJ, Getto CJ, et al: Plasma immunoreactive beta-endorphin in bulimics. Psychol Med 16:59–63, 1986

Fullerton DT, Swift WJ, Getto CJ, et al: Differences in the plasma beta-endorphin levels of bulimics. International Journal of Eating Disorders 7:191–200, 1988

Gerner RH, Sharp B: CSF beta-endorphin–immunoreactivity in normal, schizophrenic, depressed, manic and anorexic subjects. Brain Res 237:244–247, 1982

Gerner RH, Catlin DH, Gorelick DA, et al: Beta-endorphin: intravenous infusion causes behavioral change in psychiatric patients. Arch Gen Psychiatry 37:642–647, 1980

Gillberg C, Terenius L, Lonnerholm G: Endorphin activity in childhood psychosis: spinal fluid levels in 24 cases. Arch Gen Psychiatry 42:780–783, 1985

Gillman MA, Sandyk R: Opiatergic and dopaminergic function and Lesch-Nyhan syndrome (letter). Am J Psychiatry 142:1226, 1985

Gispen-de Wied CC, Westenberg HGM, Thussen JHH, et al: The dexamethasone and cortisol suppression test in depression: beta-endorphin as a useful marker. Psychoneuroendocrinology 12:355–366, 1987

Giusti M, Cavagnaro P, Torre R, et al: Endogenous opioid blockade and gonadotropin secretion: role of pulsatile luteinizing hormone–releasing hormone administration in anorexia nervosa and weight loss amenorrhea. Fertil Steril 49:797–801, 1988

Gold PW, Gwirtsman HE, Avgerinos PC, et al: Abnormal hypothalamic-pituitary-adrenal function in anorexia nervosa: pathophysiologic mechanisms in underweight and weight-corrected patients. N Engl J Med 314:1335–1342, 1986a

Gold PW, Loriaux DL, Roy A, et al: Responses to corticotropin-releasing hormone in the hypercortisolism of depression and Cushing's disease: pathophysiologic and diagnostic implications. N Engl J Med 314:1329–1335, 1986b

Grevert P, Goldstein A: Endorphins: naloxone fails to alter experimental pain or mood in humans. Science 199:1093–1095, 1978

Grossman A, Moult PJA, McIntyre H, et al: Opiate mediation of amenorrhoea in hyperprolactinaemia and in weight-loss related amenorrhoea. Clin Endocrinol (Oxf) 17:379–388, 1982

Halmi KA: Classification of the eating disorders. J Psychiatr Res 19:113–119, 1985

Herman BH, Hammock MK, Arthur-Smith A, et al: A biochemical role for opioid peptides in self-injurious behavior. Paper presented at the annual meeting of the American Academy of Child and Adolescent Psychiatry, Los Angeles, October 1986

Herman BH, Hammock MK, Arthur-Smith A, et al: Naltrexone decreases self-injurious behavior. Ann Neurol 22:550–552, 1987

Hoehn-Saric R, Masek BJ: Effects of naloxone on normals and chronically anxious patients. Biol Psychiatry 16:1041–1050, 1981

Holaday JW, Tortella FC, Long JB, et al: Endogenous opioids and their receptors: evidence for involvement in the postictal effects of electroconvulsive shock. Ann NY Acad Sci 462:124–139, 1986

Hollister LE: Drug-induced psychiatric disorders and their management. Med Toxicol 1:428–448, 1986

Holtzman SG: Behavioral effects of separate and combined administration of naloxone and *d*-amphetamine. J Pharmacol Exp Ther 189:51–60, 1974

Hudson JI, Pope HG Jr, Jonas JM, et al: Family history study of anorexia nervosa and bulimia. Br J Psychiatry 142:133–138, 1983

Jacquet YF, Marks N: The C-fragment of beta-lipotropin: an endogenous neuroleptic or antipsychotogen? Science 194:632–635, 1976

Janowsky D, Judd L, Huey L, et al: Naloxone effects on manic symptoms and growth-hormone levels (letter). Lancet 2:320, 1978

Jonas JM, Gold MS: Treatment of antidepressant-resistant bulimia with naltrexone. Int J Psychiatry Med 16:305–309, 1986–1987

Jonas JM, Gold MS: Naltrexone treatment of bulimia: clinical and theoretical findings linking eating disorders and substance abuse, in Pharmacological Issues in Alcohol and Substance Abuse. Edited by Stimmel B. New York, Haworth Press, 1988a, pp 29–37

Jonas JM, Gold MS: The use of opiate antagonists in treating bulimia: a study of low-dose versus high-dose naltrexone. Psychiatry Res 24:195–199, 1988b

Judd LL, Risch SC, Parker DC, et al: Blunted prolactin response: a neuroendocrine abnormality manifested by depressed patients. Arch Gen Psychiatry 39:1413–1416, 1982

Kaye WH, Pickar D, Naber D, et al: Cerebrospinal fluid opioid activity in anorexia nervosa. Am J Psychiatry 139:643–645, 1982

Kaye WH, Berrettini WH, Gwirtsman HE, et al: Reduced cerebrospinal fluid levels of immunoreactive proopiomelanocortin related peptides (including beta-endorphin) in anorexia nervosa. Life Sci 41:2147–2155, 1987a

Kaye WH, Gwirtsman HE, George DT, et al: Elevated cerebrospinal fluid levels of immunoreactive corticotropin-releasing hormone in anorexia nervosa: relation to state of nutrition, adrenal function, and intensity of depression. J Clin Endocrinol Metab 64:203–208, 1987b

Klein H, Jungkunz G, Nedopil N, et al: Clinical effects of the synthetic analogue of methionine-enkephaline FK33-824, in Proceedings of the Third World Congress of Biological Psychiatry. Edited by Perris C, Struwe G, Jansson B. Amsterdam, Elsevier, 1981, pp 390–393

Kleinman JE, Iadarola M, Govoni S, et al: Postmortem measurements of neuropeptides in human brain. Psychopharmacol Bull 19:375–377, 1983

Kline NS, Li CH, Lehmann HE, et al: Beta-endorphin-induced changes in schizophrenic and depressed patients. Arch Gen Psychiatry 34:1111–1113, 1977

Kraepelin E: Die psychiatrische Klinik. Leipzig, Barth, 1905

Lindstrom LH, Widerlöv E, Gunne LM, et al: Endorphins in human cerebrospinal fluid: clinical correlations to some psychotic states. Acta Psychiatr Scand 57:153–164, 1978

Luby ED, Marrazzi MA, Kinzie J: Treatment of chronic anorexia nervosa with opiate blockade (letter). J Clin Psychopharmacol 7:52–53, 1987

Margules DL: Beta-endorphin and endoloxone: hormones of the autonomic nervous system for the conservation or expenditure of bodily resources and energy in anticipation of famine or feast. Neurosci Biobehav Rev 3:155–162, 1979

Marrazzi MA, Luby ED: An auto-addiction opioid model of chronic anorexia nervosa. International Journal of Eating Disorders 5:191–208, 1986

Matthews J, Akil H, Greden J, et al: Beta-endorphin/beta-lipotropin immunoreactivity in endogenous depression: effect of dexamethasone. Arch Gen Psychiatry 43:374–381, 1986

Mitchell JE, Laine DE, Morley JE, et al: Naloxone but not CCK-8 may attenuate binge-eating behavior in patients with the bulimia syndrome. Biol Psychiatry 21:1399–1406, 1986

Moore R, Mills IH, Forster A: Naloxone in the treatment of anorexia nervosa: effect on weight gain and lipolysis. J R Soc Med 74:129–131, 1981

Morley JE, Blundell JE: The neurobiological basis of eating disorders: some formulations. Biol Psychiatry 23:53–78, 1988

Morley JE, Levine AS: Involvement of dynorphin and the kappa opioid receptor in feeding. Peptides 4:797–800, 1983

Morley JE, Levine AS, Rowland NE: Minireview: stress-induced eating. Life Sci 32:2169–2182, 1983

Naber D, Pickar D, Post RM, et al: Endogenous opioid activity and beta-endorphin immunoreactivity in CSF of psychiatric patients and normal volunteers. Am J Psychiatry 138:1457–1462, 1981

Olson GA, Olson RD, Kastin AJ: Endogenous opiates: 1987. Peptides 10:205–236, 1989

Panksepp J: A neurochemical theory of autism. Trends in Neuroscience 2:174–177, 1979

Panksepp J, Siviy SM, Normansell LA: Brain opioids and social emotions, in The Psychobiology of Attachment and Separation. Edited by Reite M, Field T. New York, Academic, 1985, pp 3–49

Petho B, Graf L, Karczag I, et al: Beta-endorphin administration to acute schizophrenic patients: a double-blind study. Ann NY Acad Sci 398:460–469, 1982

Pickar D, Davis GC, Schulz SC, et al: Behavioral and biological effects of acute beta-endorphin injection in schizophrenic and depressed patients. Am J Psychiatry 138:160–166, 1981

Pickar D, Extein I, Gold PW, et al: Endorphins and affective illness, in Endorphins and Opiate Antagonists in Psychiatric Research. Edited by Shah NS, Donald AG. New York, Plenum, 1982a, pp 375–397

Pickar D, Naber D, Post RM, et al: Endorphins in the cerebrospinal fluid of psychiatric patients. Ann NY Acad Sci 398:399–412, 1982b

Pickar D, Vartanian F, Bunney WE Jr, et al: Short-term naloxone administration in schizophrenic and manic patients. Arch Gen Psychiatry 39:313–319, 1982c

Post RM, Pickar D, Ballenger JC, et al: Endogenous opiates in cerebrospinal fluid: relationship to mood and anxiety, in Neurobiology of Mood Disorders. Edited by Post RM, Ballenger JC. Baltimore, MD, Williams & Wilkins, 1984, pp 356–368

Prior M, Werry JS: Autism, schizophrenia, and allied disorders, in Psychopathological Disorders of Childhood. Edited by Quay HC, Werry JS. New York, John Wiley, 1986, pp 156–210

Reisine TD, Rossor M, Spokes EG, et al: Opiate and neuroleptic receptor alteration in human schizophrenic brain tissue, in Receptors for Neurotransmitters and Peptide Hormones. Edited by Pepeu G, Kuhar JM, Enna SJ. New York, Raven, 1980, pp 443–450

Richardson JS, Zaleski WA: Naloxone and self-mutilation. Biol Psychiatry 18:99–101, 1983

Rimon R, Terenius L, Kampman R: Cerebrospinal fluid endorphins in schizophrenia. Acta Psychiatr Scand 61:395–403, 1980

Risch SC: Beta-endorphin hypersecretion in depression: possible cholinergic mechanisms. Biol Psychiatry 17:1071–1079, 1982

Risch SC, Cohen RM, Janowsky DS, et al: Mood and behavioral effects of physostigmine on humans are accompanied by elevations in plasma beta-endorphin and cortisol. Science 209:1545–1546, 1982

Robertson AG, Jackman H, Meltzer HY: Prolactin response to morphine in depression. Psychiatry Res 11:353–364, 1984

Ross M, Berger PA, Goldstein A: Plasma beta-endorphin immunoreactivity in schizophrenia. Science 205:1163–1164, 1979

Rubinow DR, Post RM, Pickar D, et al: Relationship between urinary free cortisol and CSF opioid binding activity in depressed patients and normal volunteers. Psychiatry Res 5:87–93, 1981

Sandman CA: Beta-endorphin disregulation in autistic and self-injurious behavior: a neurodevelopmental hypothesis. Synapse 2:193–199, 1988

Sandman CA, Datta PC, Barron J, et al: Naloxone attenuates self-abusive behavior in developmentally disabled clients. Applied Research in Mental Retardation 4:5–11, 1983

Sandman CA, Barron JL, Crinella FM, et al: Influence of naloxone on brain and behavior of a self-injurious woman. Biol Psychiatry 22:899–906, 1987

Sandyk R: Naloxone abolishes self-injuring in a mentally retarded child (letter). Ann Neurol 17:520, 1985

Shodell MJ, Reiter HH: Self-mutilative behavior in verbal and non-verbal schizophrenic children. Arch Gen Psychiatry 19:453–455, 1968

Szymanski L, Kedesdy J, Sulkes S, et al: Naltrexone in treatment of self-injurious behavior: a clinical study. Research in Developmental Disabilities 8:179–190, 1987

Tamminga CA, Tighe PJ, Chase TN, et al: Des-tyrosine-gamma-endorphin administration in chronic schizophrenics: a preliminary report. Arch Gen Psychiatry 38:167–168, 1981

Terenius L, Wahlstrom A, Lindström L, et al: Increased CSF levels of endorphins in chronic psychosis. Neurosci Lett 3:157–162, 1976

Terenius L, Wahlstrom A, Ågren H: Naloxone (Narcan) treatment in depression: clinical observations and effects on CSF endorphins and monoamine metabolites. Psychopharmacology (Berlin) 54:31–33, 1977

Verhoeven WMA, van Praag HM, van Ree JM, et al: Improvement of schizophrenic patients treated with [des-tyr^1]-gamma-endorphin (DTgammaE). Arch Gen Psychiatry 36:294–298, 1979

Vigersky RA, Loriaux DL: Anorexia nervosa as a model of hypothalamic dysfunction, in Anorexia Nervosa. Edited by Vigersky RA. New York, Raven, 1977, pp 109–123

Wagemaker H Jr, Cade R: The use of hemodialysis in chronic schizophrenia. Am J Psychiatry 134:684–685, 1977

Wagemaker H, Rogers JL, Cade R: Schizophrenia, hemodialysis, and the placebo effect: results and issues. Arch Gen Psychiatry 41:805–810, 1984

Walker JM, Matsumoto RR, Bowen WD, et al: Evidence for a role of haloperidol-sensitive sigma-"opiate" receptors in the motor effects of antipsychotic drugs. Neurology 38:961–965, 1988

Waller DA, Kiser RS, Hardy BW, et al: Eating behavior and plasma beta-endorphin in bulimia. Am J Clin Nutr 44:20–23, 1986

Weizman R, Weizman A, Tyano S, et al: Humoral-endorphin blood levels in autistic, schizophrenic and healthy subjects. Psychopharmacology (Berlin) 82:368–370, 1984

Zis AP, Haskett RF, Albala AA, et al: Opioid regulation of hypothalamic-pituitary-adrenal function in depression. Arch Gen Psychiatry 42:383–386, 1985a

Zis AP, Haskett RF, Albala AA, et al: Prolactin response to morphine in depression. Biol Psychiatry 20:287–292, 1985b

Chapter 11

Cholecystokinin in the Mammalian Central Nervous System: Review and Metabolic Analysis

K. Tanimoto, M.D.
S. Kuo, M.D.
J. N. Crawley, Ph.D.
C. A. Tamminga, M.D.

Chapter 11

Cholecystokinin in the Mammalian Central Nervous System: Review and Metabolic Analysis

Cholecystokinin (CCK) is a neurally active peptide, first described six decades ago as a gastrointestinal hormone. Not until 1975 was CCK discovered to exist in the mammalian central nervous system (CNS) (Dockray 1976; Vanderhaeghen et al. 1975). Even so, this gut-brain peptide has been found to have several unique properties in brain that suggest its potential involvement in a number of neuropsychiatric conditions. CCK can be found in high concentrations in the cerebral cortex and in some limbic system structures, whereas it exists at relatively low concentrations in the striatum and hypothalamus, and at minimal concentrations in the cerebellum and spinal cord (Crawley 1985). The peptide is colocalized with several "traditional" transmitters, implying that it may have a functional interaction with those systems. Also, several interesting behavioral actions of CCK are known. Despite these promising findings, a clear understanding of the mechanisms of CCK actions in mammalian behavior has not yet evolved. However, many discoveries have been made that provide information on the biology of CCK in brain.

BASIC CHARACTERISTICS OF NEURONAL CHOLECYSTOKININ

Cholecystokinin neurons are the most numerous of all peptidergic neurons in the CNS, with their highest concentrations occurring in the cerebral cortex and hippocampus. The cortical CCK-containing neurons are for the most part local-circuit–type neurons, but a long neuronal projection extends down from the prefrontal area to the mid-thalamus and another, from the hippocampal formation to the lateral septum (Fallon and Seroogy 1985). The CCK-containing cell bodies in the basal forebrain also appear to be local-circuit neurons. In the mesencephalon, CCK exists in cell bodies in the ventral tegmental area (VTA) and dorsal raphe, colocalized with dopamine in some of the A9 and A10 neurons. These dopamine-CCK cell bodies have long axons that project caudally to the striatum, nucleus accumbens, olfactory tubercle, septum, amygdala, and to the prefrontal anterior cingulate and piriform cortices. This latter distribution of CCK—its colocalization with DA in the A9 and A10 neurons—has stimulated a great deal of speculation about CCK's involvement with dopamine-related CNS illnesses (Fallon and Seroogy 1985). In the hippocampus, CCK stimulates pyramidal cell firing, as it does in the hypothalamus, cortex, VTA, nucleus accumbens, trigeminal nucleus, and spinal neurons.

CCK exists in several different molecular forms in brain, many of which are likely to have functional significance. Although CCKs with 58-, 39-, 33-, 12-, 8-, and 5-amino-acid residues have been detected in brain, the predominant form according to current examination is CCK-8 (Marley et al. 1984). In addition, the neurally active forms of CCK are sulfated at the tyrosine residue (Marley et al. 1984). In gut, the predominant forms appear to be CCK-58 and CCK-33.

CCK has its own receptor in brain that appears to differ from the gut receptor with respect to its affinities for the various molecular forms of the peptide. The neural CCK receptor has its highest affinity for the octapeptide, but also an equivalent affinity for the larger sequences, because they contain the exact C-terminal octapeptide sequence. Surprisingly, the C-terminal fragments of CCK-8, including both CCK-5 and CCK-4, are present in brain (Rehfeld et al. 1985) and have a sufficiently high affinity at the CCK receptor for activity (Steardo et al. 1985b). Various studies have described the degradatory pathway for CCK-8 in brain (Rose et al. 1985; Steardo et al. 1985a), and CCK-5 and CCK-4 are both probable metabolic products of the octapeptide. This finding raises the possibility that the breakdown products of CCK-8 may be active in the synapse at the CCK receptor (Steardo et al. 1985a). Thus, brain concentrations of CCK and its metabolites could potentially be pharmacologically regulated for therapeutic reasons through modification of the degradation rate.

The biosynthesis and processing of CCK derive from preprocholecystokinin (pre-pro-CCK) as translated from the CCK gene (Goltermann 1985). The cDNA for rat pre-pro-CCK has been prepared from a rat medullary tumor cell line and the sequence of the gene determined (Deschenes et al. 1985). This technique predicted a 115-amino-acid precursor to CCK (12,826 daltons). Indeed, a sequence of 96 amino acids has been identified in the mammalian CNS as the probable pre-pro-CCK. Very little is known about the intracellular proteolytic processing steps that lead from pre-pro-CCK to the smaller, biologically active, concentrated forms of CCK. However, like peptides in general, the prohormone is synthesized in the neuronal cell body on the endoplasmic reticulum from a messenger RNA (mRNA) sequence generated from nuclear DNA. Its posttranslational processing could be expected to occur, at least in part, inside the transport vesicle. The process of sulfation and cleavage of CCK occurs just outside or in the CCK terminal. A fuller knowledge of this biosynthetic process could suggest the determinants of potential CCK pathology in diseases of the brain and could also offer sites for pharmacological modulation of central CCK-8 concentrations.

CHOLECYSTOKININ AND DOPAMINE

The coexistence of CCK with dopamine-containing cells in the mesencephalic neurons was first described by Hökfelt and coworkers in colchicine-treated rat brain (Hökfelt et al. 1980). In the VTA and substantia nigra pars compacta (SNC), CCK-immunoreactive cell bodies have a distribution that is similar, even though more limited, to that of tyrosine hydroxylase–containing neurons. Also, the coexistence of CCK, dopamine, and neurotensin has been described in the VTA (Seroogy et al. 1988). In the anterior SNC and in the substantia nigra pars lateralis (SNL), many dopamine cells contain CCK; in the VTA approximately 40% of all dopamine cells contain CCK; whereas in the rest of the SNC and the substantia nigra pars reticulata (SNR), few dopamine-CCK cells exist. With respect to their projection areas, dopamine-CCK cells extend to the posterior medial nucleus accumbens, the posterior medial olfactory tubercle, the bed nucleus of the stria terminalis, the periventricular zone tail of the caudate, and the central amygdala; many dopamine projection fields contain no CCK fibers (Skirboll et al. 1981). Additional basal ganglia CCK systems exist in the SNR and in the striatum that are anatomically distinct from the dopamine-CCK cells. Lesion experiments have supported the observation of dopamine-CCK colocalization in that 6-hydroxydopamine (6-OHDA) treatment reduces both dopamine- and CCK-immunoreactive cell bodies and selectively reduces CCK in dopamine-CCK projection areas but not in dopamine-only areas (Marley et al. 1982; Studler et al. 1981). Findings in cats, monkeys, and humans are consistent with these detailed rat data.

The functional significance of the dopamine-CCK colocalization has been studied using electrophysiological, biochemical, and behavioral techniques. CCK increases the firing of neurons in areas of cells containing both CCK and dopamine, but fails to modify firing in areas with only dopaminergic neurons (Skirboll et al. 1981). CCK diminishes dopamine release in cat striatum (Markstein and Hökfelt 1984), while low concentrations may enhance dopamine release in the nucleus accumbens (Meyer and Krauss 1983). CCK also potentiates apomorphine-induced effects on dopamine cell firing, hypothesized to be an effect mediated by dopamine autoreceptors (Hommer and Skirboll 1983). Moreover, when the dopamine-CCK neurons are lesioned with 6-OHDA, CCK-8 levels are reduced (Yamamoto and Kato 1988), and neuronal response to CCK and to dopamine in the nucleus accumbens is augmented (Debonnel and DeMontigny 1988). In the nucleus accumbens, CCK potentiates dopamine-mediated behaviors, namely dopamine-induced hyperlocomotion and apomorphine-induced stereotypy. This potentiation of dopamine-related behaviors by CCK occurs in the nucleus accumbens, but not in the caudate, supporting the idea of cotransmitter-neuronal mediation. In addition, the potentiation is effectively antagonized by a CCK antagonist, proglumide, and by CCK antisera (Crawley et al. 1985).

Pathways Subserving Dopamine-CCK–Mediated Animal Behaviors

In an attempt to explore the neuronal circuit mediating CCK-potentiated dopamine-induced locomotor activity, we studied regional brain metabolism in the rat with local stereotactic administration of dopamine, CCK octapeptide (CCK-8), or dopamine and CCK-8 into the nucleus accumbens. The cerebral metabolism experiment was carried out with a dose and route of administration of these compounds already known to have reproducible behavioral activity after intercerebral administration (Crawley et al. 1985). The regional brain metabolism experiment would potentially allow visualization of the primary nucleus accumbens projection area metabolically modified by dopamine and by dopamine and CCK-8, and, perhaps, the secondary or tertiary projection sites to describe a relevant cerebral pathway for this behavior. It is useful to recognize that glucose metabolism studies provide information about regional levels of glucose utilization in specific brain areas; this utilization is generally taken to represent the level of synaptic activity of neurons in a particular location. The technique does not directly provide information about different cell populations or transmitters involved, nor whether neuronal excitation or inhibition is occurring with the synaptic discharge.

Thus, in this experiment we attempted to identify projection sites of the nucleus accumbens whose metabolism was altered by intranigral dopamine and by dopamine and CCK-8. Actual identification of this pathway would describe at least one efferent pathway of the nucleus accumbens involved in the mediation of locomotor activity in the rat.

The results (Table 11-1) failed to reveal selective metabolic alterations produced by dopamine in basal ganglia areas thought to be directly connected to the nucleus accumbens. Areas were sought whose metabolism was modified by dopamine then further altered (i.e., potentiated) by CCK-8. If found, these areas would have suggested to us the pathway that mediates the dopamine–CCK-8 motor effects. The failure to identify such a pathway may well be accounted for by the long temporal integration period of this method; these motor behaviors may require a short half-life tracer.

However, we were able to select some areas from those assessed—areas that are thought to be a part of basal ganglia circuits involved in the normal execution of rat motor behaviors—and test their relatedness statistically. The nucleus accumbens purportedly modulates rat locomotor behavior through a circuit whose first projection area is the ventral pallidum–substantia innominata. Moreover, this nucleus accumbens–ventral pallidum leg may make up a circuit involving the nucleus accumbens, ventral pallidum, dorsomedial n. thalamus, and prefrontal cortex (Figure 11-1) by which selected motor behaviors are mediated. This pathway is in contrast to the well-known pathway involving the SNC, caudate, globus pallidus, SNR, ventralis anterior/ventralis lateralis (VA/VL) n. thalamus, and premotor cortex (Figure 11-2) that is thought to subserve "extrapyramidal" motor behaviors. Our testing of these data using principal component analysis indicates four different groups of brain areas that are more uniformly affected by the treatments within themselves than between groups. Interestingly enough, the nucleus accumbens areas cluster in one factor (Figure 11-1) and include the ventral pallidum, whereas the caudate cluster includes the globus pallidus (Figure 11-2). Thus, although these treatments were unable to induce distinct metabolic patterns, they did delineate a distinction between the nucleus accumbens projection circuit (where the drugs were injected) and the caudate ("extrapyramidal") circuit.

Clinical Roles of the Dopamine-CCK Systems

Based on the experimental data suggesting that dopamine and CCK are functionally related, interest developed in exploring the actions of CCK in human diseases known to involve dopamine, such as Parkinson's disease, Huntington's chorea, and schizophrenia. Alterations in levels of CCK-8 in brain or spinal fluid have been reported in Parkinson's disease and schizophrenia (Studler et al. 1982; Verbanck et al. 1984). Further, some positive reports of therapeutic studies in

Table 11-1. Glucose utilization rates in the conscious rat with intra-accumbens drug administration

Brain area	Saline	DA	CCK	CCK + DA
Limbic circuit				
Prefrontal cortex	100.8 ± 10.8	88.3 ± 9.7	112.0 ± 9.4	111.7 ± 7.7
Anterior cingulate	103.8 ± 12.2	84.5 ± 8.3	106.0 ± 8.7	110.5 ± 9.8
Dorsomedial thalamus	92.5 ± 8.4	88.5 ± 6.7	102.4 ± 11.7	116.5 ± 8.4
Hippocampus (CA-1)	78.8 ± 13.3	70.5 ± 6.2	80.1 ± 6.9	84.8 ± 4.9
Nucleus accumbens	92.4 ± 8.1	70.5 ± 4.2	93.4 ± 13.0	83.9 ± 5.6
Ventral tegmental area	77.4 ± 6.6	66.1 ± 4.6	78.6 ± 6.7	72.0 ± 1.4
Extramyramidal circuit				
Motor cortex	111.7 ± 10.9	93.3 ± 9.4	106.2 ± 4.2	114.0 ± 4.9
VA/VL thalamus	64.0 ± 6.8	54.0 ± 9.8	56.3 ± 5.2	73.9 ± 10.3
Globus pallidus	68.1 ± 4.3	60.0 ± 2.9	72.2 ± 3.7	79.0 ± 5.8
Caudate	101.1 ± 9.2	86.4 ± 7.8	108.0 ± 10.1	114.0 ± 7.0
Substantia nigra pars reticulata	67.7 ± 6.5	60.3 ± 3.5	71.5 ± 6.0	67.0 ± 2.4
Substantia nigra pars compacta	82.7 ± 6.1	72.3 ± 5.1	88.2 ± 7.3	85.5 ± 4.1

Note. CCK = cholecystokinin; DA = dopamine; VA/VL = ventralis anterior/ventralis lateralis.

schizophrenia have been published (Moroji et al. 1982). Because the administration of drugs to man for therapeutic reasons is commonly systemic, whereas many interesting actions of CCK occur only with central administration, the question of whether or not CCK-8 penetrates into brain has arisen. CCK-8 alters dopaminergic neuronal firing in rats after systemic administration, even after vagal nerve lesion, as well as regional glucose utilization in several selected brain areas (Lucignani et al. 1984). In contrast, ^{3}H-labeled CCK injected intravenously in a chronically cannulated monkey could not be detected in the CSF even after 60 minutes (M. Knight, personal communication, April 1986). In addition, some CCK-induced behaviors with systemic administration can be blocked with vagal nerve ligation. Nonetheless, enough clinical promise was apparent in response to CCK for clinical studies to be begun by several groups in schizophrenia and Parkinson's disease.

Parkinsonian patients stabilized on L-dopa were given intramuscular injections of ceruletide (0.3–0.6 g/kg) or placebo, and the symptoms were evaluated. No change occurred in any of the chief

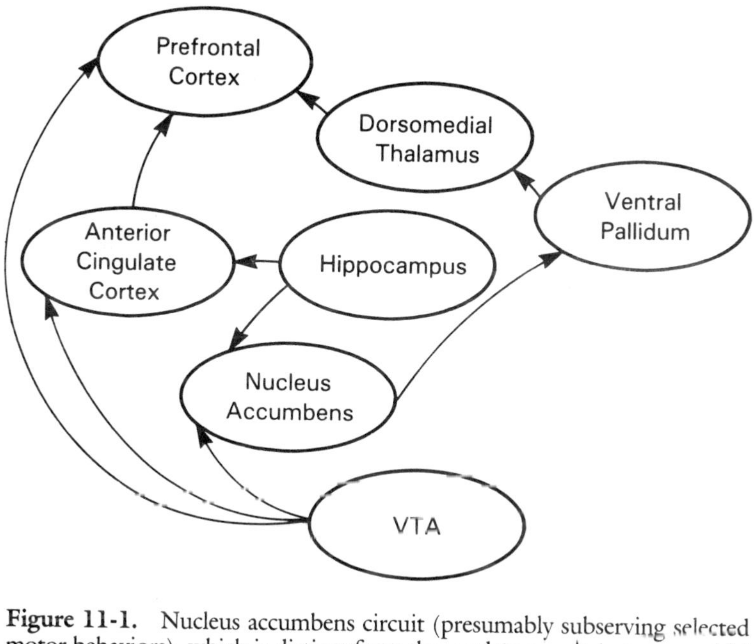

Figure 11-1. Nucleus accumbens circuit (presumably subserving selected motor behaviors), which is distinct from the caudate circuit (extrapyramidal pathway) (see Figure 11-2).

manifestations of the illness (Studler et al. 1982). In actively psychotic schizophrenic subjects otherwise drug free, ceruletide doses from 0.3 to 1.2 μg/kg did not alter any of the symptoms of schizophrenia (Bruno et al. 1985). This observation was made despite a previous report of antipsychotic efficacy. But several additional studies have now confirmed the lack of efficacy of CCK-8 and its analogue ceruletide in schizophrenia (Tamminga et al. 1986). Tamminga et al. (1986) found that ceruletide did not alter the cerebral evoked potential, suggesting that there was no central presence of a pharmacologically active substance. The conclusion from these studies is that the central activity occurring after systemic CCK administration was not sufficient to evaluate its clinical efficacy. For this reason, the actual effect of CCK in these diseases remains untested because of the lack

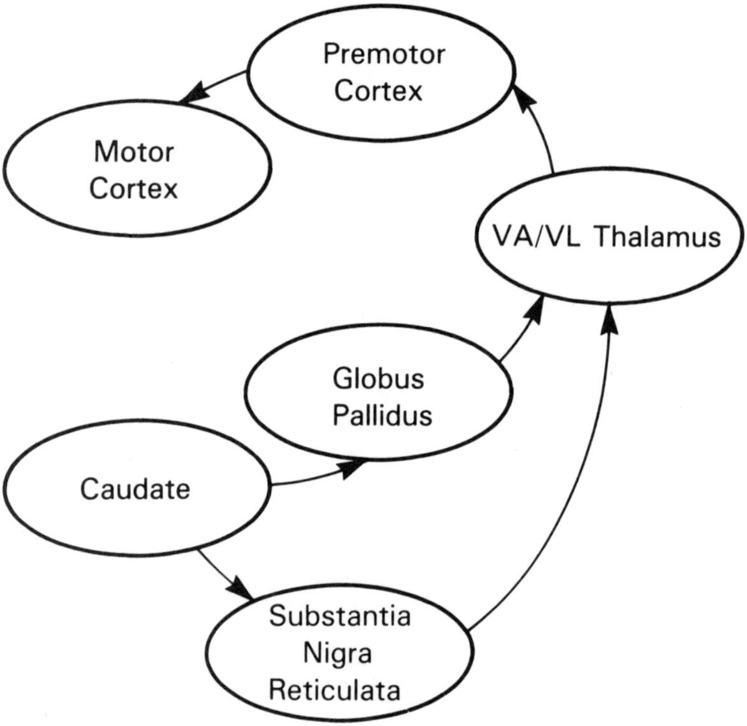

Figure 11-2. Caudate circuit or extrapyramidal pathway (presumably subserving selected motor behaviors), which is distinct from the nucleus accumbens circuit (see Figure 11-1). VA/VL = ventralis anterior/ventralis lateralis.

of any evidence suggesting that CCK or ceruletide can actually enter brain.

SUMMARY

Cholecystokinin was one of the first neurally active peptides to be vigorously studied in its relationship to human brain diseases. This early interest probably occurred because of the very early reports of its colocalization with dopamine, which suggested that CCK might regulate dopamine-mediated neuronal transmission in some way and that that knowledge might be important to illnesses such as Parkinson's disease and schizophrenia. But the pharmacologic experiments, including a number of clinical trials, began before there was a full understanding of how or even what CCK did in the mammalian CNS. Indeed, this is true of most neurally active peptides. Are these compounds neurotransmitters? neuromodulators? autocoids? or do they exert functionally different effects in different brain areas? or with respect to different peptidergic functions?

These questions are now in the process of being answered by basic research. The research so far would encourage clinicians to think that CCK system modulation might some day be a viable therapeutic strategy. However, the clinical designs carried out to date have not been able to test the outcome of central CCK system augmentation in dopamine-related illnesses. These tests will have to await some CNS peptide delivery technique of demonstrable effectiveness.

Until then, we know that CCK is a peptide that is distributed within the CNS, both by itself and colocalized with dopamine and neurotensin. CCK has its own receptors and synthetic and degradatory pathways, the former pathway involving transcription, translation, and axonal transport. CCK has effects on animal appetitive and motor behavior and satiety, and it might well have actions in the human nervous system that are of therapeutic interest to physicians.

REFERENCES

Bruno G, Ruggieri S, Chase TN, et al: Caerulein treatment of Parkinson's disease. Clin Neuropharmacol 8:266–270, 1985

Crawley JN: Comparative distribution of cholecystokinin and other neuropeptides: why is this peptide different from all other peptides? Ann NY Acad Sci 448:1–8, 1985

Crawley JN, Stivers JA, Blumstein LK, et al: Cholecystokinin potentiates dopamine-mediated behaviors: evidence for modulation specific to a site of coexistence. J Neurosci 5:1972–1983, 1985

Debonnel G, DeMontigny C: Increased neuronal responsiveness to cholecystokinin and dopamine induced by lesioning mesolimbic dopaminergic neurons: an electrophysiological study in the rat. Synapse 2:537–545, 1988

Deschenes RJ, Haun RS, Sunkel D, et al: Modulation of cholecystokinin gene expression. Ann NY Acad Sci 448:53–60, 1985

Dockray GJ: Immunochemical evidence of cholecystokinin-like peptides in brain. Nature 264:568–570, 1976

Fallon JH, Seroogy KB: The distribution and some connections of cholecystokinin neurons in the rat brain. Ann NY Acad Sci 448:121–132, 1985

Goltermann NR: The biosynthesis of cholecystokinin in neural tissue. Ann NY Acad Sci 448:76–86, 1985

Hökfelt T, Rehfeld L, Skirboll B, et al: Evidence for coexistence of dopamine and CCK in meso-limbic neurons. Nature 285:476–478, 1980

Hommer D, Skirboll L: Cholecystokinin-like peptides potentiate apomorphine-induced inhibition of dopamine neurons. Eur J Pharmacol 91:151–152, 1983

Lucignani G, Porrino LJ, Tamminga CA: Effects of systematically administered cholecystokinin-octapeptide on local cerebral metabolism. Eur J Pharmacol 101:147–151, 1984

Markstein R, Hökfelt T: Effect of cholecystokinin-octapeptide on dopamine release from slices of cat caudate nucleus. J Neurosci 4:570–575, 1984

Marley PD, Rehfeld JF: Extraction techniques for gastrins and cholecystokinins in the rat central nervous system. J Neurochem 42:1515–1522, 1984

Marley PD, Emson PC, Rehfeld JF: Effect of 6-hydroxydopamine lesions of the medial forebrain bundle on the distribution of cholecystokinin in rat forebrain. Brain Res 252:382–385, 1982

Marley PD, Rehfeld JF, Emson PC: Distribution and chromatographic characterization of gastrin and cholecystokinin in the rat central nervous system. J Neurochem 42:1536–1541, 1984

Meyer DK, Krauss J: Dopamine modulates cholecystokinin release in neostriatum. Nature 301:338–340, 1983

Moroji T, Watanabe N, Aoki N, et al: Antipsychotic effects of ceruletide (caerulein) on chronic schizophrenia. Arch Gen Psychiatry 39:485–486, 1982

Rehfeld JF, Hansen HF, Marley PD: Molecular forms of cholecystokinin in the brain and the relationship to neuronal gastrins. Ann NY Acad Sci 448:11–23, 1985

Rose C, Camus A, Schwartz JC: A serine peptidase responsible for the inactivation of endogenous cholecystokinin in brain. Proc Natl Acad Sci USA 21:8326–8330, 1985

Seroogy K, Ceccatelli S, Schalling M, et al: A subpopulation of dopamine neurons in rat ventral mesencephalon contains both neurotensin and cholecystokinin. Brain Res 455:88–98, 1988

Skirboll LR, Grace AA, Hommer DW, et al: Peptide-monoamine coexistence: studies of actions of cholecystokinin-like peptide on the electrical activity of midbrain dopamine neurons. Neuroscience 6:2111–2124, 1981

Steardo L, Knight M, Tamminga, CA, et al: $CCK_{26\text{-}33}$ degrading activity in brain and nonneural tissue: a metalloendopeptidase. J Neurochem 45:784–790, 1985a

Steardo L, Knight M, Tamminga CA, et al: Products of cholecystokinin (CCK)–octapeptide proteolysis interact with central CCK receptors. Neurosci Lett 54:319–325, 1985b

Studler JM, Simon H, Cesselin F, et al: Biochemical investigation on the localization of the cholecystokinin octapeptide in dopaminergic neurons originating from the ventral tegmental area of the rat. Neuropeptides 2:131–139, 1981

Studler JM, Javoy-Agid F, Cesselin F, et al: CCK-8 immunoreactivity distribution in human brain: selective decrease in the substantia nigra from parkinsonian patients. Brain Res 243:176–179, 1982

Tamminga CA, Littman RL, Alphs LD: Cholecystokinin: a neuropeptide in the treatment of schizophrenia. Psychopharmacology (Berlin) 22:129–132, 1986

Vanderhaeghen J-J, Signeau JC, Gepts W: New peptide in the vertebrate CNS reacting with gastrin antibodies. Nature 257:604–605, 1975

Verbanck PMP, Lotstra F, Gilles C, et al: Reduced cholecystokinin immunoreactivity in the cerebrospinal fluid of patients with psychiatric disorders. Life Sci 34:67–72, 1984

Yamamoto H, Kato T: Effects on brain cholecystokinin-8-sulfate and serotonin in adult rats after neonatal reduction of catecholamines. Neurosci Res 5:265–271, 1988

Chapter 12

Adrenocorticotropin, Interferons, and Interleukins

Lakshmi S. Kamaraju, M.D.
K. Ranga Rama Krishnan, M.D.

Chapter 12

Adrenocorticotropin, Interferons, and Interleukins

ADRENOCORTICOTROPIN

Adrenocorticotropin (ACTH) is primarily synthesized in the anterior pituitary, and its major role is the regulation of the adrenal cortex. Its role in the central nervous system (CNS) is unclear. The amount of ACTH in the CNS is less than 1% of that in the pituitary. Bioactive ACTH has been identified in the hypothalamus and amygdala. On the other hand, ACTH immunoreactivity has been identified in the neurons of the arcuate nucleus. The vast amount of immunoreactivity is in the form of $ACTH_{18-39}$. ACTH-stained nerve terminals are seen in the paraventricular nucleus, thalamic nuclei, bed nucleus, nucleus of the stria terminalis, midbrain, pons, medulla oblongata, and spinal cord (Dekloet et al. 1981; Palkovits 1980).

Behavioral Effects of ACTH

$ACTH_{1-24}$ injected into the ventricles of the brain in rats is known to induce excessive grooming behavior. This behavior is different from that induced by beta-endorphins. The grooming behavior induced by ACTH is not interrupted as much by walking and rearing activity compared with that induced by beta-endorphins. Similar behavior is induced by the administration of $ACTH_{1-24}$ into the hippocampus (Oitzl and Huston 1984). When injected into rat periaqueductal gray matter, $ACTH_{1-24}$ produces a behavioral syndrome characterized by fearful hyperactivity and explosive behavior. This syndrome is not naloxone-reversible. Further work has suggested that ACTH receptor activity may be related to the behavioral excitation seen in the opiate abstinence syndrome (Yasuko et al. 1981).

The behavioral pharmacology of ACTH fragments has been reviewed elsewhere (Bohus 1979; Dunn 1980) and will not be reviewed here other than to briefly discuss the behavioral effects of

$ACTH_{4-10}$ and $ACTH_{4-9}$ in humans (Branconnier 1981). $ACTH_{4-9}$ (ORG 2766) is a congener of $ACTH_{4-10}$. It has a longer half-life and is 1,000 times more potent behaviorally than $ACTH_{4-10}$. $ACTH_{4-10}$ is the common core heptapeptide of the proopiomelanocortin-derived hormone. $ACTH_{4-10}$, like ACTH, can ameliorate some of the behavioral deficits seen after hypophysectomy in animals.

$ACTH_{4-10}$ can affect electroencephalographic activity during stimulation but has minimal effects on spontaneous electroencephalographic activity. Unlike $ACTH_{1-24}$, $ACTH_{4-10}$ reduced state anxiety in some studies but not in others. $ACTH_{4-10}$ does not significantly and consistently affect attentional processes or memory in humans. This is in sharp contrast to the animal literature in which these compounds have been shown to produce marked effects on behavior and memory (Branconnier 1981).

Plasma ACTH concentrations are increased in patients with major depression. This elevation usually, but not always, accompanies an increase in plasma cortisol concentrations (Krishnan et al. 1988). The alteration in plasma ACTH concentration primarily reflects an activation of the hypothalamo-pituitary-adrenal (HPA) axis. Changes in cerebrospinal fluid (CSF) ACTH concentrations have not been well studied and must be considered preliminary at this juncture. In summary, little is known about the relevance of ACTH in the brain in psychiatric disorders.

An additional role for ACTH, that of immunoregulation, may also be of interest. Leukocytes possess receptors for ACTH. ACTH can either enhance or inhibit the lymphocyte proliferative response. This type of modulation induced by ACTH is donor specific. Furthermore, murine macrophages are known to produce proopiomelanocortin peptides, including ACTH. Lymphoctyes infected with the New Castle disease virus and the typhoid vaccine are also known to produce ACTH. Corticotropin-releasing factor (CRF) can also induce the production of ACTH by lymphocytes. The concentration of ACTH secreted is low and the physiological significance unclear, but this production may play a role in the neuroendocrine and neuroimmune changes seen in affective disorders.

NEUROIMMUNE REGULATION

The relationship between the nervous and endocrine systems has been well recognized. Initially the immune system was felt to be an independent entity. But now it is clearly demonstrated to be influenced by both the nervous system and the endocrine system. There are several lines of evidence indicating such a link. In animals with underdevelopment of lymphoid organs due to germ-free milieu, a concomitant hypofunctioning of the endocrine axis is observed. At the same time dwarf mice that are deficient in growth hormone and thyrotropin have impaired cellular immunity. Experimental rats, challenged with an antigen, have increased firing rates of neurons in the ventromedial nuclei of the hypothalamus at the time that plaque formation reaches its peak levels. Furthermore, manipulation of hypothalamic regions, especially the posterior hypothalamus, alters the immune reactions.

Until recently it was thought that the brain exerted its influence on immune systems through the HPA axis. But now other agents such as substance P, vasopressin, and oxytocin, and the endogenous opioid system are also implicated in neuroimmunological modulation. Recently a number of products secreted by macrophages and lymphocytes, known respectively as cytokines and lymphokines, have been added to the list of peptides that play a role in communication between and within the immune system and the CNS. In this section we will review the role of interleukins and interferons.

Interleukin 1

Interleukin 1 (IL-1) is a polypeptide that was initially shown to be secreted by mononuclear phagocytes. Subsequently, both normal and malignant cells are known to produce IL-1 (Table 12-1). Bacteria, fungi, and physiological stress induce the secretion of IL-1 (Cannon and Kluger 1983; Dinarello 1984). In addition to the human IL-1 alpha and IL-1 beta forms produced by monocytes, there exists a beta-lymphocyte–derived IL-1 form with a different amino acid sequence and function. Both IL-1 alpha (23 kilodaltons) and IL-1 beta (17 kilodaltons) are initially transcribed as precursor molecules (31-kilodalton molecular weight and 270 amino acids). Of the two, only the precursor for IL-1 alpha is capable of binding to the receptor and exerting biological activity. The active IL-1 alpha and IL-1 beta forms have 159 and 153 amino acids, respectively. When monocytes were fractionated and tested individually for IL-1 activity, the activity was recovered from cytosol, lysozymes, and plasma membranes, but not from endoplasmic reticulum. The cytosol fraction with IL-1 activity that had a 31 kilodalton molecular weight did not change much after trypsin treatment, indicating that the cytosol may contain the precursor molecule that is processed via lysosomal or prelysosomal vesicles. On the other hand, the plasma membrane–bound IL-1 activity that had a 23-kilodalton molecular weight stimulated the T cells. Proteolysis may be the mechanism by which the soluble forms of both IL-1 alpha and IL-1 beta are released. Once released, the half-life of IL-1 is relatively short because of degradation. The

Table 12-1. Effects of interleukins

System	Action	Mechanism
Central nervous system		
Hypothalmus		
Anterior hypothalamus with postpreoptic area	Fever induction	
Paraventricular nucleus	Increased release of MHPG from nonadrenergic neurons	Prostaglandin mediated
	Stimulation of CRF production	
	Stimulation of GRF production	
Intraventricular injection of IL-1	Augmentation of slow-wave sleep	
	Suppression of food and water intake	
Endocrine system		
Pituitary	Enhancement of POMC gene expression	Direct stimulation
	Increased ACTH, GH, LH, and prolactin production	Prostaglandin mediated
	Inhibition of TSH secretion	Leukotriene mediated
Adrenal cortex	Direct stimulation of the adrenal gland to induce cortisol production	Prostaglandin mediated

Pancreas	Stimulation of insulin production
Immune Systems	
T Lymphocytes	Chemotaxis and proliferation Production of IL-2
Helper Cells	Stimulation of macrophage-activating factor Colony-stimulating factor Beta cell–stimulating factor
Effector Cells	Production of interferon Chemotaxis and proliferation
Beta-lymphocytes	Activation of beta-lymphocytes
Macrophages	Generation of oxygen radicals Synthesis of prostaglandins and leukotrienes Secretion of interferon-α Increased cytotoxic activity Synthesis of tumor necrosis factor
Neutrophil	Chemotaxis and activation Induction of hydrolytic enzymes

Table 12-1. Effects of interleukins—continued

System	Action	Mechanism
Connective Tissue		
Fibroblasts	Proliferation	
Astrocytes	Proliferation and secretion of IL-1	
Glial cells	Proliferation and secretion of IL-1	
Chondrocytes	Induction of prostaglandin synthesis Degradation and reabsorption of proteoglycans and collagens	
Osteoclasts	Activation and increased resorption of bone	
Glomerular mesangial cells	Proliferation and increased production of PGE_2 and neutral proteases	
Hepatocytes	Synthesis of acute-phase reactants: serum amyloid, fibrinogen, C-reactive protein, α-1-antitrypsin	

Note. ACTH = adrenocorticotropin; CRF = corticotropin-releasing factor; GH = growth hormone; GRF = gonadotropin-releasing factor; LH = luteinizing hormone; MHPG = 3-methoxy-4-hydroxyphenylglycol; POMC = proopiomelanocortin; TSH = thyrotropin-releasing hormone.

degraded fragments with 4- and 2-kilodalton molecular weight also demonstrated biological activity (Bakouche et al. 1987; Martin and Resch 1988).

In addition to having a central role in the modulation of immune responses, IL-1 affects several other systems in the body (see Table 12-1).

Interleukin 1 and the CNS. IL-1 modulates various functions of the CNS and is produced by CNS cells such as astrocytes, glial cells, and endothelial cells. These cells secrete IL-1 in response to head trauma (Giulian and Lochman 1985). Other factors that stimulate IL-1 secretion are not known. Farrar and his colleagues (1987) have been able to map out receptors for IL-1 in different regions of the brain. Olfactory bulb, granular cells in the dentate gyrus, pyramidal cells in the hippocampal region, cerebellar cortex, and choroid plexus are some of the regions shown to have a very high density of IL-1 receptors (Farrar et al. 1987). Recently, Breder et al. (1988) identified IL-1–like immunoreactive neurons in the hypothalamus. The IL-1 immunoreactivity was high in the paraventricular, periventricular, and arcuate nuclei, median emminence, infundibulum, and in areas of the hypothalamus involved in cardiovascular regulation.

IL-1 has a variety of effects in the CNS. Bailey et al. (1976) demonstrated that injection of IL-1 into the lateral ventricles of the brain of rats, in much lower concentrations than if given systemically, induced hyperthermia, suggesting that the CNS is the primary site of action. Investigators also reported induction of slow-wave sleep coupled with fever after intraventricular infusion of IL-1 into rabbits (Walter et al. 1986). Although there was some inhibition of REM sleep, it was not very specific. However, so far there is no evidence that IL-1 plays a significant role in normal sleep. Prostaglandins are believed to be involved in both the pyrogenic activity and the soporific effects of IL-1. IL-1 beta suppresses food and water intake in rats by directly inhibiting the glucose-sensitive neurons in the hypothalamus. This effect is independent of its pyrogenicity (Plata-Salaman et al. 1988). In addition, IL-1 stimulates the production and release of CRF from the hypothalamus (Sapolsky et al. 1987). IL-1 also increases the production of MHPG in the hypothalamus, suggesting that non-adrenergic systems are involved.

Interleukin 1 and the HPA axis. IL-1 acts at multiple levels on the HPA axis. Besedovsky et al. (1986) reported an increase in ACTH and corticosterone levels in vivo after injection of supernatants from activated leukocytes. When this supernatant was pretreated with antibodies to IL-1, this capacity for induction was abolished, identifying IL-1 as the substance responsible for this effect. Besedovsky et al. also demonstrated an increase in ACTH and cortisol after direct injection of purified IL-1 into mice. This was the first indication of a role for IL-1 on the HPA axis (Besedovsky et al. 1986). When adrenal glands were perfused in situ with IL-1, there was a significant increase in corticosterone after 90 minutes. This increase was abolished by the addition of indomethacin, suggesting that the effect on the adrenals is prostaglandin mediated (Roh et al. 1987). IL-1 is also extremely potent in enhancing the expression of cytoplasmic proopiomelanocortin, both in primary pituitary cultures and in ACTH-secreting pituitary tumor cells (AtT-20) (Brown et al. 1987). IL-1 also induces ACTH release from AtT-20 cells (Woloski et al. 1985). However, there is some controversy regarding this finding, for other investigators failed to reproduce this result in their cultures (Berkenbosch et al. 1987; Uehara et al. 1987a). Lumpkin (1987) tried to address this controversy by pointing out some of the differences in the experimental settings involving sex, estrus cycle, and type of interleukin. Nonetheless, in vivo experiments clearly demonstrate stimulation of ACTH by IL-1 beta, but not by IL-1 alpha (Uehara et al. 1987b). IL-1 is now being shown to act even higher on the HPA axis. Both Sapolsky et al. (1987) and Berkenbosch et al. (1987) showed that IL-1 acts directly on the hypothalamus, stimulating the secretion of CRF. When antibody to CRF was injected prior to the administration of IL-1, rises in concentration of corticosterone were completely abolished. In fact, when Berkenbosch et al. administered colchicine, an axonal transport blocker, intracisternally along with IL-1, there was a decrease in the CRF immunofluorescence intensity, suggesting that IL-1 increased the secretory activity of CRF-producing neurons in the hypothalamus.

The significance of the effect of IL-1 on the HPA axis is not clearly understood. The interrelationship of immune and endocrine systems may be that of an "immunoregulatory feedback circuit" (Del Rey et al. 1987). Changes in glucorticoid levels in animals were shown to be proportional to immunological responses (Besedovsky et al. 1975). Various stimuli such as infections, physiological stress, and psychological stress induce the production of IL-1, which in turn stimulates the HPA axis as outlined earlier. However, cortisol secreted as a result of this stimulation has been shown to suppress the production of IL-1 in addition to other mediators of inflammation (Snyder and Unanue 1982). Similarly, IL-1 also activates the adrenergic systems both centrally and peripherally, which in turn inhibits further production of IL-1 (Koff et al. 1986). These findings raise speculation about the percise role of interleukins in stress, both physical and psychological.

Other Interleukins

In addition to IL-1, five other interleukins (IL-2, IL-3, IL-4, IL-5, IL-6) have been isolated and their immunological functions identified. Of these, IL-2 is particularly interesting in view of its effect on the CD4 receptors, the enhancement of proopiomelanocortin messenger RNA (RNA) expression, and the induction of proliferation of microglia in the CNS.

Interferons

Interferons are a family of glycoproteins that were initially isolated from cultures after infection with influenza virus. Subsequently, three types (with additional subtypes) were isolated depending on the type of cell source, inducing agent, and antigenicity. The three types are interferon-α (leukocyte derived), interferon-β (fibrocyte derived), and interferon-γ (lymphocyte derived). All three of these interferons are induced by various agents, such as viral and bacterial infections, transformed tumor cells, and synthetic compounds (Wiranowska-Stewart and Stewart 1981). The genes for interferon-α and interferon-β are situated on chromosome 9, and each has an amino acid sequence of 166 molecules. The gene for interferon-γ is located on chromosome 12, and its molecule contains 146 amino acids. Interferon is present at minimal concentrations in the resting state, and active process of secretion needs induction with an agent. For both interferon-α and interferon-β, presence of a sugar moiety on the leukocyte membrane is found to be essential, whereas interferon-γ needs macrophages that are thought to send out signals to T lymphocytes for transcription. These signals are Ca^{++} channel–activated. The exact nature of these signals from macrophages is not clear, although they are felt to consist of a lymphokine (Dianzani and Antonelli 1987; Marcus 1987). Interferon-α and interferon-β share the same receptor, whereas interferon-γ has its own receptor. After binding with the receptor, all three human interferons are internalized by endocytosis and later get degraded. Subsequently, interferon induces the synthesis of effector proteins that mediate most of its biochemical functions. Once activated, interferon-activated cells can transfer this activated state to the neighboring cells without the continued presence of interferon.

Functions of interferon. Initially the main activity of interferon was thought to be inhibition of further replication of viruses. This antiviral state was established through production of new RNA and protein. In addition to this, interferons have several other functions (see Table 12-2).

Interferon and the CNS. Effects of interferons on the CNS became noticeable during the course of treatment of patients with interferon. A great majority of patients manifested symptoms of fatigue, mental apathy, irritability, depression, anorexia, weight loss, and marked social withdrawal. Although fully alert, these patients remained very inattentive and had difficulties with concentration and memory (Adams et al. 1984). They exhibited marked poverty of thought and speech. Some patients also exhibited significant disorientation (Renault et al. 1987). These side effects disappeared after discontinuation of treatment, clearly implicating interferon as the putative agent. This also indicates that interferon, in addition to modulating the immunological functions, also affects the CNS.

Researchers began studying the effects of interferon on the CNS. Using explants from rat and kitten cerebral and cerebellar cortex, Calvet and Gresser (1979) were able to demonstrate that interferons shortened the latency, lowered the threshold to stimulation, and caused a tendency toward repetitions in neurons. These findings were replicated by other investigators, who found increased excitability of neurons in the hippocampus and sensorimotor cortex. This property was not shared by interferon-γ (Reyes-Vazquez et al. 1984). Dafny (1983) recorded high-voltage sharp waves on the EEG (in vivo experiments) that were initially seen in the ventromedial hypothalamus but later shifted to the somatosensory cortex and dorsal hippocampal regions. These changes in cerebral activity provide evidence for direct modulatory activity of interferon and explain some of the symptoms of neurotoxicity of interferon therapy.

The effects of interferon may be mediated through the neuroendocrine system. There is evidence that interferon may have neuromodulatory actions. Interferons show some of the properties of endogenous opioid systems in addition to structural relatedness. Intracerebral injection of interferon induced endorphin-like analgesia and catatonia in mice that was reversed by naloxone. Dafny et al. (1988) demonstrated attenuation of symptoms of naloxone-induced morphine withdrawal after addition of interferon. Thus, one of the effects of interferon on the CNS may be an alteration in the central opioid system. Interferons also decrease REM latency, an effect probably due to an alteration in the cholinergic system (Reite et al. 1987).

Table 12-2. Effects of interferon on various systems

Central nervous system

Increased excitability of neurons in several regions of the brain
Antiproliferation activity on glial cells
Neuromodulator activity on the CNS

Endocrine system

Pituitary
- Stimulation of secretory GH
- Stimulation of ACTH production
- Suppression of secretion of TSH

Pancreas
- Stimulation/inhibition of insulin production

Adrenal Cortex
- Stimulation of cortisol production

Cardiovascular system

Species-specific, dose-dependent increase in the beat frequency of myocardial cells

Hematopoietic system

Mediation of the differentiation of hematopoietic progenitor cells in small doses
Suppression of myeloid progenitor cells and myeloid colony formation

Musculoskeletal system

Antiviral activity
Activation of macrophages and lymphocytes
Production of cytokines
Enhancement of cytotoxicity and natural killer cell activity
Increased expression of cell membrane components, e.g., MHC antigens, Fc receptors, β_2 microglobulins
Suppression of oncogene expression
Inhibition of cell growth

Note. ACTH = adrenocorticotropin; Fc = Fc portion of immunoglobulin; GH = growth hormone; MHC = major histocompatibility antigen; TSH = thyrotropin-stimulating hormone.

Interferon and the HPA axis. Blalock and Harp (1981) showed that interferon, along with ACTH, induced steroidogenesis and melanogenesis. Once again this effect was species specific. Other investigators have also shown that interferon causes a rise in plasma cortisol concentration in patients after the infusion (Holsboer et al. 1988; Krishnan et al. 1987; Roosth et al. 1986). The actions of interferons on the HPA axis may have special significance in terms of psychiatric manifestations of interferon-treated patients. Like interleukins, interferons also have their own negative feedback control, for both ACTH and cortisol are shown to be powerful suppressors of interferon production (Cesario et al. 1986; Johnson et al. 1984).

CONCLUSIONS

We have reviewed the effects of two lymphokines (interleukin 1 and interferon) on the CNS and endocrine system and discussed how they may influence behavior. The new field of psychoneuroimmunology, which explores the relationship between the immune system and psychiatric illnesses, holds promise for having extensive clinical implications. In addition to in vitro experiments, there are numerous in vivo studies that clearly demonstrate the effect of stress on the immune systems. People who cope poorly with life stresses manifest greater anxiety levels and have a greater reduction in natural killer (NK) cell activity (Locke et al. 1984). When bereaved subjects were compared with healthy control subjects, a significant reduction in the NK cell activity was seen in the bereaved group. Similarly, depressed patients also had a marked suppression of lymphocyte mitogenic activity as well as lower NK cell activity. These clinical studies emphasize the importance and interrelationship of the immune system and psychiatric disorders. Further studies on the role of lymphokines and cytokines in behavior are warranted.

REFERENCES

Adams F, Quesada JR, Gutterman JU: Neuropsychiatric manifestations of human leukocyte interferon therapy in patients with cancer. JAMA 252:938–941, 1984

Bailey PT, Abeles FB, Hauer EC, et al: Intracerebroventricular administration of leukocytic endogenous mediators (LEM) in the rat. Proc Soc Exp Biol Med 153:419–423, 1976

Bakouche O, Brown DC, Lachman LB: Subcellular localization of human monocyte interleukin 1: evidence for an inactive precursor molecule and a possible mechanism for IL-1 release. J Immunol 138:4249–4255, 1987

Berkenbosch F, Oers JV, Del Rey A, et al: Corticotropin-releasing factor producing neurons in the rat activated by interleukin 1. Science 238:524–526, 1987

Besedovsky H, Sorkin E, Keller M, et al: Changes in blood hormone levels during the immune response. Proc Soc Exp Biol Med 150:466–470, 1975

Besedovsky H, Del Rey A, Sorkin E, et al: Immunoregulatory feedback between interleukin 1 and glucocorticoid hormone. Science 233:652–654, 1986

Blalock JE, Harp C: Interferon and adrenocorticotropic hormone induction of steroidogenesis, melanogenesis and antiviral activity. Arch Virol 67:45–49, 1981

Bohus B: Effect of ACTH-like neuropeptides on animal behavior and man. Pharmacology 18:113–122, 1979

Branconnier RJ: The human behavioral pharmacology of the common core heptapeptides. Pharmacol Ther 14:161–175, 1981

Breder CD, Dinarello CA, Saper CB: Interleukin 1 immunoreactive innervation of the human hypothalamus. Science 240:321–324, 1988

Brown SL, Smith LR, Blalock EJ: Interleukin 1 and interleukin 2 enhance proopiomelanocortin gene expression in pituitary cells. J Immunol 139:3181–3183, 1987

Calvet MC, Gresser I: Interferon enhances the excitability of cultured neurons. Nature 278:558–560, 1979

Cannon JG, Kluger MJ: Endogenous pyrogen activity in human plasma after exercise. Science 220:617–619, 1983

Cesario TC, Slater L, Poo WJ, et al: The effects of hydrocortisone on the production of interferon and other lymphokines by human peripheral blood mononuclear cells. J Interferon Res 6:337–347, 1986

Dafny N: Interferon modified EEG and EEG like activity recorded from sensory, motor and limbic structures in freely behaving rats. Neurotoxicology 4:235–240, 1983

Dafny N, Lee JR, Dougherty G: Immune response products alter CNS activity: interferon modulates central opioid functions. J Neurosci Res 19:130–139, 1988

Dekloet ER, Palkovits M, Mezery ES: Opiocortin peptides: localization, source and avenues of transport. Pharmacol Ther 12:321–351, 1981

Del Rey A, Besedovsky H, Sorkin E, et al: Interleukin 1 and glucocorticoid hormones integrate an immunoregulatory feedback circuit. Ann NY Acad Science 496:85–90, 1987

Dianzani F, Antonelli G: Mechanism of induction of gamma interferon, in The Interferon System: A Current Review to 1987. Edited by Baron S, Dianzani F, Stanton GJ, et al. Austin, TX, University of Texas Press, 1987, pp 51–61

Dinarello C: Interleukin 1. Rev Infect Dis 6:51–94, 1984

Dunn AJ: Neurochemistry of learning and memory. Ann Rev Psychol 31:343–390, 1980

Farrar WL, Kilian PL, Ruff MR, et al: Visualization and characterization of interleukin 1 receptors in the brain. J Immunol 139:459–463, 1987

Giulian D, Lochman B: Interleukin 1 stimulation of atroglial proliferation after brain injury. Science 228:497–499, 1985

Holsboer F, Stalla GC, von Bardeleban U, et al: Acute adrenocortical stimulation by recombinant gamma interferon in human controls. Life Sci 42:1–5, 1988.

Johnson HM, Torres BA, Smith EM, et al: Regulation of lymphokine (γ-interferon) production by corticotropin. J Immunol 132:246–250, 1984

Koff WC, Fann AC, Dunegan MA, et al: Catecholamine induced suppression of interleukin-1 production. Lymphokine Res 5:239–247, 1986

Krishnan KRR, Ellinwood EH, Laszlo J, et al: Effect of gamma interferon on the hypothalamic pituitary adrenal systems. Biol Psychiatry 22:1163–1166, 1987

Krishnan KRR, Ritchie JC, Manepalli AN, et al: What is the relationship between plasma ACTH and plasma cortisol in normal humans and depressed patients? in Hypothalamic-Pituitary-Adrenal Axis: Physiology, Pathophysiology and Psychiatric Complication. Edited by Nemeroff CB. New York, Raven, 1988, pp 115–127

Locke SE, Kraus L, Leserman J: Life change stress, psychiatric symptoms and natural killer cell activity. Psychosom Med 46:441–453, 1984

Lumpkin MD: The regulation of ACTH secretion by IL 1. Science 238:452–454, 1987

Marcus PJ: Interferon induction and its suppression by viruses, in The Interferon System: A Current Review to 1987. Edited by Baron S, Dianzani F, Stanton GJ, et al. Austin, TX, University of Texas Press, 1987, pp 41–49

Martin M, Resch K: Interleukin 1 more than a mediator between leukocytes. Trends in Pharmacological Sciences 9:171–177, 1988

Oitzl MS, Huston J: Electroencephalographic spreading depression and concomitant behavioral changes induced by intrahippocampal injection of $ACTH_{1-24}$ and D-Ala^2-Met-enkephalinamide in the rat. Brain Res 308:33–42, 1984

Palkovits M: Topography of chemically identified neurons in the central nervous system: progress in 1977–1979. Med Biol 58:188–227, 1980

Plata-Salaman CR, Oomura Y, Kai Y: Tumor necrosis factor and interleukin-1B: suppression of food intake by direct action in the central nervous system. Brain Res 448:106–114, 1988

Reite M, Laudenslager M, Jones J, et al: Interferon decreases REM latency. Biol Psychiatry 22:104–107, 1987

Renault P, Hoofnagle JH, Park Y, et al: Psychiatric complications of long-term interferon alpha therapy. Arch Intern Med 147:1577–1580, 1987

Reyes-Vazquez C, Prieto-Gomez B, Georgiades JA, et al: Alpha and gamma interferon's effects on cortical and hippocampal neurons: microiontophoretic application and single cell recording. J Neurosci 25:113–121, 1984

Roh MS, Drazenovich KA, Barbose JJ, et al: Direct stimulation of the adrenal cortex by interleukin 1. Surgery 102:140–146, 1987

Roosth J, Pollard RB, Brown SL, et al: Cortisol stimulation of recombinant interferon L_2. J Neuroimmunol 12:311–316, 1986

Sapolsky R, Rivier C, Yamamoto G, et al: Interleukin-1 stimulates the secretion of hypothalamic corticotropin-releasing factor. Science 238:522–524, 1987

Snyder DS, Unanue ER: Corticosteroids inhibit murine macrophage I_a expression and interleukin-1 production. J Immunol 129:1803–1805, 1982

Uehara A, Gillis S, Arimura A: Effects of interleukin-1 on hormone release from normal rat pituitary cells in primary cultures. Neuroendocrinology 45:343–347, 1987a

Uehara A, Gottschall PE, Dahl RR, et al: Stimulation of ACTH release by human interleukin 1β but not by interleukin 1Lα in conscious, freely moving rats. Biochem Biophys Res Commun 146:1286–1290, 1987b

Walter J, Davenne D, Shohan S, et al: Brain temperature changes coupled to sleep states persist during interleukin-1 enhanced sleep. Am J Physiol 250:R96–R103, 1986

Wiranowska-Stewart M, Stewart WE II: Interferon: types alpha, beta and gamma, in The Lymphokines: Biochemistry and Biological Activity. Edited by Hadden JW, Stewart WE II. Clifton, NJ, Humana Press, 1981, pp 133–145

Woloski BMRNJ, Smith EM, Meyer WJ III, et al: Corticotropin-releasing activity of monokines. Science 230:1035–1037, 1985

Yasuko F, Wolf J, Wolf G: Morphine and ACTH correlative behavioral excitation following microinjections in rat periaqueductal gray. Brain Res 219:214–218, 1981

Chapter 13

Involvement of Neuropeptide Y and Delta-Sleep–Inducing Peptide in Neuropsychiatric Illnesses

Erik Widerlöv, M.D., Ph.D.
Markus Heilig, M.D.
Anders Bjartell, M.D.
Rolf Ekman, M.D., Ph.D.

Chapter 13

Involvement of Neuropeptide Y and Delta-Sleep–Inducing Peptide in Neuropsychiatric Illnesses

Of the more than 60 neurotransmitter-neuromodulator candidates identified in the central nervous system (CNS), the vast majority belong to various polypeptide families, the so-called neuropeptides. The existence of these peptides, as well as specific receptors, has been demonstrated in most living organisms, from very primitive unicellular organisms (Csaba 1981; LeRoith et al. 1980) to the most complex ones, where they are distributed not only in the nervous tissue but also in multiple organs of the body. This seemingly universal occurrence of neuropeptides in living organisms, and the appearance of numerous biologically active peptides in the central and peripheral nervous systems, as well as in the alimentary tract and other tissues of higher organisms, suggest very basic functional roles for these compounds. In fact, these peptides serve different roles in different tissues, and throughout evolution similar peptide molecules have been adapted for different functions (for reviews, see El-Sahly 1981; Falkmer and van Noorden 1983). Two of these peptides, neuropeptide Y (NPY) and delta-sleep–inducing peptide (DSIP), are both involved in a number of CNS actions and possibly also in neuropsychiatric illnesses.

NEUROPEPTIDE Y

Neuropeptide Y is a 36-amino-acid peptide originally isolated from the porcine gut and brain (Tatemoto 1982; Tatemoto et al. 1982, 1985). NPY and the related peptide YY (PYY) belong to the pancreatic polypeptide family (Emson and de Quidt 1984; Tatemoto et al. 1982). NPY is one of the most abundant and widely distributed peptides in both the peripheral nervous system (Lundberg et al. 1982) and the CNS of mammals. In the CNS, NPY has been reported to affect the control of basic vegetative functions such as blood pressure, cardiac activity, and respiration (Fuxe et al. 1983); food intake (see below); and hormone secretion (Härfstrand et al. 1987a; Kalra and Crowley 1984; Kerkerian et al. 1985; also see below). A recent review of the central actions of NPY is presented by Wahlestedt et al. (1989).

A number of morphological, neurochemical, and functional findings prompted several groups, including our own, to study the possible involvement of NPY in neuropsychiatric illnesses and in animal behavior. As will be apparent from the following section, NPY is preferentially localized in brain regions thought to be of central importance for the regulation of emotions and for the pathogenesis of several neuropsychiatric disorders. In addition, central NPY coexists partly with noradrenaline (see below), and, using the peripheral nervous system as a model, several interactions between NPY and noradrenaline have been demonstrated (Lundberg et al. 1982). The noradrenergic pathways of the brain have been postulated to play a crucial role in the pathogenesis of affective (Siever and Davies 1985) as well as anxiety states (Redmond and Huang 1979). Finally, effects of NPY on circadian rhythm (Albers and Ferris 1984; Albers et al. 1984), on vegetative functions (see above), and on the hypothalamo-pituitary-adrenal (HPA) axis (Wahlestedt et al. 1987) have been reported after central administration of the peptide. Dysregulation of these functions is a common feature in several psychiatric illnesses, particularly in major depressive disorder.

Anatomy of Neuropeptide Y Systems in the Mammalian Brain

Regional tissue concentrations. The tissue concentrations of NPY have been determined in a number of species, including man (Adrian et al. 1983; Dawbarn et al. 1984), nonhuman primates (Khorram et al. 1987), and the rat (Y. S. Allen et al. 1983; Chronwall et al. 1985; de Quidt and Emson 1986a, 1986b). Although the numeric data vary up to one order of magnitude, presumably due to differences in extraction procedures and antibodies used, the relative contents of different regions are in good agreement between studies. In the rat, hypothalamic areas, nucleus accumbens, septum, and periaqueductal gray matter contain the highest levels of NPY. Moderately high amounts are found in cortical regions (including the hippocampus), in the thalamus, and in the basal ganglia. NPY immunoreactivity is low or absent in the pons and the cerebellum. In humans high levels of NPY are found in the basal ganglia, nucleus accumbens, amygdala, and hypothalamus. Intermediate amounts are detected in several cortical areas, and in the hippocampus, septum, and periaqueductal gray matter. Lowest levels of NPY are found in the thalamus, globus pallidus, substantia nigra, pons, and cerebellum.

Cell bodies and fiber networks. Large numbers of NPY-containing neurons have been found in the olfactory bulbs, the anterior olfactory nucleus, the olfactory tubercle, the islands of Calleja, and the piriform cortex. All these olfactory areas are also generally reported to contain high densities of NPY-positive fibers in most parts (Chronwall et al. 1985; de Quidt and Emson 1986a; Gall et al. 1986; Wahle and Meyer 1986).

NPY-containing cells and fiber networks are consistently reported in the cerebral cortex, the central part of the caudate-putamen, the medial half of the nucleus accumbens, the bed nucleus of the stria terminalis, and the amygdaloid complex (Chronwall et al. 1985; de Quidt and Emson 1986a, 1986b; Nakagawa et al. 1985; Shen 1987; Smith et al. 1985). In the neocortex, NPY neurons are small, intracortical, and nonspiny (Chan-Palay et al. 1985; Jones and Hendry 1986; Wahle et al. 1986), and seem to belong to a distinct morphological class of multipolar local circuit neurons, the members of which also contain gamma-aminobutyric acid (GABA) or acetylcholine (Jones and Hendry 1986). NPY cells are present in all hippocampal areas, and dense networks of NPY fibers innervate the entire hippocampal region (Köhler et al. 1986a, 1986b). NPY neurons are present throughout all major amygdaloid nuclei. Fiber networks are present mainly in the medial third of the central amygdaloid nucleus and in the dorsal half of the medial nucleus. This fiber distribution is similar to that of noradrenergic axons arising from the brain stem, but studies involving 6-hydroxydopamine (6-OHDA) lesions indicate that the two fiber networks are not identical (Gustafson et al. 1986). In the striatum, NPY is present in a single population of intrinsic neurons, located in zones of high acetylcholinesterase activity, and positive for NADPH-diaphorase. Fiber densities are highest in the nucleus accumbens and in the ventromedial regions of the caudate and the putamen (Christie et al. 1986; Kowall et al. 1987; Sandell et al. 1986; Smith and Parent 1986). Some NPY-positive neurons receive a GABA-ergic input (Massari et al. 1988).

Low amounts of NPY have been found in the pineal gland (Schröder 1986; Schröder and Vollrath 1986), and the sparse fibers present originate from the superior cervical ganglion (Shiotani et al. 1986). Within the thalamus, NPY-positive cells are present in the lateral geniculate body and in the olivary pretectal nucleus, while fibers are found in the thalamic paraventricular nucleus (PVN) (Chronwall et al. 1985; de Quidt and Emson 1986a; Molinari et al. 1987; Nakagawa et al. 1985). In the hypothalamus, a large population of NPY-containing perikarya in the arcuate nucleus constitutes the largest group of NPY-positive perikarya in the brain. NPY-positive cells are also present in the lateral hypothalamus and in the supramamillary nucleus. Dense plexuses of fibers are observed in the PVN, the arcuate nucleus, the internal layer of the median eminence, and the periventricular zone. Finally, at least in humans and in the cat, cell bodies are found in the median eminence and send axons along the pituitary stalk, penetrating the neural lobe (Chronwall et al. 1985; de Quidt and Emson 1986a; Hu et al. 1987; Leger et al. 1987; Pelletier et al. 1984; Sabatino et al. 1987).

NPY cells are found in the mesencephalic central gray matter, the caudal interpeduncular nucleus, and the inferior colliculus. At this level fibers are mainly confined to the dorsal raphe and the central gray matter (Chronwall et al. 1985; de Quidt and Emson 1986a).

High numbers of cells are reported in the pontine locus coeruleus and in a group of cells located adjacent to the dorsal tegmental nucleus. Low to moderate fiber densities are detected in the locus coeruleus and in the dorsal parabrachial nucleus (Chronwall et al. 1985; de Quidt and Emson 1986a).

In the medulla oblongata, cells are present in the nucleus of the solitary tract, the nucleus prepositus hypoglossi, the area postrema, the reticular formation, and the adjacent caudal facial motor nucleus. Moderate to high densities of fibers are seen within the nucleus of the solitary tract and at the border between the spinal tract of the trigeminal nerve and its nucleus (Chronwall et al. 1985; Dai et al. 1986; de Quidt and Emson 1986a; Härfstrand et al. 1987b, Yamazoe et al. 1985).

Identified pathways and patterns of innervation. NPY-containing adrenergic (C1, C2, C3) and noradrenergic (A1) cell groups within the medulla of the rat provide afferents to the hypothalamic PVN (Sawchenko et al. 1985). Another NPY-containing input to the PVN has been described to originate from the ipsilateral arcuate nucleus. The neurons that constitute this pathway do not contain catecholamines (Bai et al. 1985). The corticotropin-releasing factor (CRF) cells of the parvocellular PVN seem to be a target for this latter input (Liposits et al. 1988a; Wahlestedt et al. 1987), although vaso- pressin-containing neurons of the supraoptic nucleus are also innervated by NPY-immunoreactive fibers (Willoughby and Blessing 1987). A selective lesion of the arcuate nucleus obtained after monosodium glutamate treatment is followed by a marked decrease in the density of NPY-positive fibers in the PVN (Kerkerian and Pelletier 1986). Another NPY-containing projection from the hypothalamic arcuate nucleus has the preoptic area and/or the periaqueductal gray matter as targets (Chronwall 1985).

Neurons projecting to the dorsal vagal complex (DVC) from the paracentricular, arcuate, dorsomedial, and lateral hypothalamic areas, as well as from the central nucleus of the amygdala and the bed nucleus of the stria terminalis, are heavily innervated by NPY-containing terminals (Gray et al. 1986). Although synaptic connections at the ultrastructural level have not been demonstrated, the authors suggest a possible role of this innervation for the effects of NPY on autonomic and vegetative functions.

An NPY-containing projection from the ventrolateral geniculate nucleus (VLGN) to the suprachiasmatic nuclei (SCN) has been demonstrated in the rat (Moore et al. 1984). The neurons of this projection form both axosomatic and axodendritic synapses on cells mainly located in the ventral portion of the SCN (Ibata et al. 1988). Other studies have confirmed the existence of this projection in various species (Harrington et al. 1985, 1987), but not in monkeys (Ueda et al. 1986). Interestingly, axons of the serotonergic raphe input to the SCN converge with NPY terminals on the same perikarya and in some occasions also form axo-axonic appositions (Guy et al. 1987, 1988). The NPY-ergic VLGN-SCN projection may be related to the effects of NPY on circadian rhythms (discussed in Moore and Card 1985).

The retrohippocampal region, including the entorhinal area, receives a heavy NPY innervation of extrahippocampal as well as intrinsic hippocampal origin. The former originates from the perirhinal and piriform cortex, the endopiriform nucleus, the lateral nucleus of the amygdala, and the locus coeruleus (Köhler et al. 1986a, 1986b).

NPY is present in stria terminalis fibers projecting from the amygdala to the bed nucleus of the stria terminalis, the laterobasal septum, and the SCN (Y. S. Allen et al. 1984).

A population of epinephrine-synthesizing C1 cells in the rostral ventrolateral medulla project to the intermediolateral column of the spinal cord. Some of these cells also contain NPY. The synaptic target of this projection seems to be the cell bodies of sympathetic preganglionic neurons (SPN) (Anderson et al. 1987; Blessing et al. 1987; Krukoff 1987a). Among the sympathetic preganglionic neurons, cell bodies staining for enkephalin, neurotensin, somatostatin, and substance P are also found, and, in agreement with the finding referred to above, these cells are innervated by dense NPY-containing terminal networks (Krukoff 1987a). The innervation pattern is a diffuse one, with no apparent somatotopical or transmitter-specific organizational principle.

Although some NPY neurons have been shown ultrastructurally to make classical synaptic connections, many immunoreactive terminals exist as free endings (Hendry et al. 1984; Pelletier et al. 1984).

Colocalization of Neuropeptide Y With Other Neuromessengers and Neuronal Markers

NPY and catecholamines. The presence of NPY in catecholaminergic cell bodies was early reported in both the human and the rat medulla oblongata (Hökfelt et al. 1983a, 1983b). NPY was later located in most noradrenergic cell bodies of the A1 group in the ventrolateral medulla and in virtually all (75% to 100%) adrenergic C1, C2, and C3 cells. Many noradrenergic cell bodies in the A6 group in the locus coeruleus also contained NPY. The majority of the noradrenergic cell bodies of the A2 group, as well as A5 and A7 cells in the pons and all dopaminergic cells studied, seem to be devoid of NPY immunoreactivity (Blessing et al. 1986; Everitt et al. 1984; Sawchenko et al. 1985).

Lesions of central catecholaminergic cells with 6-OHDA leave the NPY levels unaffected in the cerebral cortex (including the hippocampus), striatum, and spinal cord. Only in the hypothalamus is the NPY content reduced by this treatment, and then only to a small extent (Schon et al. 1986). Thus, only a minority of central NPY neurons seem to be catecholaminergic as well.

NPY and somatostatin. Almost all neocortical and striatal NPY neurons also contain somatostatin. In the hippocampus and septum, this coexistence is partial, and in the hypothalamus, as well as in the bed nucleus of the stria terminalis, it is nearly absent. Except for the nucleus accumbens, the olfactory tubercle, and parts of the septum, where NPY and somatostatin cell systems show an almost complete overlap, a separate population of non-NPY–containing somatostatin neurons is also present in all of these areas (Chronwall et al. 1984; Gaspar et al. 1987; Köhler et al. 1987; Papadopoulos et al. 1987; Smith and Parent 1986). In the olfactory bulb, finally, the pattern and morphology of NPY and somatostatin neurons are identical, although coexistence in the proper sense of the word has not yet been demonstrated (Scott et al. 1987).

Cysteamine, which depletes the brain concentrations of somatostatin, does not affect staining observed with an NPY antiserum (Chattha and Beal 1987; Vecsei et al., in press). This finding is in agreement with the enzymatic mechanism of action postulated for cysteamine, that is, a chemical modification of the disulfide bridge in the somatostatin molecule (Ceccatelli et al. 1987; Chattha and Beal 1987).

In agreement with the findings indicated above, the concentrations of NPY and somatostatin, detected by radioimmunoassay, are highly correlated in the cerebral neocortex and in the striatum (r = .93–.99) of brains from monkeys or from patients with Alzheimer's dementia (Beal et al. 1986a, 1987a).

NPY and GABA. Depending on species, 90% to 100% of NPY-containing (and thus also somatostatin-containing) cells of the cortex are GABA-ergic. This coexistence is not reciprocal: other GABA-ergic cells are devoid of NPY, but contain somatostatin (Demeulemeester et al. 1988; Hendry et al. 1984).

NPY and other neuromessengers and neuronal markers. Neurons immunoreactive with antisera raised against human growth hormone–releasing hormone (GHRH) are present in the hypothalamic arcuate nucleus. About 90% of these neurons also contain NPY (Ciofi et al. 1987). A sparse colocalization of NPY and vasoactive intestinal polypeptide (VIP) has been noted in the dorsal motor nucleus of the vagal nerve (Dai et al. 1986). Some neurons containing both NPY and serotonin are observed in the nucleus raphe pallidus (Blessing et al. 1986).

The enzymatic marker NADPH-diaphorase is present in all cortical, striatal, and olfactory bulb cells containing NPY (and somatostatin), providing some evidence that these cells may constitute a homogenous class of neurons (Gonzalez and Sharp 1987; Kowall et al. 1987; Scott et al. 1987). Interestingly, the presence of NADPH-diaphorase seems to be correlated with neuronal ability to resist both chemical and surgical lesions. Further, this enzyme participates in the detoxification of quinone derivatives, including the excitotoxin quinoline (Y. S. Allen et al. 1986). Considering the role speculated for excitotoxic mechanisms in neurodegenerative disorders, the colocalization of NPY and NADPH-diaphorase may be of importance for the selective sparing of NPY immunoreactivity in these states (see below).

Neuropeptide Y and the Hypothalamo-Pituitary-Adrenal Axis

Injection of NPY into the hypothalamic PVN produces an increase in plasma adrenocorticotropin (ACTH) and corticosterone levels both in anesthetized and in conscious, freely moving rats (Wahlestedt et al. 1987). Intracerebroventricular injection of low doses of NPY seems to actually suppress corticosterone secretion, while higher doses increase both ACTH and corticosterone concentrations (Härfstrand et al. 1987a). The NPY-induced increase in ACTH and corticosterone levels may be mediated through a stimulated CRF secretion, because NPY-containing fibers innervate CRF cell bodies of the PVN (see above), and NPY administration has been demonstrated to elevate hypothalamic CRF concentrations (Haas and George 1987).

Neuropeptide Y and CNS Pathology

NPY in relation to depression and anxiety. Our group has found altered cerebrospinal fluid (CSF) concentrations of NPY-like immunoreactivity in patients with major depression (Widerlöv et al. 1988c). In that study, CSF samples were drawn from healthy volunteers and from hospitalized depressed patients. The healthy subjects (11 women, 9 men; mean age 31 years, range 20 to 50 years) had no present somatic or psychiatric disease, nor had they any personal or family history of psychiatric illness or drug abuse. Apart from oral contraceptives used by some of the females, no drugs were used by the members of this group. The depressed patients (14 women, 19 men; mean age 46 years, range 23 to 70 years) were diagnosed as suffering from major depression following the diagnostic criteria of DSM-III. At the time of the lumbar puncture they had received no antidepressant medication for at least 2 weeks. Preceding the lumbar puncture the occurrence and severity of depressive symptoms were assessed using the Hamilton Depression Rating Scale (HAM-D) (Hamilton 1967) and the Montgomery-Åsberg Rating Scale for Depression (CPRS-D) (Montgomery and Åsberg 1979). The NPY-like immunoreactivity and PYY-like immunoreactivity concentrations in CSF were determined using radioimmunological methods described in detail by Widerlöv et al. (1988c) and Ekman et al. (1986), respectively.

The depressed patients had highly reduced concentrations of NPY in the CSF when compared with the control subjects (121.8 ± 3.1 vs. 102.2 ± 2.0 pmol/l [mean ± SEM]; $P < .0001$, Student's *t* test, two-tailed). The interindividual variation was low and equal in both groups. No sex differences were observed in either group. The CSF concentrations of PYY did not differ between the control subjects and the depressed subjects (22.1 ± 1.1 pmol/l and 19.9 ± 0.8 pmol/l [mean ± SEM], respectively). No correlation was observed between the total severity of depression, as assessed by the total scores on the HAM-D or CPRS-D, and the CSF concentrations of NPY in the individual patients. Instead, significant, or nearly significant, negative correlations were found between the anxiety scores in the HAM-D and the CSF NPY concentrations (item 10, "Psychological Anxiety": $r = -.42$, $P = .06$; item 11, "Somatic Anxiety": $r = -.47$, $P = .04$; items 10 + 11, "Total Anxiety": $r = -.56$, $P = .02$) (see Widerlöv et al. 1989).

Using the antibody employed in the clinical study on rat brain tissue, we found that chronic oral treatment with the antidepressant drugs imipramine and zimelidine markedly elevated the frontal cortical concentrations of NPY-like immunoreactivity. In addition, treatment with imipramine also increased the hypothalamic levels of this material, whereas a number of other brain regions were not affected by either drug (Heilig et al. 1988; Widerlöv et al. 1988b). Electroconvulsive shocks (ECSs) similarly elevated the tissue concentrations of NPY-like immunoreactivity in both the frontal and the parietal neocortex, as well as in the hippocampus. Rats given shocks of insufficient strength for the development of generalized convulsions, as well as sham-treated animals, did not differ from untreated controls (Wahlestedt et al. 1989).

Zimelidine is thought to preferentially inhibit the neuronal reuptake of serotonin. Imipramine is rapidly and almost completely metabolized to desmethylimipramine (desipramine) after oral administration in the rat, and desipramine preferentially inhibits the reuptake of norepinephrine. The neurochemical effects of electroconvulsive therapy (ECT) are obviously numerous. The mechanism of antidepressant action of ECT and of tricyclic antidepressants remains unknown.

Thus, different treatments known to have an antidepressant effect in depressed patients seem to share an ability to elevate the cortical levels of NPY-like immunoreactivity in the rat. This observation, together with the finding of decreased levels of NPY-like immunoreactivity in the CSF of depressed patients (Widerlöv et al. 1988c), makes it tempting to hypothesize that NPY may be involved in the pathophysiology of depressive illness, as well as in the mechanism of action of various antidepressive treatments. More specifically, it may be claimed that major depression involves a deficit of central NPY-ergic functions, while antidepressant treatments bring this deficit back to normal levels.

However, in the light of an earlier preliminary study by our group (Ekman et al. 1984), this claim has to be further qualified. In the preliminary study we found significantly elevated CSF concentrations of NPY-like immunoreactivity in depressed patients, as opposed to the finding referred to above (Widerlöv et al. 1988c). The only obvious difference between the two studies was the use of two different antibodies. Thus, the role of NPY in the pathophysiology of depressive illness, if any, does not seem to be only a simple deficit. Rather, an altered processing, or metabolism, of the parent NPY molecule, or of the precursor molecule, may take place in depression, giving rise to different patterns of immunoreactive fragments in CSF of depressed patients and healthy subjects. These fragments can be recognized differently by different antibodies. In fact, HPLC analysis shows that the NPY-like immunoreactivity fragments from the CSF of depressed patients differ from those of the control subjects (Widerlöv et al. 1989). Berrettini and coworkers (1987), who found no differences in the CSF concentrations of NPY-like immunoreactivity between control subjects and patients with depression or schizophrenia, yielded only a single HPLC peak coeluting with authentic NPY. This finding clearly indicates that it is not the complete 36–amino-acid peptide itself that is altered in depression. For similar reasons, the findings of elevated brain tissue concentrations of NPY-like immunoreactivity after antidepressant treatments of rats (Heilig et al. 1988) should be regarded as preliminary until the molecular identity of the immunoreactivity material has been further characterized.

It should also be kept in mind that these results are obtained in normal, "nondepressed" animals. Therefore, it is desirable to reproduce the NPY changes found in the depressed patients in valid animal models of depression and to reexamine the effects of antidepressant drugs and ECS in these models. We have attempted to explore the usefulness of one such animal depression model, the bulbectomized rat (Jesberger and Richardson 1985), in this respect. In a preliminary experiment the concentration of NPY-like immunoreactivity in the cerebral cortex of bulbectomized rats was decreased (Widerlöv et al. 1986). In a recent study by Kataoka and coworkers (1988), bulbectomy was followed by increased levels of NPY-like immunoreactivity in the amygdala and the hypothalamus. Again, no HPLC characterization of the immunoreactive material is available. Therefore, the two contrary findings may again reflect an alteration in the turnover of NPY, as detected by the two different antibodies used. Interestingly, however, the increased NPY levels following bulbectomy reported in Kataoka et al. (1988) were brought back to normal by treatment with antidepressant drugs.

It is also possible that NPY is not primarily involved in the state of being depressed per se. As mentioned above, no correlation is found between CSF concentrations of NPY-like immunoreactivity and the degree of depression, as assessed by the total scores on the depression rating scales. Instead, significant negative correlations are present between the NPY-like immunoreactivity concentrations and the HAM-D anxiety scores obtained from the patients (see above). Because anxiety is often a prominent feature of the depressive syndrome, by selecting depressed patients we will also select patients suffering from anxiety. In this context, it can be noted that antidepressant drugs are also effective in the treatment of anxiety states (Modigh 1987).

The relationship between NPY and anxiety has been further elucidated in animal experiments. We have tested NPY for possible anxiolytic effects in two animal conflict models validated for the ability to detect anxiolytic and anxiogenic drug effects. The tests used were the elevated X-maze based on principles described by Montgomery (1958) and developed further by others (Handley and Mithani 1984; Pellow et al. 1985), and the more commonly used Vogel test (Vogel et al. 1971). The two tests share the conflict element, but otherwise differ widely. In the Vogel test we additionally controlled for interference from possible effects of NPY on pain sensitivity and thirst. In both models, NPY produced effects indistinguishable from those of well known anxiolytics. In the Vogel test neither pain sensitivity nor thirst was affected. We have therefore concluded that the behavioral effects of NPY observed in the two anxiety models are representative of an anxiolytic-like action of the peptide (Heilig et al. 1989).

As commonly seen with anxiolytic drugs, at doses higher than those required for the induction of anxiolysis, NPY seems to produce signs of sedation in experimental animals. This sedation is manifested by a suppression of locomotor activity (Heilig and Murison 1987b), and stress-protective properties of the peptide (Heilig and Murison 1987a), and correlates well with the reports of synchronizing effects of NPY on the electroencephalogram (EEG) in the rat (Fuxe et al. 1983). In this context it is interesting to note that in our clinical study (Widerlöv et al. 1988c), the degree of lassitude correlated positively ($r = .42$, $P = .025$) with the NPY-like immunoreactivity concentration in CSF of the depressed patients.

NPY and schizophrenia. The CSF concentrations of NPY- and PYY-like immunoreactivities have been determined in 35 hospitalized, drug-free patients (17 women, 18 men; mean age 28 years, range 18 to 40 years) and compared with the same immunoreactivities in 20 healthy volunteers (see above) in a study by our group (Widerlöv et al. 1988c). We did not find any difference in the NPY concentrations, whereas the PYY levels were significantly lower ($P = .001$) in the schizophrenia group. Neuroleptic treatment did not affect the CSF concentration of either peptide. The finding of similar CSF levels of NPY-like immunoreactivity in schizophrenic patients and healthy subjects is a confirmation of a previous preliminary study by our group using another NPY antibody (Ekman et al. 1984). Also, Berrettini and coworkers (1987) found no differences in the NPY concentrations in CSF of drug-free or fluphenazine-treated schizophrenic patients when compared with control subjects.

In postmortem brain studies of schizophrenic patients and control subjects, normal amounts of NPY-like immunoreactivity have been reported in the amygdala (Beal et al. 1987c) and hypothalamus (Widerlöv et al. 1988a), whereas the NPY content was reduced ($P = .003$) in the temporal cortex (Widerlöv et al. 1988a) of the schizophrenic patients.

NPY and Huntington's chorea. The striatum of patients with Huntington's chorea is severely atrophic, resulting in a substantial reduction of the number of cell bodies and also a reduction of most neuromessengers and neuronal markers. As an exception to this rule, medium-sized aspiny neurons containing NPY, somatostatin, and NADPH-diaphorase are selectively spared, resulting in increased relative tissue concentrations of NPY and somatostatin (Dawbarn et al. 1985; Ferrante et al. 1985, 1987). The mechanism behind this selective sparing is not known. In the equally atrophic amygdala of choreic patients, the NPY neurons are not spared (Zech et al. 1986).

An excitotoxin hypothesis for the pathogenesis of Huntington's chorea has been proposed. The report that quinolinic acid, but not other excitotoxins, produces NPY- and somatostatin-sparing striatal lesions closely resembling those found in the choreic patients (Beal et al. 1986b) was met with considerable interest. Subsequent studies, however, have consistently failed to replicate this finding (Boegman et al. 1987; Davies and Roberts 1987).

NPY, Alzheimer's disease, and senile dementia of the Alzheimer type. Decreased somatostatin levels have been reported in the temporal cortex of the demented brain, while NPY levels have been reported to remain normal in this area. Unlike for somatostatin, no correlation was found between tissue levels of NPY and the count of neuritic plaques in this study (Dawbarn et al. 1986), despite the fact that NPY immunoreactivity has been found in neuritic plaques of the demented brain by the same group (Dawbarn and Emson 1985). Similar dissociation between somatostatin and NPY in cortical tissue has been reported by others, who in addition found a simultaneous increase in the levels of both peptides in the substantia innominata (J. M. Allen et al. 1984). In support of these data, CSF concentrations of NPY were unaltered in patients with senile dementia of the Alzheimer type (SDAT), while the somatostatin levels were decreased (Atack et al. 1988).

In contrast, reductions in neocortical and hippocampal NPY immunoreactivity have been found by Beal and associates, who also reported unaltered NPY levels in the substantia innominata and in the striatum (Beal et al. 1986c, 1987b). Morphological examination of the hippocampus of patients with Alzheimer's disease shows a severe loss of NPY neurons and axons in areas most affected by the disease process (Chan-Palay et al. 1986). Identical morphological abnormalities were seen in the SDAT neocortex when neurons were labeled with antibodies against NPY or somatostatin (Nakamura and Vincent 1986).

Although attempted as an animal model of human dementia, excitotoxic lesions of the nucleus basalis of Meynert produce increased levels of both NPY and somatostatin in the rat cortex (Arendash et al. 1987).

NPY and Parkinson's disease. Despite a marked reduction in the concentration of somatostatin in both the neocortex and the hippocampus of patients with severe Parkinson's disease, no significant change in the concentration of NPY has been found in either region (J. M. Allen et al. 1985).

NPY and eating disorders. Recently, Kaye and coworkers (1988) found that the CSF content of NPY was significantly elevated in both underweight amenorrheic anorexic patients and the same amenorrheic patients reevaluated within 6 weeks after weight restoration. They also found an inverse relationship between CSF NPY and caloric intake in healthy volunteer women, suggesting that the elevated CSF NPY levels may reflect a homeostatic response that stimulates feeding.

The possibility of an involvement of NPY in eating behavior in humans is suggested by numerous observations of powerful effects of NPY on the regulation of food intake in experimental animals. Originally, while studying the effects of centrally administered NPY on the secretion of reproductive hormones, Clark et al. (1984) observed that ovariectomized female rats injected with NPY ate excessively. Subsequent studies confirmed this observation in intact rats and demonstrated that the effect of NPY is probably mediated through the hypothalamic PVN, while administration into other brain loci, or into the periphery, was ineffective. The magnitude of NPY-induced stimulation of feeding was higher than that induced by any pharmacological agent previously tested, and appeared to be extremely long lasting (Levine and Morley 1984; Stanley and Leibowitz 1984, 1985; Stanley et al. 1985a). NPY-induced stimulation of feeding has been reproduced in the pig (Parrott et al. 1986) and in the mouse (Morley et al. 1987a). NPY seems to specifically affect the intake of carbohydrates (Morley et al. 1987b; Stanley et al. 1985b), and its anorexigenic action does not seem to be mediated through interactions with the noradrenergic, dopaminergic, or opioid systems (Levine and Morley 1984; Morley et al. 1987b; Stanley and Leibowitz 1985).

Conclusions

The observations reviewed above suggest that NPY is a widely distributed peptide neuromessenger in the mammalian brain involved in a number of CNS functions, such as hormone secretion, cardiovascular control, regulation of food intake, and regulation of circadian rhythms. This peptide may also be involved in the pathophysiology of certain neuropsychiatric illnesses, with depression and anxiety states being the prime candidates. Whether NPY itself—or, more likely, stable nonpeptide analogues—can be used as future antidepressant or anxiolytic compounds still awaits further study.

DELTA-SLEEP–INDUCING PEPTIDE

Delta-sleep–inducing peptide was originally isolated in 1977 from cerebral venous blood in rabbits during electrical stimulation of an intralaminar thalamic area in order to induce sleep (Schoenenberger et al. 1977). Amino acid analysis and sequence determination showed that DSIP was a nonapeptide with tryptophan (Trp) at the N-terminal part of the molecule (Schoenenberger et al. 1978). The amino acid sequence is unique among neuropeptides and does not resemble any other known protein sequence.

Using radioimmunoassay, DSIP-like immunoreactivity has been described to be unevenly distributed in the CNS of several mammalian species (Kastin et al. 1978, 1981b; Nagaki and Kato 1984; Rozhanets et al. 1983). In the rat it has also been possible to measure DSIP-like immunoreactivity in extracts of peripheral organs, with the highest concentrations found in the stomach, small intestine, and kidney (Graf and Kastin 1984). In humans and some other mammals, DSIP-like immunoreactivity has also been identified in different body fluids, such as CSF, blood, urine, and milk (Banks and Kastin 1983; Ekman et al. 1983; Graf et al. 1984a, 1984b; Kastin et al. 1981a).

Using different techniques the chemical identity of DSIP-like immunoreactivity has been examined, with somewhat controversial results (Ekman et al. 1983, 1987; Graf and Kastin 1983, 1984). On the whole, both large and small forms of the molecule have been proposed to occur naturally. The peptide has also been proposed to be aggregated and/or bound to larger proteins (Graf and Kastin 1984; Kastin et al. 1981a, 1984). Various antibodies with affinities for different recognition sites on the nonapeptide have been used, and thus the concentrations of DSIP-like immunoreactivity reported in the literature have varied greatly (Graf and Kastin 1986). The precursor molecule for DSIP has not yet been characterized.

It has been shown that DSIP undergoes a rapid degradation in tissue extracts and plasma where the N-terminal Trp and alanine are easily lost (Huang and Lajtha 1978; Marks et al. 1977). The amino acid sequence of DSIP also contains serine, which can be phosphorylated, and the existence of phosphorylated DSIP has therefore been proposed. This peptide sequence has been synthesized and shown to be more potent than DSIP in exerting sleep and some other effects (Scherschlicht et al. 1984). It has been claimed that the phosphorylated form of DSIP exists naturally in tissue extracts and body fluids based on results obtained by HPLC (Graf and Kastin 1986).

DSIP has been suggested to penetrate the blood-brain barrier more easily than many other peptides (Kastin et al. 1981c, 1982). A relationship between CSF and plasma concentrations of DSIP-like immunoreactivity has also been suggested from animal experiments (Banks and Kastin 1983), but has not been confirmed in humans (Walléus et al. 1985). In addition, it has recently been proposed that the major source of DSIP may be peripheral organs and that part of the DSIP in the CNS could be of peripheral origin (Graf and Kastin 1986). Recently, it was also demonstrated that DSIP can pass into CSF but not the opposite way (Zlokovic et al. 1988).

Distribution of Delta-Sleep–Inducing Peptide

Using immunocytochemistry DSIP-like immunoreactivity has been localized in rat and rabbit brain neurons by different groups (Constantinidis et al. 1983; Feldman and Kastin 1984a, 1984b; Kato et al. 1985). Taken together, there is a rather widespread distribution in the CNS, with the hippocampus as a particularly rich source of DSIP immunoreactive neurons. So far, there are no reports on the cellular distribution of DSIP-like immunoreactivity in the human brain, but radioimmunological measurements have revealed a widespread distribution of DSIP in the rat brain and in human CSF (Kato et al. 1985; Walléus et al. 1985).

It is interesting that DSIP-like immunoreactivity occurs in high concentrations also in the hypothalamus (Kastin et al. 1978) in view of the proposed actions of DSIP to alter the release of anterior pituitary hormones (Graf et al. 1985a; Iyer and McCann 1987; Okajima and Hertting 1986; Sahu and Kalra 1986).

Whether DSIP-like immunoreactivity coexists with other messengers in brain neurons or occurs in separate systems has not yet been clarified.

Using immunocytochemistry, radioimmunoassay, and HPLC, we have recently described the occurrence of DSIP-like immunoreactivity in endocrine cells of human, porcine, rat, and mouse pituitary, adrenal medulla, and gut (Bjartell et al. 1988a, 1988b, 1989, in press a, b; manuscript submitted for publication; Ekman et al. 1987), where it coexists with other messengers such as ACTH, thyroid-stimulating hormone (TSH), epinephrine, gastrin, secretin, and PYY/glicentin.

Effects of Delta-Sleep–Inducing Peptide

A number of effects both peripherally and centrally have been attributed to DSIP. At first, DSIP was proposed to be a sleep-inducing hormone, and it has also been shown to have sleep-inducing properties following intravenous administration in a variety of species such as rabbit, cat, rat, mouse, and humans (Kafi et al. 1979; Monnier et al. 1977; Polc et al. 1978; Schneider-Helmert and Schoenenberger 1983; Schneider-Helmert et al. 1981; Ursin and Larsen 1983). Clinical trials have been performed, with successful results being reported in patients with chronic insomnia and narcolepsy (Schneider-Helmert 1984a, 1984b), although negative results have also been reported (Graf and Kastin 1986). Interestingly, DSIP seems to normalize disturbances in sleep patterns without having sedative action (Schneider-Helmert 1984a).

Many authors have described DSIP as an important factor that influences circadian cycles, such as plasma levels of pituitary hormones (growth hormone, ACTH) and the N-acetyltransferase activity in the rat pineal gland (Graf et al. 1985b; Graf and Schoenenberger 1986; Iyer and McCann 1987). Especially in the rat the plasma level of DSIP-like immunoreactivity also shows a circadian rhythm similar to that of corticosterone (Fischman et al. 1984). In healthy human subjects, or in patients with major depression, no such diurnal variation of the plasma DSIP concentrations has been observed (E. Widerlöv and R. Ekman, unpublished observation, May 1989).

DSIP also exhibits opiate agonistic effects, and withdrawal symptoms have been diminished after intravenous injections of DSIP

(Dick et al. 1984). However, the mode of action is still not fully understood, and it has been suggested that DSIP probably does not act through a modulatory effect on the opioid receptors (Taylor 1986).

At present, there is still no evidence for a specific DSIP receptor. Graf and Schoenenberger (1986) claim that DSIP could act by modulating adrenergic receptors postsynaptically as an α-receptor agonist and β-receptor antagonist. In addition, Graf and Kastin (1986) also suggest that, for example, blood pressure effects of DSIP might be explained by its influence on adrenergic transmission.

Recently, DSIP has also been suggested to be involved in the immune system regulation by altering the release of interleukins (Yehuda 1987).

Delta-Sleep–Inducing Peptide in Psychiatry

Delta-sleep–inducing peptide inhibits ACTH release after CRF stimulation in the rat (Graf et al. 1985a). Also, in humans DSIP seems to be involved in the regulation of the hypothalamo-pituitary-adrenal (HPA) axis (Bjartell et al. 1989) by inhibiting the release of ACTH following intravenous injection of DSIP into healthy male volunteers. A recent study (Lesch et al. 1988) demonstrated reduced plasma DSIP concentrations in depressed patients and elevated DSIP levels in plasma of matched healthy control subjects following CRF infusion. These findings indicate that the regulation of the HPA axis is affected differently by DSIP during depression and under normal conditions. Also, decreased concentrations of DSIP-like immunoregulation in plasma (Walléus et al. 1985) and CSF (Lindström et al. 1985; Walléus et al. 1985) have been described in patients with major depression, a condition known to be associated with hyperactivity of the HPA axis (Nemeroff et al. 1984). A reduced CSF concentration of DSIP has also been described in patients with schizophrenia (Lindström et al. 1985). It has further been shown that lithium prophylactic treatment in patients with affective disorders elevates CSF, but not plasma, levels of DSIP, suggesting that reduced CSF and plasma concentrations of DSIP may be a trait marker of affective illness (Regnell et al. 1988).

Besides sleep effects and effects on the HPA axis, DSIP has been suggested to display several other actions. In fact, Schneider-Helmert and Schoenenberger (1983) demonstrated that DSIP influences awake behavior in the direction of higher alertness, increased mental concentration, better psychomotor performance, and increased coping ability. These features are closely related to symptoms of major depression, and it is thus tempting to suggest that DSIP may be a factor involved in both the etiology and the pathogenesis of depressive disorders.

A stress-attenuating action of DSIP has also been observed in several studies (Axelrod and Reisine 1984; Schoenenberger and Schneider-Helmert 1983; Sudakov et al. 1983), and DSIP has consequently been proposed as an agent to improve stress tolerance (Graf and Kastin 1986).

Another possible indication for DSIP administration is in the treatment of drug abuse. Injections of synthetic DSIP have reduced withdrawal symptoms in alcoholic and opiate addicts, indicating that DSIP may act as an opiate agonist (Dick et al. 1984). The clinical symptoms of these patients disappeared or improved markedly following the DSIP injection. The peptide has also been given intravenously to patients with chronic pain with satisfying results (Larbig et al. 1984).

CONCLUSIONS

At present, it must be concluded that "delta-sleep–inducing peptide" is an unfortunate choice of name, because so many other effects of the peptide have been described. DSIP rather seems to be involved in the regulation of several basic homeostatic functions, of which the regulation of sleep-wakefulness was only the first one discovered. As late as 1983 some authors still claimed that DSIP could be an isolation artifact from the rabbit blood and might not correspond to a true brain hormone (Graf and Kastin 1983). Today, much evidence has accumulated that DSIP indeed should be considered a neurohormonal substance with multiple physiological effects and possibly also involved in the pathogenesis of neuropsychiatric illnesses. The fact that DSIP easily penetrates the blood-brain barrier makes it tempting to speculate whether the peptide (or more long-acting agonist or antagonist analogues) may be used as a future psychotropic drug.

REFERENCES

Adrian TE, Allen JM, Bloom SR, et al: Neuropeptide Y distribution in human brain. Nature 306:584–586, 1983

Albers HE, Ferris CF: Neuropeptide Y: role in light-dark cycle entrainment of hamster circadian rhythms. Neurosci Lett 50:163–168, 1984

Albers HE, Ferris CF, Leeman SE, et al: Avian pancreatic polypeptide phase shifts hamster circadian rhythms when microinjected into the suprachiasmatic region. Science 223:833–835, 1984

Allen JM, Ferrier IN, Roberts GW, et al: Elevation of neuropeptide Y (NPY) in substantia innominata in Alzheimer's type dementia. J Neurol Sci 64:325–331, 1984

Allen JM, Cross AJ, Crow TJ, et al: Dissociation of neuropeptide Y and somatostatin in Parkinson's disease. Brain Res 337:197–200, 1985

Allen YS, Adrian TE, Allen JM, et al: Neuropeptide Y distribution in the rat brain. Science 221:877–879, 1983

Allen YS, Roberts GW, Bloom SR, et al: Neuropeptide Y in the stria terminalis: evidence for an amygdalofugal projection. Brain Res 321:357–362, 1984

Allen YS, Bloom SR, Polak JM: The neuropeptide Y–immunoactive neuronal system: discovery, anatomy and involvement in neurodegenerative disease. Human Neurobiology 5:227–234, 1986

Anderson CR, McLachlan EM, Srb-Christie O: The relationship of terminals containing neuropeptide Y–like immunoreactivity to lumbar sympathetic vasoconstrictor neurones in the rabbit. Neurosci Lett 80:33–38, 1987

Arendash GW, Millard WJ, Dunn AJ, et al: Long-term neuropathological and neurochemical effects of nucleus basalis lesions in the rat. Science 238:952–956, 1987

Atack JR, Beal MF, May C, et al: Cerebrospinal fluid somatostatin and neuropeptide Y: concentrations in aging and in dementia of the Alzheimer type with and without extrapyramidal signs. Arch Neurol 45:269–274, 1988

Axelrod J, Reisine TD: Stress hormones: their interaction and regulation. Science 224:452–459, 1984

Bai FL, Yamano M, Shiotani Y, et al: An arcuato-paraventricular and -dorsomedial hypothalamic neuropeptide Y–containing system which lacks noradrenaline in the rat. Brain Res 331:172–175, 1985

Banks WA, Kastin AJ: CSF-plasma relationship for DSIP and some other neuropeptides. Pharmacol Biochem Behav 19:1037–1040, 1983

Beal MF, Chattha GK, Martin JB: A comparison of regional somatostatin and neuropeptide Y distribution in rat striatum and brain. Brain Res 377:240–245, 1986a

Beal MF, Kowall NW, Ellison DW, et al: Replication of the neurochemical characteristics of Huntington's disease by quinolinic acid. Nature 321:168–171, 1986b

Beal MF, Mazurek MF, Chattha GK, et al: Neuropeptide Y immunoreactivity is reduced in cerebral cortex in Alzheimer's disease. Ann Neurol 20:282–288, 1986c

Beal MF, Mazurek MF, Martin JB: A comparison of somatostatin and neuropeptide Y distribution in monkey brain. Brain Res 405:213–219, 1987a

Beal MF, Mazurek MF, McKee MA: The regional distribution of somatostatin and neuropeptide Y in control and Alzheimer's disease striatum. Neurosci Lett 79:201–206, 1987b

Beal MF, Svendsen CN, Bird ED, et al: Somatostatin and neuropeptide Y are unaltered in the amygdala in schizophrenia. Neurochem Pathol 6: 169–176, 1987c

Berrettini WH, Doran AR, Kelsoe J, et al: Cerebrospinal fluid NPY in depression and schizophrenia. Neuropsychopharmacology 1:81–83, 1987

Bjartell A, Ekman R, Sundler F, et al: Delta sleep-inducing peptide (DSIP): an overview of central actions and possible relationship to psychiatric illnesses. Nordic Psychiatric Journal 42:111–117, 1988a

Bjartell A, Ekman R, Sundler F, et al: Delta sleep-inducing peptide–like immunoreactivity in pituitary ACTH/MSH and adrenal and medullary cells. Ann NY Acad Sci 512:476–479, 1988b

Bjartell A, Ekman R, Bergquist S, et al: Reduction of immunoreactive ACTH in plasma following intravenous injection of delta sleep-inducing peptide in man. Psychoneuroendocrinology 14:347–355, 1989

Bjartell A, Castro MG, Ekman R, et al: Immunoreactive delta sleep-inducing peptide secretion from mouse dissociated anterior pituitary cells: regulation by corticotropin-releasing factor and arginine vasopressin. Neuroendocrinology (in press, a)

Bjartell A, Ekman R, Hedenbro J, et al: Delta sleep-inducing peptide (DSIP)–like immunoreactivity in gut: coexistence with known peptide hormones. Peptides (in press, b)

Blessing WW, Howe PR, Joh TH, et al: Distribution of tyrosine hydroxylase and neuropeptide Y–like immunoreactive neurons in rabbit medulla oblongata, with attention to colocalization studies, presumptive adrenaline-synthesizing perikarya, and vagal preganglionic cells. J Comp Neurol 248:285–300, 1986

Blessing WW, Oliver JR, Hodgson AH, et al: Neuropeptide Y–like immunoreactive C1 neurons in the rostral ventrolateral medulla of the rabbit project to sympathetic preganglionic neurons in the spinal cord. J Auton Nerv Syst 18:121–129, 1987

Boegman RJ, Smith Y, Parent A: Quinolinic acid does not spare striatal neuropeptide Y–immunoreactive neurons. Brain Res 415:178–182, 1987

Ceccatelli S, Hökfelt T, Hallman H, et al: Immunohistochemical analysis of the effects of cysteamine on somatostatin-like immunoreactivity in the rat central nervous system. Peptides 8:371–384, 1987

Chan-Palay V, Allen YS, Lang W, et al: Cytology and distribution in normal human cerebral cortex of neurons immunoreactive with antisera against neuropeptide Y. J Comp Neurol 238:382–389, 1985

Chan-Palay V, Lang W, Haesler U, et al: Distribution of altered hippocampal neurons and axons immunoreactive with antisera against neuropeptide Y in Alzheimer's-type dementia. J Comp Neurol 248:376–394, 1986

Chattha GK, Beal MF: Effect of cysteamine on somatostatin and neuropeptide Y in rat striatum and cortical synaptosomes. Brain Res 401:359–364, 1987

Christie MJ, Beart PM, Jarrott B, et al: Distribution of neuropeptide Y immunoreactivity in the rat basal ganglia: effects of excitotoxin lesions to caudate-putamen. Neurosci Lett 63:305–309, 1986

Chronwall BM: Anatomy and physiology of the neuroendocrine arcuate nucleus. Peptides 6 (suppl 2):1–11, 1985

Chronwall BM, Chase TN, O'Donohue TL: Coexistence of neuropeptide Y and somatostatin in rat and human cortical and rat hypothalamic neurons. Neurosci Lett 52:213–217, 1984

Chronwall BM, DiMaggio DA, Massari VJ, et al: The anatomy of neuropeptide-Y–containing neurons in rat brain. Neuroscience 15:1159–1181, 1985

Ciofi P, Croix D, Tramu G: Coexistence of hGHRF and NPY immunoreactivities in neurons of the arcuate nucleus of the rat. Neuroendocrinology 45:425–428, 1987

Clark JT, Kalra PS, Crowley WR, et al: Neuropeptide Y and human pancreatic polypeptide stimulate feeding behavior in rats. Endocrinology 115:427–429, 1984

Constantinidis J, Bouras C, Guntern R, et al: Delta sleep-inducing peptide in the rat brain: an immunohistochemical microscopic study. Neuropsychobiology 10:94–100, 1983

Csaba G: Ontogeny and phylogeny of hormone receptors. Monogr Dev Biol 15:1–172, 1981

Dai XL, Triepel J, Heym C: Immunohistochemical localization of neuropeptide Y in the guinea pig medulla oblongata: correlation with VIP and DBH. Histochemistry 85:327–334, 1986

Davies SW, Roberts PJ: No evidence for preservation of somatostatin-containing neurons after intrastriatal injections of quinolinic acid. Nature 326–329, 1987

Dawbarn D, Emson PC: Neuropeptide Y–like immunoreactivity in neuritic plaques of Alzheimer's disease. Biochem Biophys Res Commun 126:289–294, 1985

Dawbarn D, Hunt SP, Emson PC: Neuropeptide Y: regional distribution, chromatographic characterization and immunohistochemical demonstration in post-mortem human brain. Brain Res 296:168–173, 1984

Dawbarn D, De Quidt ME, Emson PC: Survival of basal ganglia neuropeptide Y–somatostatin neurones in Huntington's disease. Brain Res 340:251–260, 1985

Dawbarn D, Rossor MN, Mountjoy CQ, et al: Decreased somatostatin immunoreactivity but not neuropeptide Y immunoreactivity in cerebral cortex in senile dementia of Alzheimer type. Neurosci Lett 70:154–159, 1986

Demeulemeester H, Vandesande F, Orban GA, et al: Heterogeneity of GABAergic cells in cat visual cortex. J Neurosci 8:988–1000, 1988

de Quidt ME, Emson PC: Distribution of neuropeptide Y–like immunoreactivity in the rat central nervous system, I: radioimmunoassay and chromatographic characterisation. Neuroscience 18:527–543, 1986a

de Quidt ME, Emson PC: Distribution of neuropeptide Y–like immunoreactivity in the rat central nervous system, II: immunohistochemical analysis. Neuroscience 18:545–618, 1986b

Dick P, Costa C, Fayolle K, et al: DSIP in the treatment of withdrawal syndromes from alcohol and opiates. Eur Neurol 23:364–371, 1984

Ekman R, Larsson I, Malmquist M, et al: Radioimmunoassay of delta sleep-inducing peptide using an iodinated *p*-hydroxyphenylpropionic acid derivate as tracer. Regul Pept 6:371–378, 1983

Ekman R, Widerlöv E, Walléus H, et al: Elevated levels of NPY-like material in CSF in depression. Paper presented at the International Society of Psychoneuroendocrinology XVth International Congress, Vienna, July 15–19, 1984

Ekman R, Wahlestedt C, Böttcher G, et al: Peptide YY–like immunoreactivity in the central nervous system of the rat. Regul Pept 16:157–168, 1986

Ekman R, Bjartell A, Ekblad E, et al: Immunoreactive delta sleep-inducing peptide in pituitary adrenocorticotropin/alpha-melanotropic cells and adrenal medullary cells of the pig. Neuroendocrinology 45:298–304, 1987

El-Sahly M: On the phylogeny of the gastro-entero-pancreatic (GEP) neuroendocrine system. Acta University of Uppsala 385:1–39, 1981

Emson PC, de Quidt ME: NPY—a new member of the pancreatic polypeptide family. Trends in Neuroscience 7:31–35, 1984

Everitt BJ, Hökfelt T, Terenius L, et al: Differential co-existence of neuropeptide Y (NPY)–like immunoreactivity with catecholamines in the central nervous system of the rat. Neuroscience 11:443–462, 1984

Falkmer S, van Noorden S: Ontogeny and phylogeny of the glucagon cell, in Handbook of Experimental Pharmacology, Vol 66. Edited by Lefèbvre PJ. Berlin, Springer-Verlag, 1983, pp 81–119

Feldman SC, Kastin AJ: The distribution of neurons containing delta sleep-inducing peptide in the hippocampal formation. Brain Res Bull 13:833–837, 1984a

Feldman SC, Kastin AJ: Localization of neurons containing immunoreactive delta sleep-inducing peptide in the rat brain: an immunocytochemical study. Neuroscience 11:303–317, 1984b

Ferrante RJ, Kowall NW, Beal MF, et al: Selective sparing of a class of striatal neurons in Huntington's disease. Science 230:561–563, 1985

Ferrante RJ, Kowall NW, Beal MF, et al: Morphologic and histochemical characteristics of a spared subset of striatal neurons in Huntington's disease. J Neuropathol Exp Neurol 46:12–27, 1987

Fischman AJ, Kastin AJ, Graf MV: Circadian variation of DSIP-like material in rat plasma. Life Sci 35:2079–2084, 1984

Fuxe K, Agnati LF, Härfstrand A, et al: Central administration of neuropeptide Y induces hypotension, bradypnea and EEG synchronization in the rat. Acta Physiol Scand 118:189–192, 1983

Gall C, Seroogy KB, Brecha N: Distribution of VIP- and NPY-like immunoreactivities in rat main olfactory bulb. Brain Res 371:389–394, 1986

Gaspar P, Berger B, Lesur A, et al: Somatostatin 28 and neuropeptide Y innervation in the septal area and related cortical and subcortical structures of the human brain: distribution, relationships and evidence for differential coexistence. Neuroscience 22:49–73, 1987

Gonzalez MF, Sharp FR: Fetal frontal cortex transplanted to injured motor/sensory cortex of adult rats, I: NADPH-diaphorase neurons. J Neurosci 7:2991–3001, 1987

Graf MV, Kastin AJ: Delta sleep-inducing peptide (DSIP): a review. Neurosci Biobehav Rev 8:83–93, 1983

Graf MV, Kastin AJ: Delta sleep-inducing peptide (DSIP)–like material exists in peripheral organs of rats in large dissociable forms. Proc Soc Exp Biol Med 177:197–204, 1984

Graf MV, Kastin AJ: Delta sleep-inducing peptide (DSIP): an update. Peptides 7:1165–1187, 1986

Graf MV, Schoenenberger GA: DSIP affects adrenergic stimulation of rat pineal N-acetyltransferase in vivo and in vitro. Peptides 7:1001–1006, 1986

Graf MV, Hunter CA, Kastin AJ: Presence of delta sleep-inducing peptide–like material in human milk. J Clin Endocrinol Metab 59:127–132, 1984a

Graf MV, Kastin AJ, Fischman AJ: DSIP occurs in free form in mammalian plasma, human CSF and urine. Pharmacol Biochem Behav 21:761–766, 1984b

Graf MV, Kastin AJ, Coy DH, et al: Delta sleep-inducing peptide reduces CRF-induced corticosterone release. Neuroendocrinology 41:353–356, 1985a

Graf MV, Kastin AJ, Schoenenberger GA: Delta sleep-inducing peptide and two of its analogs reduced nocturnal increase of N-acetyltransferase activity in rat pineal gland. J Neurochem 44:629–632, 1985b

Gray TS, O'Donohue TL, Magnuson DJ: Neuropeptide Y innervation of amygdaloid and hypothalamic neurons that project to the dorsal vagal complex in rat. Peptides 7:341–349, 1986

Gustafson EL, Card JP, Moore RY: Neuropeptide Y localization in the rat amygdaloid complex. J Comp Neurol 251:349–362, 1986

Guy J, Bosler O, Dusticier G, et al: Morphological correlates of serotonin–neuropeptide Y interactions in the rat suprachiasmatic nucleus: combined radioautographic and immunocytochemical data. Cell Tissue Res 250:657–662, 1987

Guy J, Pelletier G, Bosler O: Serotonin innervation of neuropeptide Y–containing neurons in the rat arcuate nucleus. Neurosci Lett 85:9–13, 1988

Haas DA, George SR: Neuropeptide Y administration acutely increases hypothalamic corticotropin-releasing factor immunoreactivity: lack of effect in other rat brain regions. Life Sci 41:2725–2731, 1987

Hamilton M: Development of a rating scale for primary depressive illness. Br J Soc Clin Psychol 6:278–296, 1967

Handley SL, Mithani S: Effects of alpha-adrenoceptor agonists and antagonists in a maze-exploration model of "fear"-motivated behaviour. Naunyn Schmiedebergs Arch Pharmacol 327:1–5, 1984

Härfstrand A, Eneroth P, Agnati L, et al: Further studies on the effects of central administration of neuropeptide Y on neuroendocrine function in the male rat: relationship to hypothalamic catecholamines. Regul Pept 17:167–179, 1987a

Härfstrand A, Fuxe K, Terenius L, et al: Neuropeptide Y–immunoreactive perikarya and nerve terminals in the rat medulla oblongata: relationship to cytoarchitecture and catecholaminergic cell groups. J Comp Neurol 260:20–35, 1987b

Harrington ME, Nance DM, Rusak B: Neuropeptide Y immunoreactivity in the hamster geniculo-suprachiasmatic tract. Brain Res Bull 15:465–472, 1985

Harrington ME, Nance DM, Rusak B. Double labeling of neuropeptide Y–immunoreactive neurons which project from the geniculate to the suprachiasmatic nuclei. Brain Res 410:275–282, 1987

Heilig M, Murison R: Intracerebroventricular neuropeptide Y protects against stress-induced gastric erosion in the rat. Eur J Pharmacol 137:127–129, 1987a

Heilig M, Murison R: Intracerebroventricular neuropeptide Y suppresses open field and home cage activity in the rat. Regul Pept 19:221–231, 1987b

Heilig M, Wahlestedt C, Ekman R, et al: Antidepressant drugs increase the concentration of neuropeptide Y (NPY)–like immunoreactivity in the rat brain. Eur J Pharmacol 147:465–467, 1988

Heilig M, Söderpalm B, Engel JA, et al: Centrally administered neuropeptide Y (NPY) produces anxiolytic-like effects in animal anxiety models. Psychopharmacology (Berlin) 98:524–529, 1989

Hendry SH, Jones EG, DeFelipe J, et al: Neuropeptide-containing neurons of the cerebral cortex are also GABAergic. Proc Natl Acad Sci USA 81:6526–6530, 1984

Hökfelt T, Lundberg JM, Lagercrantz H, et al: Occurrence of neuropeptide Y (NPY)–like immunoreactivity in catecholamine neurons in the human medulla oblongata. Neurosci Lett 36:217–222, 1983a

Hökfelt T, Lundberg JM, Tatemoto K, et al: Neuropeptide Y (NPY)– and FMRFamide neuropeptide–like immunoreactivities in catecholamine neurons of the rat medulla oblongata. Acta Physiol Scand 117:315–318, 1983b

Hu H, Rao JK, Prasad C, et al: Localization of neuropeptide Y–like immunoreactivity in the cat hypothalamus. Peptides 8:569–573, 1987

Huang JT, Lajtha A: The degradation of a nonapeptide, sleep inducing peptide in rat brain: comparison with enkephalin breakdown. Res Commun Chem Pathol Pharmacol 19:191–199, 1978

Ibata Y, Takahashi Y, Okamura H, et al: Fine structure of NPY-containing neurons in the lateral geniculate nucleus and their terminals in the suprachiasmatic nucleus of the rat. Brain Res 439:230–235, 1988

Iyer KS, McCann SM: Delta sleep-inducing peptide (DSIP) stimulates growth hormone (GH) release in the rat by hypothalamic and pituitary actions. Peptides 8:45–48, 1987

Jesberger JA, Richardson JS: Animal models of depression: parallels and correlates to severe depression in humans. Biol Psychiatry 20:764–784, 1985

Jones EG, Hendry SH: Peptide-containing neurons of the primate cerebral cortex. Res Publ Assoc Res Nerv Ment Dis 64:163–178, 1986

Kafi S, Monnier M, Gaillard JM: The delta sleep-inducing peptide (DSIP) increases duration of sleep in rats. Neurosci Lett 13:169–172, 1979

Kalra SP, Crowley WR: Norepinephrine-like effects of neuropeptide Y on LH release in the rat. Life Sci 35:1173–1176, 1984

Kastin AJ, Nissen C, Schally A, et al: Radioimmunoassay of DSIP-like material in rat brain. Brain Res Bull 3:691–695, 1978

Kastin AJ, Castellanos PF, Banks WA, et al: Radioimmunoassay of DSIP-like material in human blood: possible protein binding. Pharmacol Biochem Behav 15:969–974, 1981a

Kastin AJ, Nissen C, Coy DH: DSIP-like immunoreactivity in the developing brain. Brain Res Bull 7:687–690, 1981b

Kastin AJ, Nissen C, Coy DH: Permeability of blood-brain barrier to DSIP peptides. Pharmacol Biochem Behav 15:955–959, 1981c

Kastin AJ, Banks WA, Castellanos PF, et al: Differential penetration of DSIP into rat brain. Pharmacol Biochem Behav 17:1187–1191, 1982

Kastin AJ, Castellanos PF, Fischman AJ, et al: Evidence for peptide aggregation. Pharmacol Biochem Behav 21:969–973, 1984

Kataoka Y, Ushio M, Koizumi S, et al: Changes in the concentration of brain neuropeptide Y (NPY)–like immunoreactivity following olfactory bulbectomy and effects of antidepressants in rats. Society of Neuroscience Abstracts 114:11, 1988

Kato N, Nagaki S, Takahashi Y, et al: DSIP-like material in rat brain, human cerebrospinal fluid, and plasma as determined by enzyme immunoassay, in Endogenous Sleep Substances and Sleep Regulation. Edited by Inoue S, Borbely AA. Utrecht, The Netherlands, VNU Science Press, 1985, pp 141–153

Kaye WH, Berrettini W, Gwirtsman H, et al: Altered cerebrospinal fluid neuropeptide Y (NPY) in anorexia nervosa and peptide YY (PYY) in normal weight bulimia: relationship to appetite behaviour and menstrual function. Abstracts of the 27th annual meeting of the American College of Neuropsychopharmacology, 108, December 1988

Kerkerian L, Pelletier G: Effects of monosodium L-glutamate administration on neuropeptide Y containing neurons in the rat hypothalamus. Brain Res 369:388–390, 1986

Kerkerian L, Guy J, Lefévre G, et al: Effects of neuropeptide Y (NPY) on the release of anterior pituitary hormones in the rat. Peptides 6:1201–1204, 1985

Khorram O, Roselli CE, Ellinwood WE, et al: The measurement of neuropeptide Y in discrete hypothalamic and limbic regions of male rhesus macaques with a human NPY-directed antiserum. Peptides 8:159–163, 1987

Köhler C, Eriksson L, Davies S, et al: Neuropeptide Y innervation of the hippocampal region in the rat and monkey brain. J Comp Neurol 244:384–400, 1986a

Köhler C, Smialowska M, Eriksson LG, et al: Origin of the neuropeptide Y innervation of the rat retrohippocampal region. Neurosci Lett 65:287–292, 1986b

Köhler C, Eriksson LG, Davies S, et al: Co-localization of neuropeptide tyrosine and somatostatin immunoreactivity in neurons of individual subfields of the rat hippocampal region. Neurosci Lett 78:1–6, 1987

Kowall NW, Ferrante RJ, Beal MF, et al: Neuropeptide Y, somatostatin, and reduced nicotinamide adenine dinucleotide phosphate diaphorase in the human striatum: a combined immunocytochemical and enzyme histochemical study. Neuroscience 20:817–828, 1987

Krukoff TL: NPY-containing nerve terminals and fibers in close association with peptidergic sympathetic preganglionic neurons. Neurosci Lett 77:1–4, 1987a

Krukoff TL: Neuropeptide Y–like immunoreactivity in cat spinal cord with special reference to autonomic areas. Brain Res 415:300–308, 1987b

Larbig W, Gerber WD, Kluck M, et al: Therapeutic effects of delta sleep-inducing peptide (DSIP) in patients with chronic pronounced pain episodes. Eur Neurol 23:372–385, 1984

Leger L, Charnay Y, Danger JM, et al: Mapping of neuropeptide Y–like immunoreactivity in the feline hypothalamus and hypophysis. J Comp Neurol 255:283–292, 1987

LeRoith D, Shiloach J, Roth J, et al: Evolutionary origins of vertebrate hormones: substances similar to mammalian insulins are native to unicellular eukaryotes (*Tetrahymena/Neurospora*). Proc Natl Acad Sci USA 77:6184–6188, 1980

Lesch KP, Widerlöv E, Ekman R, et al: Delta sleep-inducing peptide response to human corticotropin-releasing hormone (CRH) in major depressive disorder: comparison with CRH-induced corticotropin and cortisol secretion. Biol Psychiatry 24:162–172, 1988

Levine AS, Morley JE: Neuropeptide Y: a potent inducer of consummatory behavior in rats. Peptides 5:1025–1029, 1984

Lindström LH, Ekman R, Walléus H, et al: Delta sleep-inducing peptide in cerebrospinal fluid from schizophrenics, depressives and healthy volunteers. Prog Neuropsychopharmacol Biol Psychiatry 9:83–90, 1985

Liposits Z, Sievers L, Paull WK: Neuropeptide-Y and ACTH-immunoreactive innervation of corticotropin releasing factor (CRF)–synthesizing neurons in the hypothalamus of the rat: an immunocytochemical analysis at the light and electron microscopic levels. Histochemistry 88:227–234, 1988

Lundberg JM, Terenius L, Hökfelt T, et al: Neuropeptide Y (NPY)–like immunoreactivity in peripheral noradrenergic neurons and effects of NPY on sympathetic function. Acta Physiol Scand 116:477–480, 1982

Marks N, Stern F, Kastin AJ, et al: Degradation of delta sleep-inducing peptide (DSIP) and its analogs by brain extracts. Brain Res Bull 2:491–493, 1977

Massari VJ, Chan J, Chronwall BM, et al: Neuropeptide Y in the rat nucleus accumbens: ultrastructural localization in aspiny neurons receiving synaptic input from GABAergic terminals. J Neurosci Res 19:171–186, 1988

Modigh K: Antidepressant drugs in anxiety disorders. Acta Psychiatr Scand 76 (suppl 335):51–71, 1987

Molinari M, Hendry SH, Jones EG: Distributions of certain neuropeptides in the primate thalamus. Brain Res 426:270–289, 1987

Monnier M, Dudler L, Gaechter R, et al: Delta sleep-inducing peptide (DSIP): EEG and motor activity in rabbits following intravenous administration. Neurosci Lett 6:9–13, 1977

Montgomery KC: The relation between fear induced by novel stimulation and exploratory behaviour. J Comp Physiol Psychol 48:254–260, 1958

Montgomery S, Åsberg MA: A new depression scale designed to be sensitive to change. Br J Psychiatry 134:382–389, 1979

Moore RY, Card JP: Visual pathways and the entrainment of circadian rhythms. Ann NY Acad Sci 453:123–133, 1985

Moore RY, Gustafson EL, Card JP: Identical immunoreactivity of afferents to the rat suprachiasmatic nucleus with antisera against avian pancreatic polypeptide, molluscan cardioexcitatory peptide and neuropeptide Y. Cell Tissue Res 236:41–46, 1984

Morley JE, Hernandez EN, Flood JF: Neuropeptide Y increases food intake in mice. Am J Physiol 253:R516–R522, 1987a

Morley JE, Levine AS, Gosnell BA, et al: Effect of neuropeptide Y on ingestive behaviors in the rat. Am J Physiol 252:R599–R609, 1987b

Nagaki S, Kato N: Delta sleep-inducing peptide–like material in rat brain as determined by enzyme immunoassay: effect of sleep deprivation. Neurosci Lett 51:253–257, 1984

Nakagawa Y, Shiosaka S, Emson PC, et al: Distribution of neuropeptide Y in the forebrain and diencephalon: an immunohistochemical analysis. Brain Res 361:52–60, 1985

Nakamura S, Vincent SR: Somatostatin- and neuropeptide Y–immunoreactive neurons in the neocortex in senile dementia of Alzheimer's type. Brain Res 370:11–20, 1986

Nemeroff CB, Widerlöv E, Bisette G, et al: Elevated cerebrospinal fluid concentrations of corticotropin-releasing factor–like immunoreactivity in major depression. Science 226:1342–1344, 1984

Okajima T, Hertting G: Delta sleep-inducing peptide (DSIP) inhibited CRF-induced ACTH secretion from rat anterior pituitary gland in vitro. Hormone Metab Res 18:497–498, 1986

Papadopoulos GC, Parnavelas JG, Cavanagh ME: Extensive coexistence of neuropeptides in the rat visual cortex. Brain Res 420:95–99, 1987

Parrott RF, Heavens RP, Baldwin BA: Stimulation of feeding in the satiated pig by intracerebroventricular injection of neuropeptide Y. Physiol Behav 36:523–525, 1986

Pelletier G, Desy L, Kerkerian L, et al: Immunocytochemical localization of neuropeptide Y (NPY) in the human hypothalamus. Cell Tissue Res 238:203–205, 1984

Pellow S, Chopin P, File SE, et al: Validation of open:closed arm entries in an elevated plus-maze as a measure of anxiety in the rat. J Neurosci Methods 14:149–167, 1985

Polc P, Schneeberger I, Haefely W: Effects of the delta sleep-inducing peptide (DSIP) in the sleep-wakefulness cycle of cats. Neurosci Lett 9:33–36, 1978

Redmond DE, Huang YH: New evidence for a locus coeruleus–norepinephrine connection with anxiety. Life Sci 25:2149–2162, 1979

Regnell G, Widerlöv E, Ekman R: Delta sleep-inducing peptide in CSF of patients with affective illness is elevated by lithium treatment. Biol Psychiatry 24:112–116, 1988

Rozhanets VV, Yukkananov RY, Chizhevskaya MA, et al: Regional distribution of delta sleep-inducing peptide (DSIP)–like immunoreactivity in rat brain and other organs. Neurokhimiia 2:353–363, 1983

Sabatino FD, Murnane JM, Hoffman RA, et al: Distribution of neuropeptide Y–like immunoreactivity in the hypothalamus of the adult golden hamster. J Comp Neurol 257:93–104, 1987

Sahu A, Kalra SP: Delta sleep-inducing peptide (DSIP) stimulates LH release in steroid-primed ovariectomized rats. Life Sci 40:1201–1206, 1986

Sandell JH, Graybiel AM, Chesselet MF: A new enzyme marker for striatal compartmentalization: NADPH diaphorase activity in the caudate nucleus and putamen of the cat. J Comp Neurol 243:326–334, 1986

Sawchenko PE, Swanson LW, Grzanna R, et al: Colocalization of neuropeptide Y immunoreactivity in brainstem catecholaminergic neurons that project to the paraventricular nucleus of the hypothalamus. J Comp Neurol 241:138–153, 1985

Scherschlicht R, Aeppli L, Polc P, et al: Some pharmacological effects of delta-sleep–inducing peptide (DSIP). Eur Neurol 23:346–352, 1984

Schneider-Helmert D: DSIP in insomnia. Eur Neurol 23:358–363, 1984a

Schneider-Helmert D: Effects of DSIP on narcolepsy. Eur Neurol 23:353–357, 1984b

Schneider-Helmert D, Schoenenberger GA: Effects of DSIP in man. Neuropsychobiology 9:197–206, 1983

Schneider-Helmert D, Gnirss F, Monnier M, et al: Acute and delayed effects of DSIP on human sleep behaviour. Int J Clin Pharmacol Ther Toxicol 19:341–345, 1981

Schoenenberger GA, Schneider-Helmert D: Psychophysiological functions of DSIP. Trends in Pharmacological Sciences 4:307–310, 1983

Schoenenberger GA, Maier PF, Tobler KJ, et al: A naturally occurring delta-EEG enhancing nonapeptide in rabbits: final isolation, characterization and activity test. Pflügers Arch 369:99–109, 1977

Schoenenberger GA, Maier PF, Tobler KJ, et al: The delta-EEG (sleep)–inducing peptide (DSIP), XI: amino-acid analysis, sequence, synthesis and activity of the nonapeptide. Pflügers Arch 376:119–129, 1978

Schon F, Allen JM, Yeats JC, et al: The effect of 6-hydroxydopamine, reserpine and cold stress on the neuropeptide Y content of the rat central nervous system. Neuroscience 19:1247–1250, 1986

Schröder H: Neuropeptide Y (NPY)–like immunoreactivity in peripheral and central nerve fibres of the golden hamster (*Mesocricetus auratus*), with special respect to pineal gland innervation. Histochemistry 85:321–325, 1986

Schröder H, Vollrath L: Neuropeptide Y (NPY)–like immunoreactivity in the guinea pig pineal organ. Neurosci Lett 63:285–289, 1986

Scott JW, McDonald JK, Pemberton JL: Short axon cells of the rat olfactory bulb display NADPH-diaphorase activity, neuropeptide Y–like immunoreactivity, and somatostatin-like immunoreactivity. J Comp Neurol 260:378–391, 1987

Shen CL: Distribution of neuropeptide Y immunoreactivity in the forebrain of the rat. Proc Natl Sci Counc Repub China [B] 11:115–127, 1987

Shiotani Y, Yamano M, Shiosaka S, et al: Distribution and origins of substance P (SP)–, calcitonin gene–related peptide (CGRP)–, vasoactive intestinal polypeptide (VIP)– and neuropeptide Y (NPY)–containing nerve fibers in the pineal gland of gerbils. Neurosci Lett 70:187–192, 1986

Siever LJ, Davies KL: Overview: towards a dysregulation hypothesis of depression. Am J Psychiatry 142:1017–1031, 1985

Smith Y, Parent A: Neuropeptide Y–immunoreactive neurons in the striatum of cat and monkey: morphological characteristics, intrinsic organization and co-localization with somatostatin. Brain Res 372:241–252, 1986

Smith Y, Parent A, Kerkerian L, et al: Distribution of neuropeptide Y immunoreactivity in the basal forebrain and upper brainstem of the squirrel monkey (*Saimiri sciureus*). J Comp Neurol 236:71–89, 1985

Stanley BG, Leibowitz SF: Neuropeptide Y: stimulation of feeding and drinking by injection into the paraventricular nucleus. Life Sci 35:2635–2642, 1984

Stanley BG, Leibowitz SF: Neuropeptide Y injected in the paraventricular hypothalamus: a powerful stimulant of feeding behavior. Proc Natl Acad Sci USA 82:3940–3943, 1985

Stanley BG, Chin AS, Leibowitz SF: Feeding and drinking elicited by central injection of neuropeptide Y: evidence for a hypothalamic site(s) of action. Brain Res Bull 14:521–524, 1985a

Stanley BG, Daniel DR, Chin AS, et al: Paraventricular nucleus injections of peptide YY and neuropeptide Y preferentially enhance carbohydrate ingestion. Peptides 6:1205–1211, 1985b

Sudakov KV, Ivanow VT, Koplik EV, et al: Delta sleep-inducing peptide (DSIP) as a factor facilitating animals' resistance to acute emotional stress. Pavlov J Biol Sci 18:1–5, 1983

Tatemoto K: Neuropeptide Y: complete amino acid sequence of the brain peptide. Proc Natl Acad Sci USA 79:5485–5489, 1982

Tatemoto K, Carlquist M, Mutt V: Neuropeptide Y—a novel brain peptide with structural similarities to peptide YY and pancreatic polypeptide. Nature 296:659–660, 1982

Tatemoto K, Siimesmaa S, Jörnvall H, et al: Isolation and characterization of neuropeptide Y from porcine intestine. FEBS Lett 179:181–184, 1985

Taylor JE: Delta sleep-inducing peptide does not compete with the in vitro binding of ^{3}H naloxone and ^{3}H DADLE on opioid receptors. IRCS Med Sci 14:1122, 1986

Ueda S, Kawata M, Sano Y: Identification of neuropeptide Y immunoreactivity in the suprachiasmatic nucleus and the lateral geniculate nucleus of some mammals. Neurosci Lett 68:7–10, 1986

Vecsei L, Ekman R, Alling C, et al: Influence of cysteamine and cysteine on open-field behavior, and on brain concentrations of catecholamines, somatostatin, neuropeptide Y, and corticotropin-releasing hormone in the rat. J Neural Transm (in press)

Vogel JR, Beer B, Clody DE: A simple and reliable conflict procedure for testing anti-anxiety agents. Psychopharmacology (Berlin) 21:1–7, 1971

Wahle P, Meyer G: The olfactory tubercle of the cat, II: immunohistochemical compartmentation. Exp Brain Res 62:528–540, 1986

Wahle P, Meyer G, Albus K: Localization of NPY-immunoreactivity in the cat's visual cortex. Exp Brain Res 61:364–374, 1986

Wahlestedt C, Skagerberg G, Ekman R, et al: Neuropeptide Y (NPY) in the area of the hypothalamic paraventricular nucleus activates the pituitary-adrenocortical axis in the rat. Brain Res 417:33–38, 1987

Wahlestedt C, Ekman R, Widerlöv E: Neuropeptide Y (NPY) and the central nervous system: distribution, effects and possible relationship to neurological and psychiatric disorders. Prog Neuropsychopharmacol Biol Psychiatry 13:31–54, 1989

Walléus H, Widerlöv E, Ekman R: Decreased concentrations of delta sleep-inducing peptide in plasma and cerebrospinal fluid from depressed patients. Nordic Psychiatric Journal 39 (suppl 11):63–67, 1985

Widerlöv E, Wahlestedt C, Hakanson R, et al: Altered brain neuropeptide function in psychiatric illnesses—with special emphasis on NPT and CRF in major depression. Clin Neuropharmacol 9 (suppl 4):572–574, 1986

Widerlöv E, Gottfries CG, Lindström L, et al: Brain and CSF neuropeptide alterations in schizophrenia. Neurochemistry International 13 (suppl 1): 66, 1988a

Widerlöv E, Heilig M, Ekman R, et al: Possible relationship between neuropeptide Y (NPY) and major depression—evidence from human and animal studies. Nordic Psychiatric Journal 42:131–137, 1988b

Widerlöv E, Lindström LH, Wahlestedt C, et al: Neuropeptide Y and peptide YY as possible cerebrospinal markers for major depression and schizophrenia, respectively. J Psychiatr Res 22:69–79, 1988c

Widerlöv E, Heilig M, Ekman R, et al: Neuropeptide Y: possible involvement in depression and anxiety, in Nobel Conference on NPY. Edited by Mutt V, Fuxe K, Hökfelt T, et al. New York, Raven, 1989, pp 331–342

Willoughby JO, Blessing WW: Neuropeptide Y injected into the supraoptic nucleus causes secretion of vasopressin in the unanesthetized rat. Neurosci Lett 75:17–22, 1987

Yamazoe M, Shiosaka S, Emson PC, et al: Distribution of neuropeptide Y in the lower brainstem: an immunohistochemical analysis. Brain Res 335:109–120, 1985

Yehuda S: Effects of DSIP, 5-HTP and serotonin on the lymphokine system: a preliminary study. Int J Neurosci 33:185–197, 1987

Zech M, Roberts GW, Bogerts B, et al: Neuropeptides in the amygdala of controls, schizophrenics and patients suffering from Huntington's chorea: an immunohistochemical study. Acta Neuropathol (Berl) 71:259–266, 1986

Zlokovic BV, Segal MB, Davson H, et al: Passage of delta sleep-inducing peptide (DSIP) across the blood–cerebrospinal fluid barrier. Peptides 9:533–538, 1988

Chapter 14

Neurotransmitter Receptor Imaging Techniques

Errol B. De Souza, Ph.D.

Chapter 14

Neurotransmitter Receptor Imaging Techniques

The concept that most drugs and endogenous substances, such as hormones and neurotransmitters, produce their biological effects by interaction with specific molecular sites, termed *receptors*, is fundamental to the science of biology and pharmacology. While receptors have been studied for several decades using intact isolated organ preparations, the advent of radiolabeled ligands for directly labeling receptor binding sites has revolutionized our understanding of the biochemical aspects and heterogeneity of receptors. At the same time, major advances have been made in understanding the nature of the interactions between receptor binding sites and their associated second-messenger effector mechanisms (e.g., enzymes, ion channels), the molecular composition of the receptors themselves, and the uses of receptor measurements in the characterization and/or detection of disease states.

The goal of this chapter is to discuss and critically evaluate the techniques that are available to study receptors (see Table 14-1). The main emphasis will be on the use of radioligand-binding techniques to study receptors, since this approach dominates the field at this time. However, other methods such as the use of antibody and molecular biological techniques that represent the future directions for studying receptors will also be discussed. Finally, the techniques available to study the role of receptors in human disease will be addressed.

I am indebted to Dr. Michael J. Kuhar for his help with all aspects of the chapter, to Dr. Peter J. Whitehouse for helpful discussions and suggestions on the use of autoradiographic techniques to study receptors in neurodegenerative disease, and to Dr. Dean Wong for valuable information on the use of PET scanning techniques to study receptors in health and in disease. I thank Sharon Amos for manuscript preparation.

TECHNIQUES USED TO STUDY RECEPTORS

Radioligand Binding Methods

Detailed strategies for the identification, characterization, and quantification of receptors in homogenates (termed "grind and bind") have been described (Bennett and Yamamura 1985). Briefly, homogenates of discrete areas of brain or other tissues are incubated under optimal conditions with radioactive ligand that is specific for a given neurotransmitter receptor; the specificity of the radioactive ligand for a given neurotransmitter receptor is defined by coincubating with an unlabeled drug that has high specificity for the receptor of interest. The "radiotagged" receptor in the membrane can then be separated from the free radioactive ligand by one of several techniques, including filtration, centrifugation, or precipitation. (The details of the optimal conditions to label receptors and methods to separate membrane-bound receptors are beyond the scope of this chapter and are described in detail elsewhere [Bennett and Yamamura 1985].) The relative ease of this technique lends itself well to studying the kinetic characteristics, pharmacological specificity, and modulation of receptors following in vitro or in vivo treatments. The major disadvantage of this approach is its lack of anatomical resolution and its relative lack of sensitivity (i.e., it is difficult to measure a very small concentration of receptor). These disadvantages can be overcome by using *receptor mapping techniques*, as described below.

The fundamental advantages of microscopic receptor mapping are increased anatomical resolution and greatly increased sensitivity of

Table 14-1. Techniques used to study neurotransmitter receptors

Radioligand binding methods
"Grind and bind": biochemical characterization of receptors in homogenates
In vitro autoradiography
In vivo autoradiography
Positron emission tomography (PET)
Immunocytochemistry using antibodies for receptors
In situ hybridization histochemistry using probes for receptor mRNA and cDNA

measurement when compared to the "biochemical" (i.e., grind-and-bind) approaches described above. The increase in anatomical resolution is obvious because these mapping approaches are microscopic techniques that always have greater resolution than microdissection techniques. The greater sensitivity in measurement derives from the fact that one can measure receptor densities in very small, microscopic regions. This increase in sensitivity can be orders of magnitude greater than that found in biochemical studies. Thus, receptor mapping will be useful in any situation requiring receptor measurement in small regions or in situations where overall quantities (but not necessarily densities) of receptors are low.

In general, there are two important principles that one must keep in mind when carrying out receptor-mapping experiments. The first principle is *selective or preferential labeling of receptors.* The development of large numbers of radioactive ligands and the availability of extensive pharmacological studies on many receptors using primarily radioligand binding in homogenates (see above) have provided the ability to define, quite precisely, the type of receptor to which binding is occurring. The second principle is the *selection of appropriate methods of visualization.* This is important because one does not visualize the receptor directly, but rather the radioligand that binds to it. Thus, one must produce an autoradiogram or image in such a way that one prevents or minimizes the diffusion of the ligand away from the receptor. The latter is not an important issue when dealing with irreversibly binding ligands. However, the vast majority of available ligands are reversible binding agents, and the autoradiography must be done in a way that takes into account the diffusible nature of the signal (Barnard 1979; Roth and Stumpf 1969; Young and Kuhar 1979). There are two main experimental approaches to receptor mapping experiments: in vitro labeling procedures and in vivo labeling procedures. Various aspects of receptor mapping have been previously reviewed (Kuhar 1985; Kuhar et al. 1986).

In vitro labeling autoradiography. The details of many of these procedures and examples of in vitro receptor binding studies have been presented elsewhere (Kuhar 1985; Kuhar et al. 1986). In in vitro labeling procedures, slide-mounted tissue sections are incubated with radioactive ligands so that the receptors are labeled under very controlled conditions (Young and Kuhar 1979). Following receptor labeling, the slide-mounted tissue sections can be rinsed in buffer to remove nonreceptor-bound drug and improve the specific-to-nonspecific binding ratios. Once the slide-mounted tissue sections have been prepared so that selective receptor labeling has occurred, autoradiograms can be generated, usually by apposition techniques. The slide-mounted tissue sections with labeled receptors are apposed to emulsion-coated glass coverslips (Kuhar 1985; Young and Kuhar 1979), plastic coverslips (Kuhar 1985), or tritium-sensitive Ultrofilm (LKB, Gaithersburg, MD) (Kuhar 1985). The emulsions and Ultrofilm are developed by standard methods after adequate exposure. The exposure time depends on the quantity of radioactivity in the tissues, which in turn is determined by the number of receptors labeled and the specific activity of the radioactive ligand.

In vivo labeling autoradiography. Detailed strategies for carrying out in vivo labeling experiments and some examples of in vivo receptor binding studies have been described elsewhere (Kuhar 1985; Kuhar et al. 1986). The term *in vivo receptor labeling* refers to the procedure in which receptors are labeled in intact living tissues in vivo after systemic administration of the ligand or drug. If the ligand has a very high affinity for the receptor, tracer quantities of the drug can be injected into the animal, and after a relatively short time interval the drug is carried to the brain by the blood, diffuses into the brain, and binds to the receptors. The nonreceptor-bound drug is then removed from the brain and other tissues by various excretory processes. The high affinity of the drug for the receptor causes the retention of the drug in the vicinity of the receptor molecule. As mentioned above, the autoradiograms can be produced by apposition of the slide-mounted tissue sections to emulsion. The generation of autoradiograms for the in vivo labeling procedures is identical to the procedure described above for in vitro autoradiography.

Imaging receptors in vivo: PET scanning techniques. Recent developments have utilized positron-emitting ligands to image and quantify neurotransmitter receptor distributions in living humans using emission tomographic techniques (Frost et al. 1985; Wagner et al. 1983; Wong et al. 1984, 1986). In vivo–labeling autoradiography (see above) has been important in the development of positron-emission tomography (PET) scanning images of receptors because of the feasibility of labeling certain neurotransmitter receptors in vivo. PET is a technique providing a computerized image reconstruction in which the distribution of positron-emitting compounds is revealed. In this technique a ligand containing a radioactive isotope that decays by emitting a positron (positive electron) is injected into an animal or human. If the ligand is suitable, then receptors in brain will be preferentially labeled (see above). Emitted positrons will immediately combine with an electron, and the two are mutually annihilated. The annihilation results in the emission of two gamma rays that go out in very nearly opposite directions, pass through the tissue, and are detected outside the subject by a circular array of detectors. The signals are transformed by a computer, which rapidly reconstructs the spatial distribution of the radioactivity and displays a resulting image on a cathode-ray screen. The great advantage of this approach is that it is a noninvasive method whereby receptors can be quantitatively and spatially detected in humans.

Advantages and limitations of the various receptor mapping techniques. In vitro labeling procedures have many advantages over in vivo labeling procedures. The in vitro labeling procedures provide greater specificity and efficiency. Inhibitors can be added to prevent metabolism of the labeling ligand, and ligands including many peptides that will not cross the blood-brain barrier in in vivo labeling procedures can be used. Various receptor distributions can be easily compared because it is possible to use different ligands with consecutive sections of tissue. Also, this approach has a relatively low cost because an entire animal does not have to be labeled with the drug. It is also possible to carry out studies with human postmortem tissue. An additional advantage of in vitro labeling is that one can quite precisely define the receptor type that one is studying because of parallel biochemical experiments that can be carried out with the slide-mounted tissue sections. In spite of all the disadvantages of in vivo labeling, this technique is still quite important. Perhaps a main advantage of in vivo labeling is that receptors can be labeled and then imaged by various noninvasive techniques such as PET.

The disadvantage of in vivo labeling procedures using PET scanning techniques is that they are expensive procedures that require a large team with a complicated technology. A cyclotron is necessary to produce the radioactive isotope, and nuclear chemists are required to rapidly synthesize the short–half-life isotopes into receptor-specific ligands. Another difficulty, compared to autoradiographic methods, is that PET scans are of lower resolution; a resolution unit is on the average just 1 cubic centimeter. Nevertheless, despite some limitations, great opportunities for information are available through PET scanning.

In vitro autoradiography, with all of its advantages (see above), still has significant limitations. Although one can use ligands with a lower affinity than is necessary for in vivo labeling autoradiography, low-affinity sites are still not easily identified because the dissociation rate of the ligand is rapid enough that there is a large diffusion of the ligand away from the receptor during the washing necessary after the incubation step. Another limitation is that the preparation of tissue, which involves dissection and freezing, may destroy some receptors and may produce morphological defects in the tissue. Also, the techniques of in vitro and in vivo autoradiography are primarily light microscopic and lack the ultrastructural resolution necessary for a complete picture of the distribution of receptors at the level of membranes.

Immunocytochemistry Using Antibodies for Receptors

The availability of antibodies for receptors provides an important alternative to radioligand-binding techniques: the localization of receptors using immunocytochemistry. In addition, immunoneutralization of the receptors using antibodies could provide insights into functions mediated by the receptors. The antibodies could be used to localize receptors at the light microscopic level using fluorescent markers. Also, for light or electron microscopy, an enzymatic reaction product can be deposited locally; a commonly employed enzyme is peroxidase, which is linked to the receptor by an antibody bridge. For electron microscopy, electron-dense labels can be attached to the antibodies; ferritin, hemocyanase, or colloidal gold are possible labels. Important successes have been made in localizing a variety of neurotransmitter receptors in brain by immunocytochemistry, including nicotinic cholinergic receptors (Lentz and Chester 1977; Swanson et al. 1983), dopamine receptors (Goldsmith et al. 1979), β–adrenergic receptors (Strader et al. 1982), and a GABA-benzodiazepine receptor complex (Richards et al. 1986). More recently, antibodies directed against specific peptides and monoamines have been used to immunize animals and generate anti-idiotypic antibodies that in turn may have an affinity for the same receptor as the original antigen. Anti-idiotypic antibodies have been generated for a variety of receptors, including insulin (Schechter et al. 1982), opioid (Ng and Isom 1985), prolactin (Amit et al. 1986), vasopressin (Knigge et al. 1987), corticotropin-releasing factor (CRF) (Piekut and Knigge 1988), dopamine (Schreiber et al. 1983), and a β-adrenergic ligand (Guillet et al. 1984).

Immunohistochemical techniques have some advantages over autoradiographic techniques because emulsion development is not required. Also, these techniques may be useful under experimental conditions where tissue morphology is better preserved. An important advantage of immunocytochemical studies is that cell bodies containing receptors are clearly delineated (Richards et al. 1986; Swanson et al. 1983); this is not the case with autoradiography. Finally, ultrastructural techniques with antibodies have better electron microscopic resolution than those with autoradiography (see Barnard 1979). A major disadvantage of immunohistochemical approaches is that the results are not easily quantifiable, at least when compared with receptor autoradiography.

Molecular Biological Approaches Used in Studying Receptors

Major advances have been made over the past few years in the development of molecular biological techniques and their application to the study of receptors. Gene cloning techniques to identify the structures of protein macromolecules that comprise receptors for neurotransmitters are currently being used. For example, genes for the various subunits of the nicotinic cholinergic receptor (Mishina et al. 1984), the β-adrenergic receptor (Dixon et al. 1986), and the D_2 dopamine receptor (Bunzow et al. 1988) have been cloned. In parallel, rapid advances have been made in the use of molecular biological probes to quantify and localize messenger RNA (mRNA) levels using Northern analysis and in situ hybridization histochemical techniques, respectively. The application of these techniques to quantify and localize message levels for cloned receptors will provide new insights into the synthesis rates of receptors as well as the turnover of these receptor macromolecules. Recently, nicotinic receptor mRNA was detected in high concentrations in rat hypothalamus, hippocampus, habenula, cerebellum, and adrenal gland using both Northern blot analysis and in situ hybridization techniques (Boulter et al. 1986; Goldman et al. 1986). The use of molecular biological techniques to study receptors in combination with "traditional" radioligand binding techniques will allow us to better define the mechanisms (synthesis and/or degradation) underlying changes in receptors following experimental manipulations or drug treatments, and/or as a result of disease.

USES OF RECEPTOR MAPPING

Some of the uses of receptor mapping are summarized in Table 14-2. Receptor maps provide powerful insights into the mechanism of drug

Table 14-2. Uses of receptor mapping

Mechanism of drug action
Complement to neurotransmitter histochemical maps
Target sites for other experiments
Neuropathology

action by identifying those brain regions that have the receptors and, therefore, those areas that are affected by drug administration. For example, administration of opiate drugs causes a variety of physiological effects, including analgesia, pupillary constriction, respiratory depression, and suppression of various visceral reflexes. Perhaps the only way this wide range of physiological action can be fully understood is to associate the various physiological effects with receptors in those various neuronal circuits that mediate the effects. In other words, identifying the neuronal circuits that have the receptors and that will be affected by drug administration may provide an understanding of how the drug produces its effect.

Receptor mapping is also a valuable complement to neurotransmitter mapping. Receptor maps help complete our view of the biochemical organization of the brain. For example, studies on CRF receptors (De Souza et al. 1984, 1985) (see Figure 14-1) have shown that these receptors are found in many regions in the brain where endogenous CRF-containing neurons have been identified (De Souza et al. 1984, 1985).

Other uses of receptor maps include providing needed data for a variety of additional types of experiments, such as locating targets for experiments involving direct drug injections. A major use of receptor maps involves identifying changes in receptors in neuropathological conditions and in neuropsychiatric disorders. This latter aspect of the use of receptor maps and the role of receptors in a variety of diseases are described in greater detail in the following section.

THE ROLE OF RECEPTORS IN DISEASE

Changes in specific neurotransmitter systems play a key role in the pathophysiology of various neurodegenerative and neuropsychiatric disorders. Among the different neuronal synaptic components altered in disease are neurotransmitter receptors. The application of the various techniques described above for studying the role of receptors in disease will be elaborated in this section.

Neurodegenerative disorders, such as Parkinson's disease, Huntington's disease, Alzheimer's disease, and amyotrophic lateral sclerosis, are characterized by loss of neurons in specific regions of the central nervous system. Specific neurotransmitter receptors are localized to certain neurons in brain and thus provide good markers for specific neuronal populations. Dysfunction or loss of specific neuronal systems in brain as a consequence of disease states should result in changes in neurotransmitter receptors that are localized to these populations. For example, there is a marked loss in dopamine-containing neurons of the substantia nigra in Parkinson's disease.

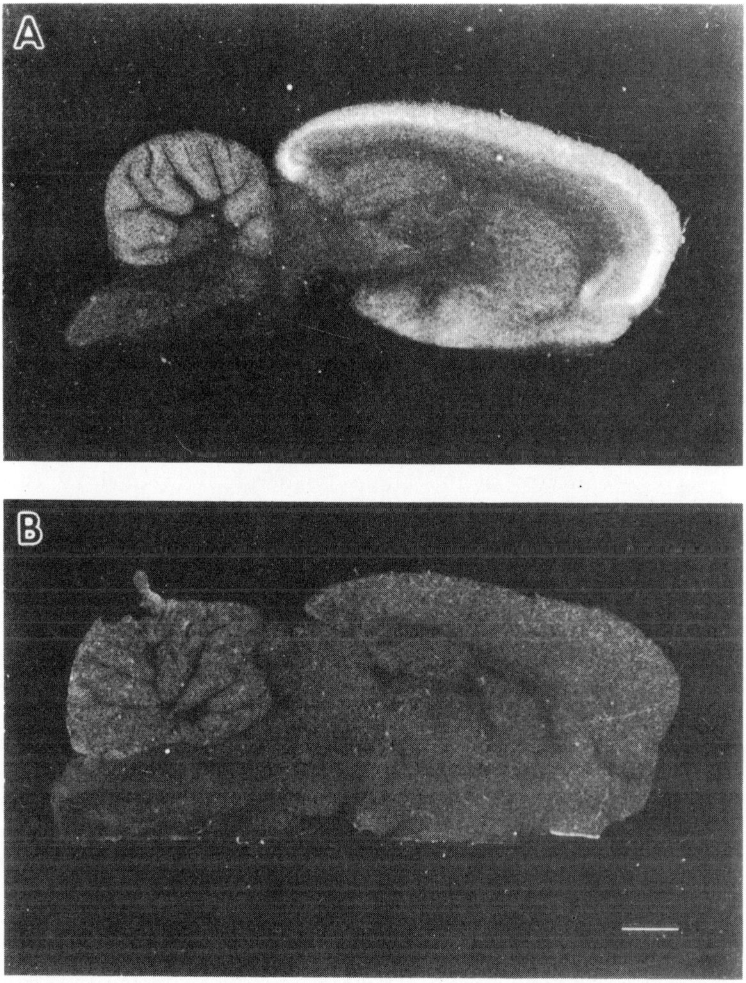

Figure 14-1. Autoradiographic distribution of corticotropin-releasing factor (CRF) receptor binding sites in rat brain, labeled with [^{125}I]Tyr^{o}-ovine-CRF. A and B are the distribution of autoradiographic grains in sagittal sections of rat brain. In dark-field illumination the autoradiographic grains (i.e., binding sites) appear as white spots and the tissue is not visible. Thus, the brightest areas have the highest concentration of binding sites. A shows the "total" binding and B shows the absence of specific receptor binding when 1 μM unlabeled rat-human CRF is included in the incubation buffer (blank). Bar = 2 mm.

Homogenate binding and autoradiographic studies have demonstrated that substantia nigra dopamine, neurotensin, and GABA-benzodiazepine receptors are depleted in Parkinson's disease (Lloyd et al. 1977; Quik et al. 1979; Uhl et al. 1984). These data not only are useful in defining the cell loss in the disease, but by providing a "natural" lesion, are also useful in defining the neurotransmitters that may regulate the cells in question. In vitro labeling autoradiography using postmortem human tissue has been particularly useful in defining receptor alterations in neurodegenerative disorders (see Whitehouse 1985). In amyotrophic lateral sclerosis, a disease characterized by loss of motor neurons, there are major reductions in a variety of neurotransmitter receptor densities (loss of muscarinic, cholinergic, benzodiazepine, and glycine receptors) in Rexed layer IX in association with the degeneration of motor neurons in this region of the spinal cord (Whitehouse et al. 1983). Other examples of neurotransmitter receptors as specific markers for neuronal populations are seen in a loss of muscarinic cholinergic (Enna et al. 1976; Wastek and Yamamura 1976; Whitehouse et al. 1985), benzodiazepine, and dopamine (Reisine et al. 1977; Whitehouse et al. 1985) receptors in the caudate nucleus in Huntington's disease and a loss of muscarinic cholinergic (Mash et al. 1985), nicotinic cholinergic (Whitehouse et al. 1986), serotonergic (Reynolds et al. 1984), and somatostatin (Beal et al. 1985) receptors in the amygdala and cerebral cortex in Alzheimer's disease.

PET scanning techniques have been very useful in visualizing and quantifying loss in neurotransmitter receptors associated with age or with disease. For example, reductions in levels of D_2 dopamine and S_2 serotonin receptors with ^{11}C-labeled 3-N-methylspiperone were seen in the caudate nucleus, putamen, and cerebral cortex over the age span studied (19 to 73 years) (Wong et al. 1984). More recently, alterations in D_2 dopamine receptors have been examined using PET scanning techniques in schizophrenic patients utilizing both [^{11}C]-3-N-methylspiperone (Wong et al. 1986) and ^{11}C-labeled raclopride (Farde et al. 1987) as radioligands. A significant increase in the density of ^{11}C-3-N-methylspiperone–labeled D_2 dopamine receptors was reported in the basal ganglia in both drug-naive and drug-treated schizophrenic patients when compared with the distribution in healthy human volunteers (Wong et al. 1986). However, in another study no significant alterations in either the affinity or density of caudate [^{11}C]raclopride-labeled D_2 dopamine receptors were noted in schizophrenic patients when compared with healthy control subjects (Farde et al. 1987).

Neurotransmitter receptors are good "functional" neuronal

markers in that they provide an accurate index of synaptic connectivity. A loss of neurotransmitter innervating the receptor would be expected to up-regulate (increase the density of) the neurotransmitter receptor, while an increase in neurotransmitter may be expected to down-regulate the neurotransmitter receptor. An example of an up-regulation of the receptor in a disease state is provided by a recent study in which we reported selective up-regulation of CRF receptors in Alzheimer's disease in cerebral cortical areas that had reductions in the concentration of the neurotransmitter itself (De Souza et al. 1986). These data not only provide insight into the role of this neurotransmitter in Alzheimer's disease but also suggest that CRF-receptive cells are maintained in the disease and may provide target sites for therapies that may be useful in treatment of the disease. In Huntington's disease, increases in benzodiazepine receptor density have been reported in the cerebral cortex, globus pallidus, substantia nigra, and cerebellum (Penney and Young 1982; Reisine et al. 1979; Whitehouse et al. 1985), which may be caused by denervation supersensitivity occurring as a result of loss of GABA-ergic neurons. These examples of denervation supersensitivity not only provide markers of synaptic connectivity (or its loss) but are important in

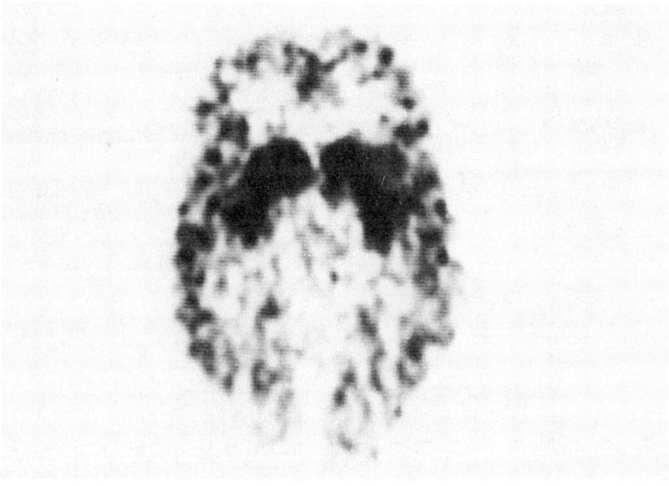

Figure 14-2. PET scan of a human subject (29-year-old male) following intravenous injection of ^{11}C-labeled 3-N-methylspiperone to label D_2 dopamine and S_2 serotonin receptors in brain. The dark areas represent regions of high receptor density. Note the high accumulation of activity in the basal ganglia relative to the rest of the brain. (Courtesy of D. Wong.)

defining the neurotransmitter specificity of the input to the cell demonstrating changes in receptors.

In some disorders the disease process may be a consequence of direct effects on the receptor. A primary example is myasthenia gravis, in which autoimmune attack on nicotinic cholinergic receptors can be linked to muscle weakness (Drachman 1983). Finally, receptors are primary target sites for neuroactive drugs that produce their effects by stimulating or blocking receptors; an in-depth understanding of changes in receptors in various disorders is crucial to designing therapies to treat these diseases. Studies have demonstrated that neurotensin receptors up-regulate after chronic administration of antipsychotic drugs (Uhl and Kuhar 1984), indicating the involvement of neurotensin in the nigrostriatial system and possibly in systems involved in schizophrenia. These studies suggest that drugs aimed at neurotensin receptors might be useful in treating movement disorders or emotional disorders associated with dopaminergic systems. A study of receptors in human autopsy tissues using the techniques described above, PET scanning studies in living patients, and in vivo and in vitro studies in animal models of disease should help elucidate the role of receptors in disease.

REFERENCES

Amit T, Barkley RJ, Gavish M, et al: Anti-idiotypic antibodies raised against anti-prolactin (PRL) antibodies recognize the PRL receptor. Endocrinology 118:835–843, 1986

Barnard EA: Visualization and counting of receptors at the light and electron microscopic levels, in The Receptor, Vol 1: General Principles and Procedures. Edited by O'Bried RD. New York, Plenum Press, 1979, pp 247–310

Beal MF, Mazurek MF, Tran VT, et al: Reduced numbers of somatostatin receptors in the cerebral cortex in Alzheimer's disease. Science 229:289–291, 1985

Bennett JP Jr, Yamamura HI: Neurotransmitter, hormone, or drug receptor binding methods, in Neurotransmitter Receptor Binding. Edited by Yamamura HI, Enna SJ, Kuhar MJ. New York, Raven, 1985, pp 61–89

Boulter J, Evans K, Goldman D, et al: Isolation of a cDNA clone encoding for a possible neural nicotinic acetylcholine receptor-subunit. Nature 319:368–374, 1986

Bunzow JR, Van Tol HHM, Grandy DK, et al: Cloning and expression of a rat D_2 dopamine receptor cDNA. Nature 336:783–787, 1988

De Souza EB, Perrin MH, Insel TR, et al: Corticotropin-releasing factor receptors in rat forebrain: autoradiographic identification. Science 224:1449–1451, 1984

De Souza EB, Insel TR, Perrin MH, et al: Corticotropin-releasing factor receptors are widely distributed within the rat central nervous system: an autoradiographic study. J Neurosci 5:3189–3203, 1985

De Souza EB, Whitehouse PJ, Kuhar MJ, et al: Reciprocal changes in corticotropin-releasing factor (CRF)–like immunoreactivity and CRF receptors in cerebral cortex of Alzheimer's disease. Nature 319:593–595, 1986

Dixon RAF, Kobilka BK, Strader DJ, et al: Cloning of the gene and cDNA for mammalian beta-adrenergic receptor and homology with rhodopsin. Nature 321:75–79, 1986

Drachman DB: Myasthenia gravis: immunobiology of a receptor disorder. Trends in Neuroscience 6:446–451, 1983

Enna SJ, Bennett JP Jr, Bylund DB, et al: Alterations of brain neurotransmitter receptor binding in Huntington's chorea. Brain Res 116:531–537, 1976

Farde L, Wiesel FA, Hall H, et al: No D_2 receptor increase in PET study of schizophrenia. Arch Gen Psychiatry 44:671–672, 1987

Frost JJ, Wagner HN, Dannals RF, et al: Imaging opiate receptors in the human brain by positron tomography. J Comput Tomogr 9:231–236, 1985

Goldman D, Simmons D, Swanson LW, et al: Mapping of brain areas expressing RNA homologous to two different acetylcholine receptor-subunit cDNAs. Proc Natl Acad Sci USA 83:4076–4080, 1986

Goldsmith PC, Cronin MJ, Weiner RI: Dopamine receptor sites in the anterior pituitary. J Histochem Cytochem 27:1205–1207, 1979

Guillet JG, Chamat S, Hoebeke J, et al: Production and detection of monoclonal anti-idiotype antibodies directed against a monoclonal anti-β-adrenergic ligand antibody. J Immunol Methods 74:163–171, 1984

Knigge KM, Piekut DT, Berlove D, et al: Staining of magnocellular neurons of the supraoptic and paraventricular nuclei with vasopressin anti-idiotype antibody: a potential method for receptor immunocytochemistry. Molecular Brain Research 2:69–78, 1987

Kuhar MJ: Receptor localization with the microscope, in Neurotransmitter Receptor Binding. Edited by Yamamura HI, Enna SJ, Kuhar MJ. New York, Raven Press, 1985, pp 153–176

Kuhar MJ, De Souza EB, Unnerstall JR: Neurotransmitter receptor mapping by autoradiography and other methods. Annu Rev Neurosci 9:27–59, 1986

Lentz TL, Chester J: Localization of acetylcholine receptors in central synapses. J Cell Biol 75:258–267, 1977

Lloyd KG, Shemen L, Hornykiewicz O: Distribution of high affinity sodium independent [^{3}H]-gamma-aminobutyric acid (^{3}H-GABA) binding in human brain: alterations in Parkinson's disease. Brain Res 127:269–278, 1977

Mash DC, Flynn DD, Potter LT: Loss of muscarinic receptors in the cerebral cortex in Alzheimer's disease and experimental cholinergic denervation. Science 228:1115–1117, 1985

Mishina M, Kurosaki T, Tobimatsu T, et al: Expression of functional acetylcholine receptor from cloned cDNA's. Nature 307:604–608, 1984

Ng DDS, Isom GE: Anti-morphine anti-idiotypic antibodies: opiate receptor binding and isolated tissue responses. Biochem Pharmacol 34:2853–2858, 1985

Penney JB, Young AB: Quantitative autoradiography of neurotransmitter receptors in Huntington's disease. Neurology 32:1391–1395, 1982

Piekut DT, Knigge KM: Immunocytochemistry in rat forebrain using a CRF anti-idiotypic antibody. Society of Neuroscience Abstracts 14:271–274, 1988

Quik M, Spokes EG, Mackay AVP, et al: Alterations in ^{3}H-spiperone binding in human caudate nucleus, substantia nigra and frontal cortex in the Shy-Drager syndrome and Parkinson's disease. J Neurol Sci 43:429–437, 1979

Reisine TD, Fields JZ, Stem LZ, et al: Alterations in dopaminergic receptors in Huntington's disease. Life Sci 21:1123–1128, 1977

Reisine TD, Wastek GJ, Speth RC, et al: Alterations in the benzodiazepine receptor of Huntington's diseased human brain. Brain Res 165:183–187, 1979

Reynolds GP, Arnold L, Rossor MN, et al: Reduced binding of ^{3}H-ketanserin to cortical $5HT_2$ receptors in senile dementia of the Alzheimer type. Neurosci Lett 44:47–51, 1984

Richards G, Mohler H, Haefely W: Mapping benzodiazepine receptors in the CNS by radiohistochemistry and immunohistochemistry, in Neurology and Neurobiology, Vol 16: Neurohistochemistry—Modern Methods and Applications. Edited by Panula P, Paivarinta H, Soinila S. New York, Alan R Liss, 1986, pp 629–677

Roth LJ, Stumpf WE: Autoradiography of Diffusible Substances. New York, Academic, 1969

Schechter Y, Maron R, Elias D, et al: Autoantibodies to insulin receptor spontaneously develop as anti-idiotypes in mice immunized with insulin. Science 216:542–545, 1982

Schreiber M, Fogelfeld L, Souroujon MC, et al: Autoantibodies to spiroperidol and their anti-idiotypes as probes for studying dopamine receptors. Life Sci 33:1519–1526, 1983

Strader CD, Pickel VM, Joh TH, et al: Antibodies to the beta-adrenergic receptor: functional characterization and receptor immunolocalization in brain. Society of Neuroscience Abstracts 8:526, 1982

Swanson LW, Lindström J, Tzartos S, et al: Immunohistochemical localization of monoclonal antibodies to the nicotinic acetylcholine receptor in chick midbrain. Proc Natl Acad Sci USA 80:4532–4536, 1983

Uhl GR, Kuhar MJ: Chronic neuroleptic treatment enhances neurotensin receptor binding in human and rat substantia nigra. Nature 309:350–352, 1984

Uhl GR, Whitehouse PJ, Price DL, et al: Parkinson's disease: depletion of substantia nigra neurotensin receptors. Brain Res 308:186–190, 1984

Wagner HN, Burns HD, Dannals RF, et al: Imaging dopamine receptors in the human brain by positron tomography. Science 221:1264–1266, 1983

Wastek G, Yamamura HI: Biochemical characterization of muscarinic cholinergic receptors in human brain. Life Sci 19:1033–1040, 1976

Whitehouse PJ: Receptor autoradiography: applications in neuropathology. Trends in Neuroscience 8:434–437, 1985

Whitehouse PJ, Wamsley JK, Zarbin MA, et al: Amyotrophic lateral sclerosis: alterations in neurotransmitter receptors. Ann Neurol 14:8–16, 1983

Whitehouse PJ, Trifiletti RR, Jones BE, et al: Neurotransmitter receptor alterations in Huntington's disease: autoradiographic and homogenate studies with special reference to benzodiazepine receptor complexes. Ann Neurology 18:202–210, 1985

Whitehouse PJ, Martino AM, Antuono PG, et al: Nicotinic acetylcholine binding sites in Alzheimer's disease. Brain Res 371:146–151, 1986

Wong DF, Wagner HN Jr, Dannals RF, et al: Effects of age on dopamine and serotonin receptors measured by positron tomography in the living human brain. Science 226:1393–1396, 1984

Wong DF, Wagner HN, Tune LE, et al: Positron emission tomography reveals elevated D_2 dopamine receptors in drug-naive schizophrenics. Science 234:1558–1563, 1986

Young WS III, Kuhar MJ: A new method for receptor autoradiography: ^{3}H-opioid receptor labeling in mounted tissue sections. Brain Res 179:255–270, 1979

Chapter 15

Neuroendocrine and Peptide Challenge Tests in Primary and Secondary Depression

Dwight L. Evans, M.D.
Robert A. Stern, Ph.D.
Robert N. Golden, M.D.
John J. Haggerty, Jr., M.D.
Diana O. Perkins, M.D.
Jeffrey S. Simon, M.D.
Charles B. Nemeroff, M.D., Ph.D.

Chapter 15

Neuroendocrine and Peptide Challenge Tests in Primary and Secondary Depression

The role of neuroendocrine function in relation to psychiatric illness in general and major affective disorder in particular has been the subject of considerable study in recent years. The hypothalamo-pituitary-adrenal (HPA) (Carroll et al. 1968; Stokes 1966) and the hypothalamo-pituitary-thyroid (HPT) (Gold et al. 1981; Prange et al. 1972) axes have received the most intense investigation in psychoneuroendocrinological research. Alterations in both the HPA and HPT axes have been well described in patients with major affective disorder. The majority of the available studies have focused on patients with primary affective disorders. However, there are a number of recent studies of the activity of the HPA and HPT axes in patients with secondary affective illnesses.

Our research group at the University of North Carolina at Chapel Hill has been studying the clinical and biological characteristics of primary and secondary psychiatric disorders, with a focus on affective disorders in psychiatric and medical populations. We have studied the similarities and differences in clinical features and neuroendocrine characteristics between psychiatric patients with primary depression and those with secondary depression (vitamin B_{12} deficiency, thyroid disorder, dementia), as well as in medical patients with secondary depression (cancer, stroke) (Evans 1988a; Evans and Golden 1987; Evans and Nemeroff 1983, 1984, 1987; Evans et al. 1983a, 1983b, 1984, 1986; Haggerty et al. 1987; Nemeroff et al. 1985; Stern and Bachman 1989).

This work was supported in part by National Institute of Mental Health (NIMH) Grants MH-42625-02 and MH-33127-10 (to D.L.E.) and NIMH Grants MH-42088 and MH-40159 (to C.B.N.). The authors are grateful to Steven J. Austin for preparation of this manuscript.

We will review here our clinical findings as well as findings using neuroendocrine and peptide challenge tests in patients with primary and secondary affective disorders with and without organic factors presumed to be etiologic in the affective syndromes.

CLINICAL AND NEUROENDOCRINE FINDINGS

Primary Depression

In our clinical research on primary depression we have examined the descriptive diagnostic characteristics of major affective disorders and have assessed the activity of the HPA axis using the overnight (1 mg) dexamethasone suppression test (DST) in DSM-III subtypes of major affective disorder (Evans and Nemeroff 1987). In a study of psychiatric patients hospitalized on our inpatient psychiatry service, 66 of 104 patients with major depression (63%) exhibited nonsuppression of serum cortisol (≥5 μg/dl at 4 or 11 P.M criterion) following dexamethasone. Five of 36 psychiatric control patients with depressive symptoms (14%) showed dexamethasone nonsuppression (Table 15-1). We found a progressively increasing rate of DST nonsuppression across the diagnostic continuum, from minor depressive symptoms, to major depression without melancholia, to major depression with melancholia, and finally to major depression with psychosis. A similar pattern was found for the postdexamethasone serum cortisol concentrations; an increasing degree of postdexamethasone serum cortisol nonsuppression was observed across the same diagnostic continuum of depression subtypes (Figure 15-1).

It should be noted that we followed the DSM-III classification in reserving the major depression with melancholia subtype for the more severely depressed patients. Furthermore, the patients with psychotic depression were severely depressed and in many cases melancholic.

Table 15-1. Rates of dexamethasone nonsuppression in psychiatric inpatients

Diagnostic group	*n*	% DST nonsuppression (≥ 5 μg/dl)
Psychiatric controls with depressive symptoms	36	14
Major depression (total)	104	63
Without melancholia	62	48
With melancholia	23	78
With psychosis	19	95

Thus, our findings of both an increasing rate and a greater degree of HPA axis hyperactivity as measured by the DST across this diagnostic continuum may represent an increasing severity of depression and/or a more biologically distinct subtype of depression (Evans 1988a; Evans and Nemeroff 1987). These findings are in accord with those of both Schatzberg et al. (1983), who found the highest rates and greatest degree of nonsuppression in patients with psychotic depression, and Meador-Woodruff et al. (1987), who found significant

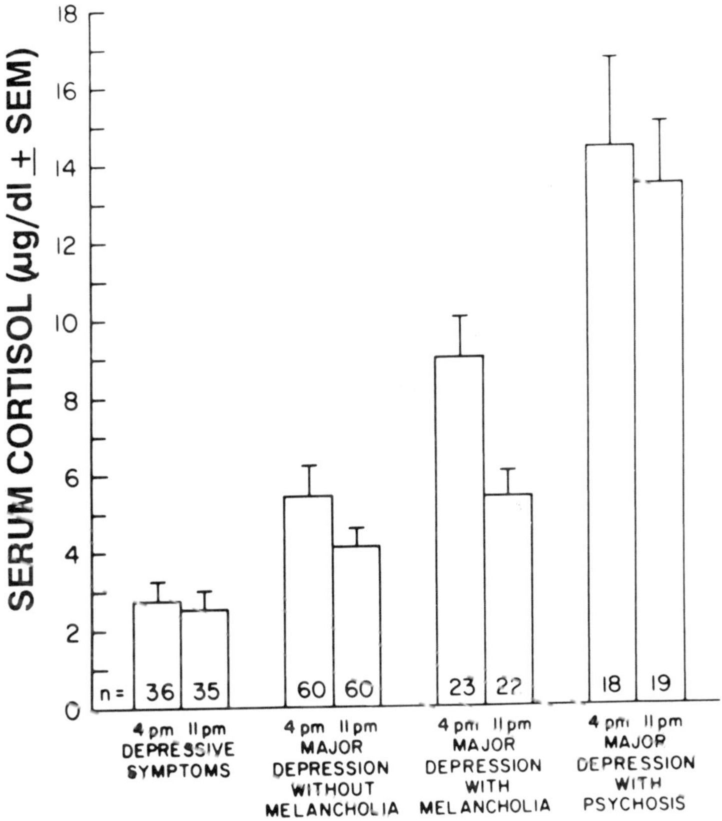

Figure 15-1. Mean serum cortisol concentrations after dexamethasone in different diagnostic subgroups.

correlations between postdexamethasone serum cortisol levels and severity of depression as measured by the Hamilton Depression Rating Scale (Hamilton 1960).

In additional studies we have confirmed early reports that DST nonsuppression resolves with treatment (Albala et al. 1981; Brown and Shuey 1980; Greden et al. 1980) and may predict the relative risk of relapse after treatment (Goldberg 1980a, 1980b; Greden et al. 1980). We found the DST to be a state marker for depression, and normalization of the DST (conversion from nonsuppression to suppression) occurred with successful antidepressant treatment (Evans and Nemeroff 1984). DST normalization was associated with greater clinical improvement and decreased risk of relapse. We found a similar relationship between DST normalization and clinical response in a small series of patients with mixed bipolar disorder (Evans and Nemeroff 1983) and in patients with secondary depression (Evans and Nemeroff 1984), as will be discussed below.

Secondary Depression

Organic factors presumed etiologic. The DST has received considerable study in a wide variety of psychiatric conditions. However, the use of the DST to measure HPA axis activity in patients with organic affective syndrome has been limited. Our group has studied patients with organic affective syndrome secondary to vitamin B_{12} deficiency and to thyroid disease. These patients met Feighner criteria (Feighner et al. 1972) and Research Diagnostic Criteria (RDC) (Spitzer et al. 1988) for secondary depression, although their clinical profiles included some similarities and some differences compared to psychiatric patients with primary depression. Unlike most patients with primary depression, these patients can exhibit marked cognitive deficits and show physiological alterations such as diffuse slowing on the electroencephalogram (EEG). However, they can also exhibit the full range of DSM-III major depressive symptoms, including psychosis (Evans and Nemeroff 1984; Evans et al. 1983b, 1984). Furthermore, in a small series of patients with secondary depression, we found dysregulation of the HPA axis similar to that found in patients with primary depression (Evans and Nemeroff 1984, 1987). Four of the six patients with organic affective syndrome (67%) exhibited DST nonsuppression, and postdexamethasone serum cortisol concentrations were similar to those found in patients with primary depression. Although we treated with psychiatric medication the majority of these patients with secondary depression, it should be noted, as discussed below, that treatment of an underlying organic condition may be sufficient for resolution of the psychiatric state in some patients (Evans and Nemeroff 1984; Evans et al. 1983b, 1984).

Because thyroid alterations have been associated with affective disorder (Gold et al. 1981; Loosen and Prange 1982; Nemeroff and Evans 1989; Whybrow and Prange 1981), we have also studied aspects of HPT axis function in a large series of psychiatric patients with affective symptoms (Haggerty et al. 1987; Nemeroff et al. 1985). Although some patients with marginal hypothyroidism may exhibit neuropsychiatric deficits (Haggerty et al. 1986), patients with symptomless autoimmune thyroiditis (presence of antimicrosomal thyroid or antithyroglobulin antibodies) do not characteristically exhibit cognitive deficits. However, symptomless autoimmune thyroiditis does occur frequently in psychiatric patients with affective symptoms (Extein et al. 1981; Gold et al. 1981). In a series of 45 consecutively hospitalized patients with significant depressive symptoms, we found that 20% had evidence of symptomless autoimmune thyroiditis as measured by detectable titers of antithyroid antibodies (Nemeroff et al. 1985). This rate is considerably higher than the rate of 5% to 10% often cited in healthy subjects (see, for example, Doniach et al. 1980; Pinchera et al. 1979). In an extension of our initial study we found a 17% rate of positive thyroid antibody titers in a large series of psychiatric patients hospitalized with affective symptoms, confirming our earlier findings (Nemeroff et al. 1985) and those of others (Gold et al. 1981; Reus et al. 1986). Thyroid antibody status was unrelated to DST status in these patients, but there was a significant association between the finding of an elevated basal thyroid-stimulating hormone (TSH) concentration (a marker of subclinical hypothyroidism) and DST nonsuppression. This association suggests a possible relationship between dysregulation of the HPT and the HPA axes in these patients with subclinical hypothyroidism. Expanding the HPT axis evaluation to include thyrotropin-releasing hormone (TRH) stimulation testing will help delineate the interrelationship between these two neuroendocrine axes in patients with depression secondary to marginal hypothyroidism. These patients with marginal, occult hypothyroidism may have abnormal tissue sensitivity to thyroid hormones and may, as discussed below, require thyroid hormone replacement for treatment of this subtle thyroid failure and the accompanying psychiatric symptomatology.

In addition to B_{12} deficiency and thyroid disease, we have also studied HPA axis activity as measured by the DST in a small number of patients with dementia and depressive pseudodementia (pseudodementia, $n = 2$; dementia, $n = 3$; depression superimposed upon dementia, $n = 4$) (Evans 1988b). The DST was abnormal in both patients with pseudodementia, and the DST normalized following successful antidepressent treatment. Three of the four patients with depression superimposed upon dementia exhibited an abnormal DST that normalized after successful treatment. One of the three patients with dementia without major depression had an abnormal DST. It should be noted that a considerable number of studies have found abnormal DST findings in patients with advanced dementia (Greenwald et al. 1986; Grunhaus et al. 1983; Raskind et al. 1982; Spar and Gerner 1982). Although our preliminary findings in this small series of patients suggest that the DST may identify major depression in patients with early and/or mild to moderate dementia, further controlled study of larger populations is necessary.

We have also studied the effects of focal structural brain lesions on depression (Stern and Bachman 1989). As in prior studies of poststroke depression (Robinson et al. 1984; Sinyor et al. 1986), we found that approximately 50% of our 52 unilateral stroke patients exhibited some degree of depression. The symptoms were not associated with severity of physical disability or other similar variables, supporting the argument that the depressive symptomatology following stroke is not merely a natural grief reaction to loss of function. Symptoms were assessed with modified self-report instruments and observer rating so as to diminish the confounding effects of other cognitive and behavioral changes associated with cerebral infarctions (e.g., aphasia, dysprosody). Our data indicated that certain depressive symptoms, especially dysphoric mood and insomnia, are associated with specific lesion locations, as assessed by computed tomography (CT) scan. Multivariate analyses showed significant interactions among inter- (right-left) and intrahemispheric (dorsal-ventral, frontal-nonfrontal) lesion dimensions.

Because depression has been found to hamper rehabilitation outcome following stroke (Sundet et al. 1988), accurate diagnosis and appropriate treatment are crucial. Ross and Rush (1981) have proposed that the DST may be an effective diagnostic tool in poststroke depression, one that avoids the difficulties inherent in the use of standardized psychiatric inventories with this population.

Although we did not study our poststroke patients with neuroendocrine challenge tests, a review of the use of the DST in identifying depression in poststroke patients includes several interesting preliminary reports (Evans and Golden 1987). DST specificity in this population has ranged from 70% to 87%, with sensitivity ranging from 47% to 67%. One study indicated that the DST may serve as a marker of antidepressant medication treatment response (Finklestein et al. 1982). Interpretation of DST results in poststroke patients may be affected by a variety of factors, however. For example, the size and location of the lesion may alter DST results (Evans and Nemeroff

1985; Feibel et al. 1983; Lipsey et al. 1985), possibly indicating that the neurological damage may directly affect neuroendocrine regulation without concomitant development of depressive symptomatology (Bauer et al. 1983). Finally, some authors argue that DST sensitivity and specificity in poststroke patients would improve if diagnostic criteria of depression were modified specifically for this population (Ross et al. 1986). If the DST proves to be specific for major depression in the poststroke patient, this neuroendocrine challenge test would have general clinical utility in this population of patients with secondary depression (Evans and Golden 1987).

Organic factors not presumed etiologic. Although there is considerable evidence suggesting that depression is found in a high percentage of patients with cancer (Buckberg et al. 1984; Petty and Noyes 1981), it has been proposed that secondary depression in cancer patients may differ from the depressive syndrome as seen in psychiatric patients with primary depression. In order to assess the similarities and differences in clinical and biological characteristics of primary and secondary depression, we have studied a uniform population of patients with recently diagnosed, nonovarian, gynecologic cancer (Evans et al. 1986). We studied 83 patients and found that 47% had evidence of significant depression: 23% of the patients met DSM-III criteria for major depression, 24% met criteria for minor depression, 7% met criteria for other diagnoses, and 46% did not fulfill criteria for any psychiatric diagnosis.

The clinical characteristics of major depression in these cancer patients resembled the clinical features seen in the subgroup of major depressed psychiatric patients reported on above (Evans and Nemeroff 1987). The cancer patients with major depression did not exhibit symptoms of the DSM-III melancholic subtype of major depression (anhedonia, marked psychomotor retardation, excessive guilt, early morning awakening, a diurnal mood variation). Furthermore, thoughts of suicide were rare, and none of the cancer patients were acutely suicidal, nor did they exhibit psychosis. Thus, the clinical characteristics of depression in cancer patients appear to resemble the characteristics of acutely ill psychiatric inpatients who have the less severe form of DSM-III major depression without melancholic or psychotic features (Evans et al. 1986). These clinical findings describing a less severe form of major depression among cancer patients are consistent with the findings of other investigators (Buckberg et al. 1984; Lansky et al. 1987; Plumb and Holland 1977).

In order to assess neuroendocrine characteristics of depression associated with cancer, we have studied two neuroendocrine challenge tests, the DST and the TRH stimulation test, in 83 patients with gynecologic cancer (Evans et al. 1986). These neuroendocrine studies suggest further similarity between subtypes of primary depression and secondary depression as manifested in cancer patients. Six of the 15 cancer patients with major depression (40%) showed hypercortisolism as measured by the DST. This rate of nonsuppression of serum cortisol following dexamethasone is very similar to the nonsuppression rate we found in the nonmelancholic, depressed psychiatric patients with primary depression reported above (Evans and Nemeroff 1987). The postdexamethasone serum cortisol concentrations at 4 P.M. and 11 P.M. were also similar in the nonmelancholic, depressed psychiatric patients and in the depressed cancer patients. The sensitivity and the specificity of the DST for the diagnosis of depression in these two patient groups are summarized in Table 15-2.

The TSH response to exogenously administered TRH is abnormal in some depressed psychiatric patients (Prange et al. 1972), and approximately 25% of patients with primary depression exhibit a blunted TSH response to TRH (Extein et al. 1981; Loosen 1987; Loosen and Prange 1982). Using the TRH stimulation test, we found a blunted TSH response in 29% of the cancer patients with major depression compared to 8% of the cancer patients with no psychiatric diagnosis. We found no relationship between the DST results and the TRH test results, a finding consistent with earlier observations (Loosen and Prange 1982). It should be noted that our sample size was relatively small, so these TRH stimulation test findings should be viewed as preliminary. If similar TRH test results were obtained in a larger sample of cancer patients, this would represent further evidence suggesting a similar neuroendocrine profile in primary depression and secondary depression as manifested in patients with cancer.

Table 15-2. Sensitivity and specificity of the dexamethasone suppression test in primary and secondary depression

Diagnostic group	Sensitivity	Specificity
Cancer		
Major depression without melancholia	40%	88%
Psychiatric		
Major depression without melancholia	48%	86%

Summary

In summary, these preliminary neuroendocrine results coupled with the clinical findings suggest a similar neuroendocrine alteration as well as a clinical similarity of depression in patients with primary depression and secondary depression with and without organic factors presumed to be etiologic. We have observed the greatest similarity between nonmelancholic depressed psychiatric patients and major depressed gynecologic oncology patients. It should be noted that we believe it is premature to recommend that these neuroendocrine challenge tests be used routinely in depressed cancer patients; the medical exclusion rate was quite high in our study, and the combined effect of tumor load and weight loss may affect interpretation of the DST and TRH tests (Evans et al. 1986). However, to the extent that some forms of secondary depression share clinical and biological characteristics of primary depression, these forms of secondary depression might be likely to have a treatment response similar to that seen in primary depression. In the section that follows, we will review findings regarding the use of neuroendocrine and peptide challenge tests for the selection of pharmacotherapy in primary depression, and we will also review our recent findings regarding biological treatments of secondary depression.

TREATMENT OF PRIMARY AND SECONDARY DEPRESSION

Primary Depression

Early investigations suggested that hyperactivity of the HPA axis as measured by the DST might be a predictor of antidepressant medication response (Brown and Shuey 1980) and a predictor of response to specific antidepressant medications with relatively selective neurotransmitter activity (Amsterdam et al. 1982; Beckmann et al. 1984; Brown and Qualls 1981; Brown et al. 1980; Greden et al. 1981; Nelson et al. 1982). In a pilot study of 34 consecutively admitted patients with DSM-III diagnoses of major depression, we randomly assigned patients to antidepressant treatment with maprotiline (chosen for its relatively selective action on norepinephrine reuptake) or trazodone (chosen as a relatively selective serotonergic agent). We found a trend for a greater response rate among DST nonsuppressors (87% responded) compared to DST suppressors (68% responded) (Simon et al. 1987). There was no difference between the maprotiline and trazodone treatment groups: 76% of the patients in each group responded to treatment. Furthermore, there was no significant treatment effect on the response rate for DST suppressors compared with nonsuppressors: 86% of the nonsuppressors responded to maprotiline and 88% of the nonsuppressors responded to trazodone, while 76% of the suppressors responded to maprotiline and 67% of the suppressors responded to trazodone. The findings of this study and those of the earlier investigations suggest that it is premature to state that a patient's DST status can be used as a predictor of response to antidepressant treatment in general or of response to specific antidepressant treatment. If the DST can be used to identify biochemically distinct depressive subtypes (e.g., "noradrenergic" vs. "serotonergic" depressions), it will not necessarily follow that specific treatments can be targeted for these subtypes; relatively specific norepinephrine uptake inhibitors affect central serotonergic along with norepinephrinergic systems, and specific serotonin (5-hydroxytryptamine [5-HT]) uptake inhibitors alter norepinephrine and serotonergic systems (Potter et al. 1985). Still, the concept that neuroendocrine challenge studies can identify biologically distinct subtypes of major depression remains attractive.

It should be noted that there has been little study regarding the use of the TRH stimulation test to identify subtypes of depression that are preferentially responsive to specific antidepressant treatments. We have observed that patients with antithyroid antibodies or with low normal thyroid function have diminished response to antidepressant medication (Haggerty et al. 1988; Prange et al., in press). Triiodothyronine (T3) has been used to both accelerate the treatment effects of antidepressants (Prange et al. 1969) and supplement tricyclic antidepressant treatment in patients with refractory depression (Goodwin et al. 1982). The use of neuroendocrine challenge tests such as the TRH test to identify patients who would respond to thyroid hormone supplementation awaits further investigation. However, Targum et al. (1984) found that many refractory depressed patients who respond to thyroid supplementation have preexisting subclinical hypothyroidism when tested by TRH infusion.

Secondary Depression

There are relatively few systematic studies regarding the treatment of secondary depression. Certainly, correction of the underlying organic factor that is presumed etiologic in producing or contributing to the depressive syndrome should be accomplished. Although it is not known if correction of the underlying organic factor is sufficient to bring about full resolution of the depressive illness, there is anecdotal evidence to suggest that treatment of the underlying organic condition may result in resolution of the depression (Evans and Nemeroff 1984; Evans et al. 1983b, 1984; Kronfol et al. 1982). For example, in a small series of patients with organic affective syndrome (Evans and Nemeroff 1984), one patient with B_{12} deficiency received B_{12} replacement and within days showed symptomatic improvement. Over a 4-week period this patient went on to show complete resolution of psychotic depression and cognitive impairment. Thus, correction of the underlying organic factor was sufficient for the successful treatment of this individual's depression. However, we treated with psychiatric medication the remaining five patients in this small series of patients with organic affective syndrome because we believed the major affective disorder was sufficiently severe to warrant treatment with psychotropic medications in addition to treatment of the abnormal organic condition. These patients responded successfully to this combined treatment. Controlled treatment trials will be necessary to determine if psychotropic medications are necessary for more rapid or more complete resolution of depression than would occur only from correction of the underlying organic condition.

These considerations may be relevant to the rapidly expanding field of acquired immunodeficiency syndrome (AIDS) research. Recent evidence indicates that human immunodeficiency virus (HIV)–infected patients may develop psychiatric symptoms as a consequence of direct CNS action of HIV, similar to other organic psychiatric syndromes such as thyroid disease, vitamin B_{12} deficiency, or cerebral infarction, where an organic factor is presumed to play an etiologic role in the development of the psychiatric symptoms. Just as treatment of the underlying organic condition may be necessary for resolution of the psychiatric syndrome, anti-HIV treatment may treat or prevent the development of organic psychopathology. We have preliminary observational data from five HIV-infected patients suggesting that depressive symptoms may be responsive to zidovudine treatment. The most dramatic case was that of a young, asymptomatic HIV-positive hemophilia patient who met criteria for DSM-III-R major depression, but who did not respond to a 4-week trial of the antidepressant doxepine. The patient was placed on zidovudine and experienced a clear remission of his major depressive symptoms, including depressed mood, insomnia with early morning awakening, anorexia and weight loss, hopelessness, decreased energy, and anhedonia (Perkins and Evans, in press). Although anecdotal, these findings suggest that zidovudine may be effective in treating or preventing the development of depressive syndromes in HIV-infected patients. As discussed above, the need for psychotropic medication treatment in addition to the antiviral treatment will require assessment in controlled research trials.

As reviewed above, our clinical and neuroendocrine findings in depressed cancer patients suggest a similarity to those in depressed, nonmelancholic psychiatric patients. If depression secondary to cancer is similar to primary depression, then a similar response to antidepressant medication treatment might be expected in the depressed cancer patient. Remarkably, the use of antidepressant medication treatment in depressed cancer patients has received little systematic investigation (Costa et al. 1985; Noyes and Kathol 1986).

Our group has preliminary results from a pilot study suggesting that depressed cancer patients who receive adequate antidepressant treatment have significant improvement in depression and better psychosocial adjustment to their cancer after antidepressant treatment (Evans et al. 1988). This study was an extension of the larger neuroendocrine study described above (Evans et al. 1986). We assessed the response to antidepressant treatment by evaluating the degree of depression and the quality of life in patients who were referred for antidepressant medication treatment. Depressed patients who received antidepressant treatment were compared with those patients who received inadequate antidepressant medication. We studied 22 patients who either met DSM-III criteria for major depression (12 patients) or had significant depressive symptoms (minor depression; 10 patients). All 22 patients were referred for antidepressant medication treatment, but two comparison groups emerged: a treated group ($n = 12$) and an untreated group ($n = 10$). The tumor load (cancer stage at the time of initial assessment) was equally distributed within the treated and untreated groups. All 22 patients were reevaluated after discharge (mean [± SD] = 8.6 ± 4.8 months). Each patient received both a Hamilton Depression Rating Scale and a Psychosocial Adjustment to Illness Scale (PAIS) (Derogatis 1986). No significant difference existed between initial Hamilton depression scores for the treated and untreated groups. The mean posttreatment Hamilton depression score was significantly lower for the treated group when compared with that of the untreated group. In addition, the PAIS score was significantly lower for the group receiving treatment.

These preliminary findings suggest that depressed cancer patients who receive adequate antidepressant treatment have an improvement in depression similar to that of patients with primary depression. Furthermore, these findings suggest that antidepressant treatment produces better psychosocial adjustment to cancer. Interestingly, the patients with minor depression who received treatment had levels of adaptation similar to those of major depressed patients who received adequate antidepressant treatment. Further controlled study will be necessary to confirm the benefits of antidepressants in cancer patients with major as well as minor depression. Furthermore, the use of neuroendocrine and peptide challenge tests to identify a type of depression that is more responsive to treatment or to specific treatments also awaits further study.

SUMMARY

Our group has systematically investigated clinical and biological characteristics of primary and secondary psychiatric disorders, with a focus on affective illness. Findings from these investigations suggest both similarities and differences in the symptom profiles of primary and secondary depression. Findings from neuroendocrine and peptide challenge tests suggest similarities between primary depression and secondary depression as seen in patients with cancer. Subtyping the secondary depressions into those conditions with a presumed organic etiology (e.g., vitamin B12 deficiency, thyroid disorder, stroke) and those with no apparent organic etiology (e.g., cancer) suggests different organopathophysiologies of the psychiatric disorders and, therefore, may suggest condition-specific treatment (e.g., vitamin or hormone replacement, antidepressant medications). These findings may be important in conceptualizing and adopting research strategies to study secondary depression as well as the psychological and biological treatments of secondary depression.

REFERENCES

Albala AA, Greden JF, Tarika J, et al: Changes in serial dexamethasone suppression tests among unipolar depressives receiving electroconvulsive treatment. Biol Psychiatry 16:551–560, 1981

Amsterdam JD, Winokur A, Caroff SN, et al: The dexamethasone suppression test in outpatients with primary affective disorder and healthy control subjects. Am J Psychiatry 139:287–291, 1982

Bauer M, Gans JS, Harley JP, et al: Dexamethasone suppression test and depression in a rehabilitation setting. Arch Phys Med Rehabil 64:421–422, 1983

Beckmann H, Holzmüller B, Fleckstein P: Clinical investigations into antidepressive mechanisms, II: dexamethasone suppression test predicts response to nomifensine or amitriptyline. Acta Psychiatr Scand 70:341–353, 1984

Brown WA, Qualls CB: Pituitary-adrenal distribution in depression: marker of a subtype with characteristic clinical features and response to treatment? Psychiatry Res 4:115–128, 1981

Brown WA, Shuey I: Response to dexamethasone and subtype of depression. Arch Gen Psychiatry 37:747–751, 1980

Brown WA, Haier RJ, Qualls CB: Dexamethasone suppression test identifies subtypes of depression which respond to different antidepressants. Lancet 1:928–929, 1980

Buckberg J, Penman D, Holland JC: Depression in hospitalized cancer patients. Psychosom Med 46:199–212, 1984

Carroll BJ, Martin FIR, Davies BM: Resistance to suppression by dexamethasone of plasma 11-OHCS levels in severe depressive illness. Br Med J 3:285–287, 1968

Costa D, Mogos I, Toma T: Efficacy and safety of mianserin in the treatment of women with cancer. Acta Psychiatr Scand 72 (suppl 320):85–92, 1985

Derogatis LR: The psychosocial adjustment to illness scale. J Psychosom Res 30:77–91, 1986

Doniach D, Bottazzo GF, Khoury EL: Prospects in human autoimmune thyroiditis, in Autoimmune Aspects of Endocrine Disorders. Edited by Pinchera A, Doniach D, Fenzi GF, et al. New York, Academic, 1980, pp 25–38

Evans DL: Depression in the cancer patient: antidepressant treatment response, endocrine and immune relationships. CALGB Psychiatry Cable 1(2):5–7, 1988a

Evans DL: Use of the dexamethasone suppression test in clinical psychiatry, in The Hypothalamic-Pituitary-Adrenal Axis: Physiology, Pathophysiology, and Psychiatric Implications. Edited by Schatzberg AF, Nemeroff CB. New York, Raven, 1988b, pp 133–155

Evans DL, Golden RN: The dexamethasone suppression test: a review, in Handbook of Clinical Psychoneuroendocrinology. Edited by Nemeroff CB, Loosen PT. New York, Guilford, 1987, pp 313–335

Evans DL, Nemeroff CB: Use of the dexamethasone suppression test using DSM-III criteria on an inpatient psychiatric unit. Biol Psychiatry 18:505–511, 1983

Evans DL, Nemeroff CB: The dexamethasone suppression test in organic affective syndrome. Am J Psychiatry 141:1465–1467, 1984

Evans DL, Nemeroff CB: The DST and organic affective disorder: reply. Am J Psychiatry 142:992, 1985

Evans DL, Nemeroff CB: The clinical use of the dexamethasone suppression test in DSM-III affective disorders: correlation with the severe depressive subtypes of melancholia and psychosis. J Psychiatr Res 21:185–194, 1987

Evans DL, Burnett GB, Nemeroff CB: The dexamethasone suppression test in the clinical setting. Am J Psychiatry 140:586–589, 1983a

Evans DL, Edelsohn GA, Golden RN: Organic psychosis without anemia or spinal cord symptoms in vitamin B12 deficient patients. Am J Psychiatry 140:218–221, 1983b

Evans DL, Edelsohn GA, Golden RN: Mental symptoms of vitamin B12 deficiency (letter). Am J Psychiatry 141:146–147, 1984

Evans DL, McCartney CF, Nemeroff CB, et al: Depression in women treated for gynecological cancer: clinical and neuroendocrine assessment. Am J Psychiatry 143:447–452, 1986

Evans DL, McCartney CF, Nemeroff CB, et al: Depression in cancer patients: diagnostic and treatment considerations. NC Med J 49:546–548, 1988

Evans DL, Golden RN, Nemeroff CB, et al: Clinical aspects of neuropeptide research, in Neuropsychopharmacology. Edited by Bunney WE, Hippins H, Laakmann G, et al. Berlin, Springer-Verlag (in press)

Extein I, Pottash ALC, Gold MS, et al: The thyrotropin-releasing hormone test in the diagnosis of unipolar depression. Psychiatry Res 5:311–316, 1981

Feibel J, Kelly M, Lee L, et al: Loss of adrenocorticol suppression after acute brain injury: role of increased intracranial pressure and brain stem function. J Clin Endocrinol Metab 57:1245–1250, 1983

Feighner JP, Robins E, Guze SB, et al: Diagnostic criteria for use in psychiatric research. Arch Gen Psychiatry 26:57–63, 1972

Finklestein S, Benowitz L, Baldessarini R, et al: Mood, vegetative disturbance, and the dexamethasone suppression test after stroke. Ann Neurol 12:463–468, 1982

Gold MS, Pottash ALC, Extein I, et al: Diagnosis of depression in the 1980's. JAMA 245:1562–1564, 1981

Goldberg IK: Dexamethasone suppression test as indicator of safe withdrawal of antidepressant therapy. Lancet 1:376, 1980a

Goldberg IK: Dexamethasone suppression tests in depression and response to treatment. Lancet 2:92, 1980b

Goodwin FK, Prange AJ, Post RM: Potentiation of antidepressant effects by L-triiodothyronine in tricyclic nonresponders. Am J Psychiatry 139:34–38, 1982

Greden JF, Albala AA, Haskett RF, et al: Normalization of dexamethasone suppression test: a laboratory index of recovery from endogenous depression. Biol Psychiatry 15:449–458, 1980

Greden JF, Kronfol Z, Gardner R, et al: Dexamethasone suppression test and selection of antidepressant medications. J Affective Disord 3:389–396, 1981

Greenwald BS, Mather AA, Mohs RC, et al: Cortisol and Alzheimer's disease, II: dexamethasone suppression, dementia severity, and affective symptoms. Am J Psychiatry 143:442–446, 1986

Grunhaus L, Dilsaver S, Greden JF, et al: Depressive pseudodementia: a suggested diagnostic profile. Biol Psychiatry 18:215–225, 1983

Haggerty JJ, Evans DL, Prange AJ: Organic Brain Syndrome associated with marginal hypothyroidism. Am J Psychiatry 143:785–786, 1986

Haggerty JJ, Simon JS, Evans DL, et al: Relationship of serum TSH concentration and antithyroid antibodies and DST response in psychiatric inpatients. Am J Psychiatry 144:1491–1493, 1987

Haggerty JJ, Browne J, Evans DL, et al: Antidepressant response in autoimmune thyroiditis. Abstract of paper presented at the 141st annual meeting of the American Psychiatric Association, Montreal, Quebec, May 1988

Hamilton M: A rating scale for depression. J Neurol Neurosurg Psychiatry 23:56–62, 1960

Kronfol Z, Greden JP, Condon M, et al: Application of biological markers in depression secondary to thyrotoxicosis. Am J Psychiatry 139:1219–1322, 1982

Lansky SB, List MA, Ritter-Sterr C: Recognizing depression in oncology patients. Abstract of paper presented at the 140th annual meeting of the American Psychiatric Association, Chicago, IL, May 1987

Lipsey JR, Robinson RG, Pearlson GD, et al: The dexamethasone suppression test and mood following stroke. Am J Psychiatry 141:318–323, 1985

Loosen PT: The TRH stimulation test in psychiatric disorders: a review, in Handbook of Clinical Psychoneuroendocrinology. Edited by Loosen PT, Nemeroff CB. New York, Guilford, 1987, pp 336–360

Loosen PT, Prange AJ: Serum thyrotropin response to thyrotropin-releasing hormone in psychiatric patients: a review. Am J Psychiatry 139:405–416, 1982

Meador-Woodruff JH, Haskett RF, Grunhaus L, et al: Post dexamethasone plasma cortisol and β-endorphin levels in depression: relationship to severity of illness. Biol Psychiatry 22:1137–1150, 1987

Nelson WH, Orr WW, Stevenson JM, et al: Hypothalamic-pituitary-adrenal axis activity and tricyclic response in major depression. Arch Gen Psychiatry 39:1033–1036, 1982

Nemeroff CB, Evans DL: Thyrotropin-releasing hormone (TRH). Ann NY Acad Sci 553:304–310, 1989

Nemeroff CB, Simon JS, Haggerty JJ, et al: Anti-thyroid antibodies in depressed patients. Am J Psychiatry 142:840–843, 1985

Noyes R, Kathol RG: Depression and cancer. Psychiatr Dev 4:77–100, 1986

Perkins DO, Evans DL: HIV-related major depression: response to AZT treatment. Psychosomatics (in press)

Petty F, Noyes R: Depression in cancer. Biol Psychiatry 16:1203–1221, 1981

Pinchera A, Fenzi GF, Bartalena L, et al: Antigen-antibody systems involved in thyroid autoimmunity, in Autoimmune Aspects of Endocrine Disorders. Edited by Pinchera A, Doniach D, Fenzi GF, et al. New York, Academic, 1979, pp 57–72

Plumb MM, Holland J: Comparative studies of psychological function in patients with advanced cancer, I: self-reported depressive symptoms. Psychosom Med 39:264–276, 1977

Potter WZ, Scheinin M, Golden RN, et al: Selective antidepressants and cerebrospinal fluid: lack of specificity on norepinephrine and serotonin metabolites. Arch Gen Psychiatry 42:1171–1177, 1985

Prange AJ, Wilson IC, Rabon AM, et al: Enhancement of imipramine antidepressant activity by thyroid hormone. Am J Psychiatry 126:457–469, 1969

Prange AJ, Wilson IC, Lara PP, et al: Thyrotropin-releasing hormone in depression. Lancet 2:999–1002, 1972

Prange AJ, Haggerty JJ, Browne JL, et al: Marginal hypothyroidism in mental illness: preliminary assessments of prevalence and significance. Neuropsychopharmacology (in press)

Raskind M, Peskind E, Rivard ME, et al: Dexamethasone suppression test and cortisol circadian rhythm in primary degenerative dementia. Am J Psychiatry 139:1468–1471, 1982

Reding M, Orto L, Willensky P, et al: The dexamethasone suppression test: an indicator of depression in stroke but not a predictor of rehabilitation outcome. Arch Neurol 42:209–212, 1985

Reus VI, Berlant J, Galante M, et al: Autoimmune thyroiditis in female depressives. Paper presented at the 41st annual meeting of the Society of Biological Psychiatry, Washington, DC, May 1986

Robinson RG, Starr LB, Price TR: A two-year longitudinal study of mood disorders following stroke: prevalence and duration at 6 months follow-up. Br J Psychiatry 144:256–262, 1984

Ross ED, Rush AJ: Diagnosis and neuroanatomical correlates of depression in brain-damaged patients: implications for a neurology of depression. Arch Gen Psychiatry 38:1344–1354, 1981

Ross ED, Gordon WA, Hibbard M, et al: The dexamethasone suppression test, post-stroke depression and the validity of DSM-III diagnostic criteria. Am J Psychiatry 143:1200–1201, 1986

Schatzberg AF, Rothchild AJ, Stahl JB, et al: The dexamethasone suppression test: identification of subtypes of depression. Am J Psychiatry 140:88–91, 1983

Simon JS, Evans DL, Nemeroff CB: The dexamethasone suppression test and antidepressant response in major depression. J Psychiatr Res 21:313–317, 1987

Sinyor D, Jacques P, Kaloupek DG, et al: Poststroke depression and lesion location. Brain 109:537–546, 1986

Spar JE, Gerner R: Does the dexamethasone suppression test distinguish dementia from depression? Am J Psychiatry 139:238–240, 1982

Spitzer RL, Williams JB, Gibbon M, et al: Structured clinical interview for DSM-III disorders (SCID) and SCID-NP. New York, New York State Psychiatric Institute, 1988

Stern RA, Bachman DL: Dysphoric mood and vegetative disturbance following stroke: patterns of lesion localization (abstract). J Clin Exp Neuropsychol 11:97–98, 1989

Stokes PE: Pituitary suppression in psychiatric patients, in Abstracts of the 48th Meeting of the Endocrine Society. Bethesda, MD, Endocrine Society, 1966, p 101

Sundet K, Finset A, Reinvang I: Neuropsychological predictors in stroke rehabilitation. J Clin Exp Neuropsychol 10:363–379, 1988

Targum SD, Greenberg RD, Harmon RL: Thyroid hormone and the TRH stimulation test in refractory depression. J Clin Psychiatry 45:345–346, 1984

Whybrow PC, Prange AJ: A hypothesis of thyroid-catecholamine-receptor interaction: its relevance to affective illness. Arch Gen Psychiatry 38:106–113, 1981